Textbook of Immunology

THE AUTHOR

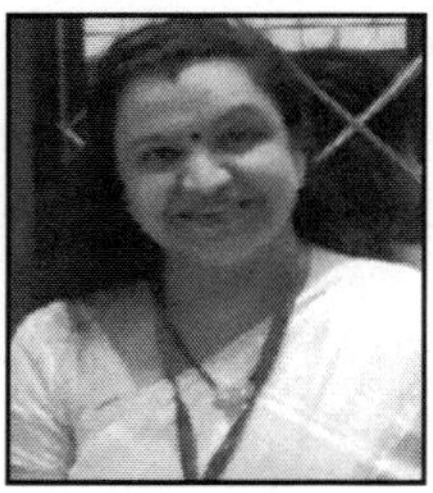

Dr. Latika Bhatia is an Assistant Professor in Department of Microbiology and Bioinformatics in Atal Bihari Vajpayee Vishwavidyalaya, Bilaspur, CG, India. She has 20 years of teaching experience working in University. She did her Ph.D. from ITM University, Gwalior, on Biofuels. She is a recipient of IASc-INSA-NASI Summer Research Fellowship. She has awards and honours in her credit. She has been invited to deliver a technical talk in All India Institute of Medical Sciences (AIIMS, New Delhi) and in many national and international conferences. She has published more than 30 research articles in peer-reviewed journals of an international repute, 05 book chapters and 03 monographs, 02 books, with citation index more than 200. Recently, Dr. Bhatia has organized Indian Council of Medical Research (ICMR) sponsored workshop on Medical lab Technology: Recent Advances in Lab Diagnostics. She has successfully completed many consultancy and research projects.Dr. Bhatia is reviewer of PLOS, Sugar Tech (Springers), Springer Nature, Chemical Engineering & Technology (Wiley, Germany) and member of national advisory committee of eminent universities. Dr. Bhatia has developed online certificate course on immunology, in collaboration with Commonwealth Educational Media Center for Asia (CEMCA), available on Web-portal-"e-atalgyansangum", on UGC's specified 4 quadrant approaches.

Textbook of Immunology

Latika Bhatia

2021

Daya Publishing House®

A Division of

Astral International Pvt. Ltd.

New Delhi – 110 002

Cataloging in Publication Data--DK

Courtesy: D.K. Agencies (P) Ltd. <docinfo@dkagencies.com>

Bhatia, Latika, author.

Textbook of immunology / Latika Bhatia.

pages cm

Includes bibliographical references.

ISBN 9789390435883

1. Immunology--Textbooks. I. Title.

LCC QR181.B43 2021 | DDC 616.079 23

Published by : **Daya Publishing House®**
A Division of
Astral International Pvt. Ltd.
– ISO 9001:2015 Certified Company –
4736/23, Ansari Road, Darya Ganj
New Delhi-110 002
Ph. 011-43549197, 23278134
E-mail: info@astralint.com
Website: www.astralint.com

Printed at : **Replika Press Pvt Ltd**

Dedicated to my beloved Parents, Sister and Husband

Preface

Immunology as a science probably began with the observations by Metchnikoff in 1882 that starfish when pierced by a foreign object (a rose thorn) responded by coating it with cells (later identified as phagocytes). Immunology- the study of the way in which the body defends itself against invading organisms or internal invaders (tumors)- has developed rapidly over the last 50 years, and more recently with the advent of molecular techniques has contributed critical tools for research and diagnosis, and therapeutics for treatment of wide range of human diseases.

Immunology has thus become an integral part of human and life science courses as well as medical studies. Immunology is potentially an intimidating subject for new students. Not only does it appear to have a language all of its own, including plenty of obscure Latin terminology, but it covers a bewilderingly wide range of material. The present book on Immunology is written to cater the beginners in microbiology and biotechnology. The syllabus mainly covers common core syllabus of B.Sc. and M.Sc. Microbiology students of most of the Universities in India and it also meets the requirements of pharmacy and basic biotechnology of many Indian Universities.

Every effort is made to make the subject matter simple. The language written is lucid supported by clear diagrams. The necessary information is précised in tabular form. The review questions are given at the end of every chapter for self-evaluation and to learn the subject perceptibility. About 300 multiple choice questions are provided at the end of the chapter. This will support the students aspiring for various competitive exams like CSIR NET, GATE, PSC, and other medical entrance exams.

The present book on Immunology is first in series written to cater the beginners in microbiology. The present book is designed to cater the needs of B.Sc. and M.Sc. students of Microbiology, Biotechnology and Pharmacy. The basic concepts of Immunology such as antigen, antibody, serological reactions, hypersensitivity are discussed concisely for better understanding of the students and form a source material to the teachers. Immunohematology, autoimmune disease and immunodeficiency are also covered precisely. The subject matter is written in simple language keeping in view of student's standard and very well illustrated with clear diagrams.

We are fully conscious of the fact that science subject is never final and it changes with more and more studies. We hope that students find this approach to be logical and useful. I have benefited enormously from my own experience of teaching students, both of microbiology and biotechnology. We earnestly request the students and teachers alike for their constructive criticism and valuable suggestions, which will help to make the book perfect and acceptable to one and all, and serve the student community for long time to come. Most of all I hope that atleast some students will be fascinated by this subject, and will see this text as their first step on the road to Immunology related career.

I am greatly indebted to my family members who always are the source of my inspiration. I am thankful to my colleagues, well wishers and friends, in particulars Dr. Anuj Chandel, Scientist, Engineering School of Lorena (EEL), University of Sao Paulo, Lorena, Brazil and Dr. Prakash Sarangi, Directorate of Research Central Agricultural University Imphal and Prof. O. N. Tiwari, Scientist, Indian Council of Agricultural Research, New Delhi, who always encouraged me by discussions over the issues related to research, publications and contemporary biology. I acknowledge the assistance of my students particularly Akansha, Nidhi, Aditi, Vikas, Jyoti, Abha for making clear diagrams for this book and for their support during proof reading of the manuscript.

The work of this magnitude needs an unstinted cooperation from different persons who deserve our whole-hearted thanks and gratitude. One person who has been instrumental for initiation of this book and who has rendered his whole hearted support at all times for successful completion of this book is none other than Prof. G. D. Sharma, honourable founder Vice Chancellor, Bilaspur University. I owe him my heartfelt gratitude. The support of Atal Bihari Vajpayee University, Bilaspur in my academic endeavours is sincerely acknowledged. I thank the team of Astral International Pvt. Ltd. for their sustained interest in the publication of this book neatly and timely.

I am extremely happy to contribute this book to the academia at the time when Atal Bihari Vajpayee University is celebrating its 10th establishment year.

Last but not least, I am greatly indebted to Shree SAI for his blessings and making my path smooth.

Dr. Latika Bhatia

Contents

CHAPTER 1

History and Development of Immunology

Introduction

The discipline of immunology grew out of the observation that individuals who had recovered from certain infectious diseases were thereafter protected from the disease. It had been observed from very early days that persons surviving an attack of small pox did not develop this disease when exposed to the infection. Thus, the human body resists the invasion of pathogens and their toxic products and this resistance forms the basis of the subject immunology.

Immunology is a branch of biology. It is concerned with immunity. It is a resistance of living organisms to infection of microorganisms. Immunology is a broad branch of biomedical science, which covers the study of all aspects of immune system. Immunology deals with the physiological function of immune system in state of both health and disease, and malfunction of the immune systems in immunological disorders. The different areas of immunology include classical immunology, development immunology, immunotherapy, diagnostic immunology, evolutionary immunology, medical immunology and reproductive immunology. Some of the milestones in the development of immunology are précised. The Latin term *immunis,* meaning "exempt/ freedom from," is the source of the English word immunity, meaning the state of protection from infectious disease. In ancient times, the term immunity was used only to mean 'exemption' from military service or taxes and later it was introduced into medicine to refer to human beings who do not get further attacks of diseases like small pox or plague, once they contact those diseases. Immunology deals with the study of processes by which the body defends itself from the invasion and attack of foreign organisms.

In the process of evolution of individual, organisms developed the property of distinguishing self is accepted and nonself (foreign) is rejected or degraded. For this purpose, body has developed a versatile defense system called as immune system that operates via different mechanisms, which is called as immunity or resistance. The immunity operates against non-self agents and is called immune response. Immunity is of two types:

1. Innate (Non-specific or natural)
2. Acquired (Specific or adaptive)

Immunity is more highly-evolved system of specific responses, and it recognizes and selectively eliminates specific microbial pathogens or foreign substances. Substances that are recognized by the immune system as foreign and provoke immune response are called antigens. The special substances (proteins) that are generated by an antigen are called as antibodies (immunoglobulin). These proteins bind to the specific cells that generate antibodies. There are also some other cells of immune system that destroy the foreign invaders. Both these immunities work together and provide protection to the body repeatedly. Following milestones are prominent in the development of science of Immunology-

1. Development of vaccination

According to Stanley A. Plotkin, the three greatest discoveries of medicine in the last 200 years are antisepsis, antibiotics, and vaccines. Since the time of the ancient Greeks, it has been recognized that people who have recovered from plague, smallpox, yellow fever, and various other infectious diseases rarely contract the diseases again. The first recorded attempts to induce immunity deliberately were performed by the Chinese and Turks in the fifteenth century. Various reports suggest that the dried crusts derived from smallpox pustules were either inhaled into the nostrils or inserted into small cuts in the skin (a technique called *variolation*). In 1718, Lady Mary Wortley Montagu, the wife of the British ambassador to Constantinople, observed the positive effects of variolation on the native population and had the technique performed on her own children.

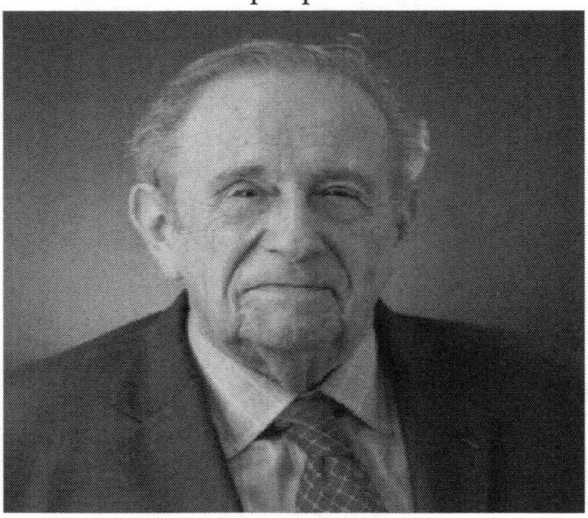

Stanley A. Plotkin

The first scientific attempts at artificial immunizations were made in the late eighteenth century by Edward Jenner (1749–1823): a country doctor from Berkley, Gloucestershire, England. Jenner investigated the basis for the widespread belief of the English peasants that anyone who had vaccinia (cowpox) never contracted smallpox. Smallpox was often fatal—10 to 40% of the victims died—and those who recovered had disfiguring pockmarks. Yet most English milkmaids, who were readily infected with cowpox, had clear skin because cowpox was a relatively mild infection that left no scars. It was on May 14, 1796, that Jenner extracted the contents of a pustule from the arm of a cowpox-infected milkmaid, Sarah Nelmes, and injected it into the arm of eight-year-old James Phipps. As Jenner expected, immunization with the cowpox virus caused only mild symptoms in the boy. When he subsequently inoculated the boy with smallpox virus, the boy showed no symptoms of the disease. Jenner then inoculated large numbers of his patients with cowpox pus, as did other physicians in England and on the European continent.

By 1800 the practice known as vaccination had begun in America, and by 1805 Napoleon Bonaparte had ordered all French soldiers to be vaccinated.

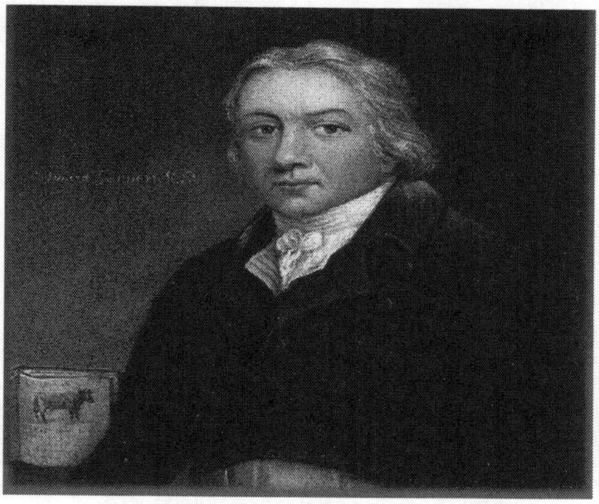

Edward Jenner

Louis Pasteur, in 1880, isolated the bacterium responsible for chicken cholera and grew it in pure culture. During the course of experiments, Pasteur noticed that chicken cholera bacterium lost its disease-causing ability or virulence when the bacterial culture was incubated for longer interval between transfers. Such bacteria are called as attenuated bacteria. When such attenuated culture was inoculated to the healthy chicken, it did not develop disease symptoms; instead exhibited ability to resist the pathogen. These experiments of Louis Pasteur clearly established that most of the animals possess a mechanism by which they are able to resist pathogens. Pasteur called the attenuated cultures as vaccines in honor of Edward Jenner because many years before the Pasteur experiments, Jenner had used material from cowpox lesions for vaccination to protect the people against smallpox. Shortly after this, Pasteur and Chamberland developed an attenuated anthrax vaccine in two ways: by treating cultures with potassium bichromate and by incubating the bacteria at 42 to 43°C.

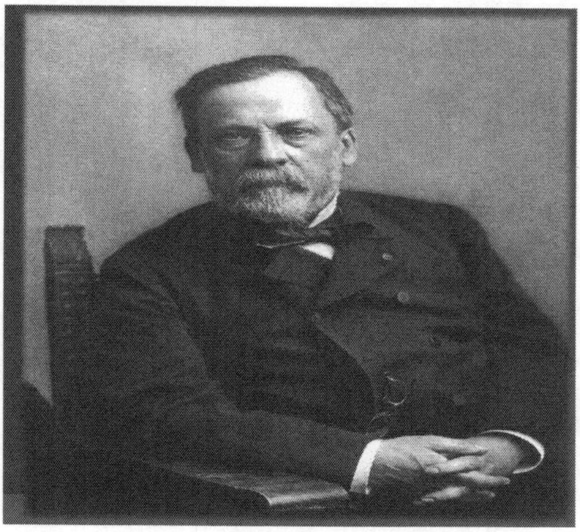

Louis Pasteur

Pasteur also developed a dead vaccine for rabies. He attenuated rabies pathogen by growing it in the rabbit brain. The brain and spinal cord of the infected rabbit was excised and dried for several days, pulverized and mixed with glycerin. This vaccine was given to Joseph Meister, a nine-year old boy, who had been bitten by a rabid dog repeatedly for 13 times over a period of 10 days with increasingly virulent preparations of the attenuated culture, Joseph Meister survived. Pasteur was as surprised as anyone else. Joseph Meister did not die even after several weeks of crucial trails. Having convinced people all over the world contributed liberally for the construction of the development of vaccines.

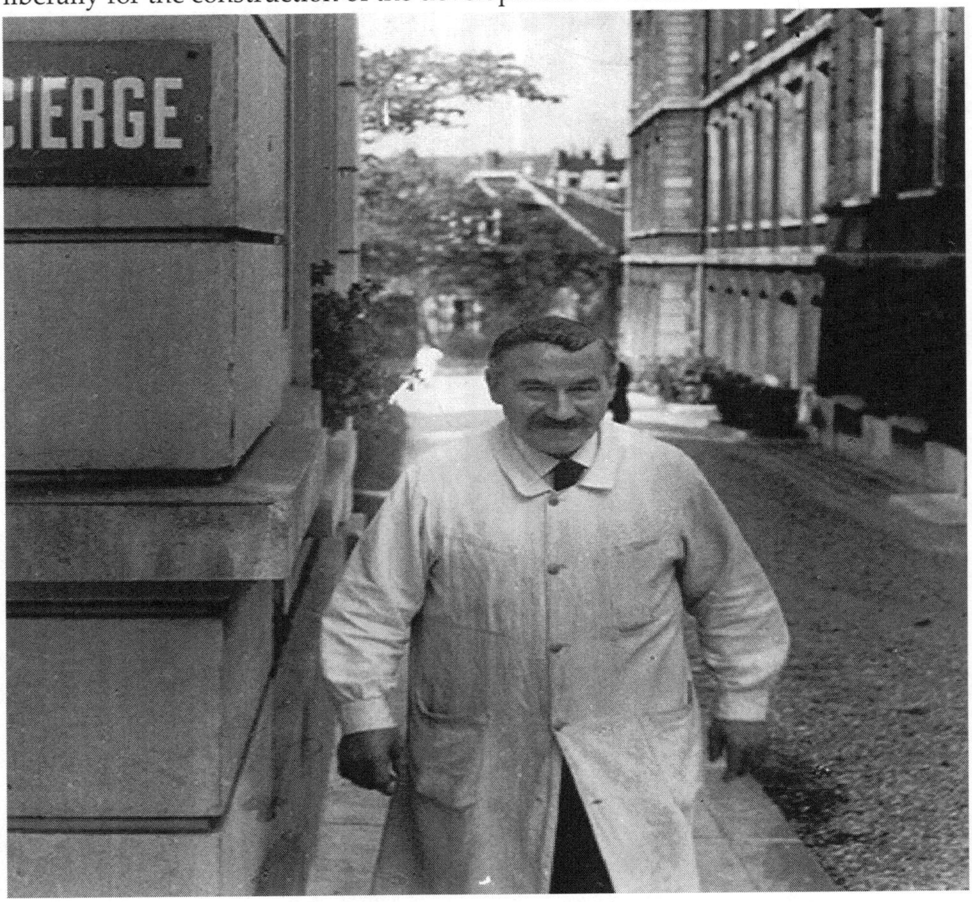

Joseph Meister

Pasteur's development of vaccines for cholera, anthrax and rabies though successful, the mechanism of protection provided by them remained obscure and different persons interpreted the involved mechanism differently. Nuttal (1988) observed that defabrinated blood had a bactericidal effect. Buncher (1989) observed involvement of a heat-labile bactericidal factor called alexine, while Behring and Kitasato (1890) explained the involvement of humoral factor or antibody. Elie Metchnikoff (1880) observed that certain leukocytes present in the blood could swallow disease-causing bacteria. He called these cells as phagocytes and the phenomenon as phagocytosis. Wright (1903) demonstrated the phenomenon as phagocytes and antibodies in neutralizing the antigens. Pfeffer (1893) demonstrated lysis of live cholera Vibrios. Bordet (1895) explained the participation of two components in the lysis of live cholera vibrios; the first being heat stable and found in immune sera (later called as antibody), and the second being heat labile and identical with Buchner's alexine, which was named subsequently as complement. Further studies reported other processes in which antibodies react with antigens such as agglutination, precipitation, complement fixation and neutralization.

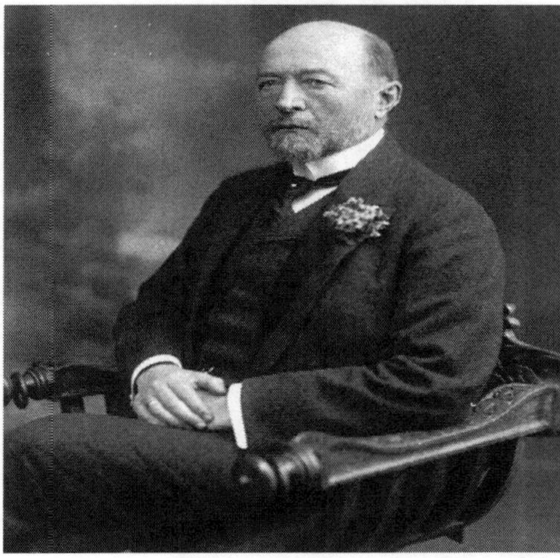

Emil Adolf von Behring

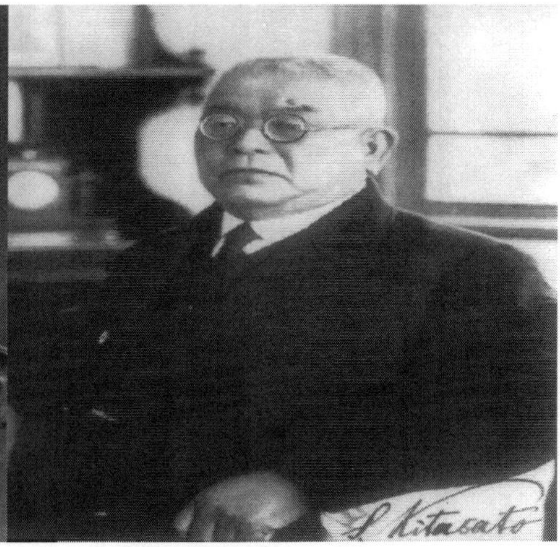

Kitasato Shibasaburo

2. Discovery of humoral and cell mediated immunity

Emil Von Behring and Kitasato Shibasaburo (1890) injected inactivated diphtheria toxin into rabbits stimulating them to produce antitoxin in the blood cells. This antitoxin would inactivate the toxin produced by the diphtherial bacterium and would protect the animal from diphtheria disease. Von Behring and Kitasato demonstrated that (the liquid, noncellular component of coagulated blood) from animals previously immunized to diphtheria could transfer the immune state to unimmunized animals. They have also developed tetnus antitoxin. These toxins are used even now in the prevention of diphtheria and tetanus respectively.

The antitoxin work provided evidence that immunity could result from soluble substances in the blood which are now called as antibodies. Because immunity was mediated by antibodies contained in body fluids (known at the time as humors), it was called humoral immunity. This has resulted in the development of concept of humoral immunity mediated by non-cellular body fluids for which Behring was awarded Nobel prize in 1901. However, humoral immunity was fully realized only by the work of Elvin A. Kabat and other workers during 1930 who demonstrated that a fraction of serum, called gamma globulin, was responsible for immunity acquired following immunization.

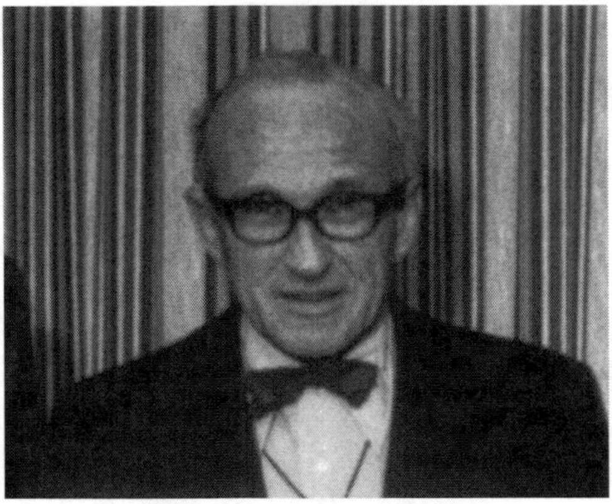

Elvin A. Kabat

Elie Metchnikoff (1940) discovered that certain leukocytes present in the blood could swallow disease-causing bacteria. He further observed that these phagocytes were more active in immunized animal and contributed to the immune state. Metchnikoff hypothesized that the cells were the major effector of immunity and he gave the concept of cell-mediated immunity. It became clear that blood cells were also important in immunity. Noting that these phagocytic cells were more active in animals that had been immunized, Metchnikoff hypothesized that cells, rather than serum components, were the major effector of immunity. The active phagocytic cells identified by Metchnikoff were likely blood monocytes and neutrophils.

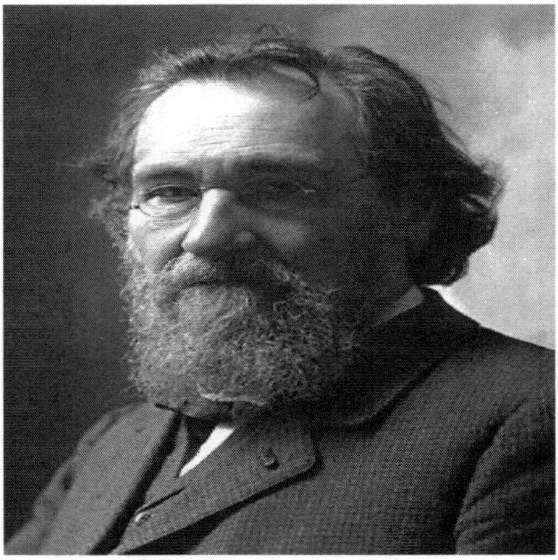

Elie Metchnikoff

A great deal of controversy developed between the supporters of cell-mediated immunity and of humoral immunity. It was later shown that both are correct—immunity requires both cellular and humoral responses. Concepts of humoral immunity developed rapidly due to ready availability of blood while it was difficult to study the activities of immune cells. With the development of tissue culture techniques, cell-mediated immunity also got acceptance during 1940. Subsequent studies during 1950 proved that both the types of immunity are interrelated. The identification of lymphocytes as the responsible cells for both cell-mediated and humoral immunity resulted in the end of controversy. Bruce Glick (1950) demonstrated two types of lymphocytes; T lymphocytes derived from the thymus mediated cellular immunity, and B lymphocytes from the bursa of Fabricius (an outgrowth of the cloaca in birds) were involved in humoral immunity.

In the early 1930s Rebecca Lancefield (1895–1981) recognized the importance of serological tests. She developed a classification system for the streptococci based on the antigenic nature of cell wall carbohydrates. Her system is now known as the Lancefield system in which each different serotype is a Lancefield group and identified by a letter (A through T). This scheme is based on specific antibody agglutination reactions with cell wall carbohydrate antigens (C polysaccharides) extracted from the streptococci. Lancefield also showed that further subdividing of the group A streptococci into specific serological types was possible, based on the presence of type-specific M (protein) antigens. Jules Border demonstrated that immunity can also be caused by any non-pathogenic organisms or organic substances from other animals. Karl Landsteiner and others have demonstrated that inoculating an animal with almost any organic substance induces production of antibodies. The discovery of blood groups (ABO) by Landsteiner (1930) led to the successful blood transfusion in humans. This sensational discovery won Landsteiner a Nobel prize in 1930. His studies demonstrated that antibodies have a capacity for an almost unlimited range of reactivity, including responses to compounds that had only recently been synthesized in the laboratory and had not previously existed in nature. In addition, it was shown that molecules differing in the smallest detail could be distinguished by their reactivity with different antibodies. The selective theory was proposed to account for this specificity.

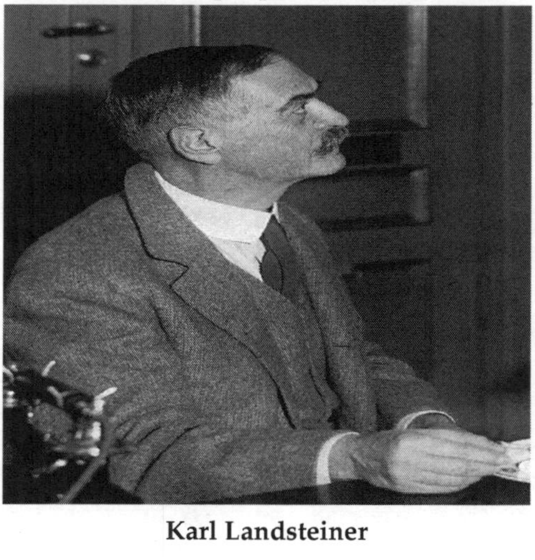

Karl Landsteiner

3. Selective theory

Paul Ehrlich (1900) proposed the concept of selective theory, which states that cells in the blood possesses variety of receptors on their surface. He called these receptors as side-chain receptors that react specifically with pathogenic organisms and kill them. Borrowing a concept used by Emil Fischer in 1894 to explain the interaction between an enzyme and its substrate, Ehrlich proposed that binding of the receptor to an infectious agent was like the fit between a lock and key.

In addition, such cells also produce more receptors with same specificity. Thus, he demonstrated specificity between antigen and the receptors. According to Ehrlich's theory, the specificity of the receptor was determined before its exposure to antigen, and the antigen selected the appropriate receptor. This concept was further refined by subsequent workers such as David Talmadge and Macfarlance Burnet during 1950, and named it as clonal selection theory. Burnet was awarded the Nobel prize along with Sir Peter Medawar. According to this theory, an individual lymphocyte expresses membrane receptors that are specific for a distinct antigen. This unique receptor specificity is determined before the lymphocyte is exposed to the antigen. Binding of antigen to its specific receptor activates the cell, causing it to proliferate into a clone of cells that have the same immunologic specificity as the parent cell. The clonal selection theory has been further refined and is now accepted as the underlying paradigm of modern immunology. Subsequently, Neilijerne (1984) was also awarded a Nobel prize for his contribution to the development of clonal expression and evaluation of the idiotype network in the regulation of immune responses.

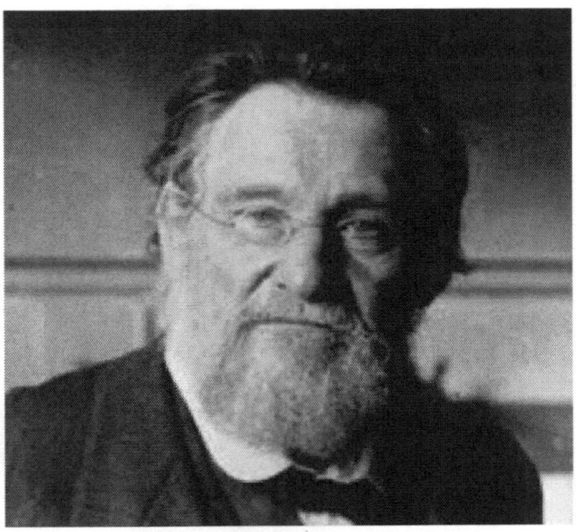

Paul Ehrlich

4. Structure of an antibody

Rodery Porter and Gerald M. Edleman (1972) elucidated the structure of antibody (immunoglobulin) with the help of enzymes. The immunoglobulin polypeptide chain can be cleaved into 3-4 pieces i.e., two antibody fragments (fab) and one crystallizable fragment (FC). These people were awarded for Nobel prize in 1972 for this work. Wu and Kabat (1972) demonstrated the hypervariable region in antibody molecule. The early experiments of Kabat and Tiselius resolved serum proteins into three majors non albumin peaks— α, β and γ. The presence of a serum component responsible for allergic reactions was first demonstrated in 1921 by K. Prausnitz and H. Kustner, who injected serum from an allergic person intradermally into a nonallergic individual. When the appropriate antigen was later injected at the same site, a wheal and flare reaction (analogous to hives) developed there. This reaction, called the P-K reaction (named for its originators, Prausnitz and Kustner), was the basis for the first biological assay for IgE activity. Actual identification of IgE was accomplished by K. and T. Ishizaka in 1966. Peter Gorer proposed a concept of rejection of a foreign tissue in responses to cell surface molecules regulated by the genes. These molecules were identified to be four groups of genes (group 1 to 4) that encoded blood cell antigens. They further confirmed that group 2 genes participated in the rejection of transplanted tumours and other tissue. Snell called these genes as histocompatible genes. For this work, Snell along with Dausset and Benacerraf, who worked on Human Leucocyte Antigen (HLA) complexes, were awarded Nobel prize in 1980.

5. Somatic hybridization

In 1975, Georges Köhler and Cesar Milstein devised a method for preparing monoclonal antibody, which quickly became one of immunology's key technologies. This technique was called somatic hybridization by which homozygous monoclonal antibodies could be developed. By fusing a normal activated, antibody-producing B cell with a myeloma cell (a cancerous plasma cell), they were able to generate a hybrid cell, called a hybridoma, that possessed the immortal growth properties of the myeloma cell and secreted the antibody produced by the B cell. The resulting clones of hybridoma cells, which secrete large quantities of monoclonal antibody, can be cultured indefinitely. Kohler and Milstein were awarded Nobel prize in 1984 for this achievement. Later this technique got popularity by the name 'hybridoma technology'.

Invasion by a microorganism or presence of an antigen did not always result in the beneficial effect of immunity or protection. Sometimes, it caused the opposite effect. Koch (1890) had noticed that when the tubercle bacillus or its protein was injected into guinea pig, an abnormal reaction took place, known as Koch phenomenon. This was later on known as hypersensitivity reaction. Charles Richet and Paul Portier (1902) made the at range observation while studying the effect of toxic extract of sea anemones in dogs. According to their observation, dogs, which had prior contact with the toxins, were abnormally sensitive even to minute quantities of the toxin. Portier and Richet coined the term *anaphylaxis,* loosely translated from Greek to mean the opposite of *prophylaxis,* to describe this overreaction. Richet was subsequently awarded the Nobel Prize in Physiology or Medicine in 1913 for his work on anaphylaxis. Later, many similar reactions were observed, both experimentally and in nature of injury, disease or even death resulting from repeated contacts with antigen. The importance of this phenomenon in the pathogenesis of many human diseases led to the development of the discipline of allergy.

Scope of immunity

Till recently, a generalized concept of immunity prevailed. It was considered as a protective mechanism intended to defend the body against invading microorganisms. Based on the original suggestion of Thomas (1954), Burnet (1967) developed the concept of immunological surveillance. According to this concept, the primary function of the immune system is to preserve the integrity of the body by identifying and destroying all foreign antigens whether autogenous (internal) or external in origin. Malignancy was visualized as a failure of immunological surveillance, and the scope of immunity was enlarged to include natural defense against cancer.

Another aspect of the role of immunity is in the rejection of homograft. It was possible to understand the immunological basis of organ transplantation by the works of Medawar and Burnet. This concept was made possible with the elective immunosuppression and proper selection of donors based on histocompatibility. The history of transplantation, thus, parallel to the history of blood transfusion, which was unsuccessful and even fatal before the discovery of blood groups by Landstainer (1900).

The last two decades have witnessed an explosion of conceptual and technical advances in immunology. Immunological processes in health and disease are now better understood following the identification of the two components of immunity i.e., the humoral or antibody-mediated processes and the cellular or cell-mediated processes, which are developed and manifested in separate pathways.

Possibility of culturing of different types of cells in vitro and to clone these cells to get a population of cells with identical genetic makeup helped to investigate cellular interactions and gene inactivation. The role of a number of gene products has been elucidated by producing transgenic animals and studying the effect of the introduced genes.

Many new techniques developed by immunologists such as monoclonal antibodies revolutionized immunoassays and detection systems that employ antibodies. Potentials of these substances are infinite in the treatment of infectious diseases, cancers, organ transplant, etc. In addition to antibodies, other immunologically-important molecules have been produced and are being developed as therapeutic agents. The flow cytometry has revolutionized the analysis of the populations, and PCR has increased the sensitivity of the detection of microorganism.

The interactions between the cells and molecules of the immune system is extremely complex, and intricacies of immune recognition are far from the understanding. Some molecules play different functions depending on the location and presence of other molecules, which need to be exploited not only in the elimination of pathogens, but also the cancer cells. It may also enable us to treat the immune-diseases, allergies and tumours. It will also help us to develop new strategies to reduce transplant rejection.

Talk W. Mak and Mark M. Davis (1984) characterized T-cell receptor. They further cloned and sequenced, a gene expressed and rearranged in T-cells, but not in B-cells. They further revealed that many of the T-cell receptor sequences were homologous to those of immunoglobulin genes. Peter Dobety and Rolf M.

Zinkernagel (1955) reported that these T-cells from mice infected with meningitis virus were destroyed. Virus infected cells only from the same strain of mice showed that T-cells must recognize two signals on an infected cell; one from the virus and other from the cell's own antigen to destroy it. For these observations, Mak and Davis, and Dobety and Zinkernagel shared Nobel Prize in 1996. Thus, various developments in the fields of Medical Microbiology such as organ and tissue transplantation, vaccinology and molecular biology had great effect on overall development of mankind.

Knowledge of the immunological process underlying the reactions of the body to infectious agents, tumours, and transplanted tissues and organs has advanced significantly by the use of modern techniques, which have enabled the identification of gene coding for molecules such as cell receptors and MHC molecules. The genes coding for immunologically-important molecule have been cloned and relatively large amounts of recombinant proteins have been produced.

The field of immunology continues to fascinate and frustrate the researchers all over the world, and many lead to the better understanding of tumour immunology, autoimmunity and responses to immunization. It could also help to develop strategies for protection against many crippling diseases. Immunity is a powerful tool created by nature to ensure the continued survival of the human beings and could perhaps be manipulated to yield a better quality of life.

Question Bank

1. Very short answer type questions
   (a) Who characterized the T-Cell receptors?
   (b) Who discovered the blood groups?
   (c) Who developed the concepts of immunological surveillance?
   (d) Who coined the term anaphylaxis?
   (e) Who gave the technique of hybridoma technology?
   (f) Who gave structure of antibody?
   (g) Who was awarded Nobel Prize for HIA complex?
   (h) Who gave selective theory?
   (i) Who gave lance field system?
2. Short answer type questions
   (a) What is Koch phenomenon?
   (b) What is hybridoma technology?
   (c) What is hybridoma?
   (d) What is P-k reaction?
   (e) What is selective theory?
   (f) What is Lancefield system?
   (g) What are the contributions of Elie Metchnikofff?
   (h) What short note on discovery of humoral and cell mediated immunity?
   (i) Define variolation.

(j) Define immunology.

3. Long answer type questions
   (a) Describe in detail the scope of immunity and immunology.
   (b) Describe in detail the contribution of various researchers in development of immunology.
   (c) Give in detail the important contributions of Louis Pasteur in field of immunology.
   (d) What are important contributions of Edward Jenner in development of immunology.
   (e) Describe in detail the development of vaccination.
   (f) Describe in detail the discovery of humoral and cell mediated immunity.
   (g) Describe in detail the development of somatic hybridization.

Multiple Choice Questions

1. A state in which the organism persists in small numbers in tissue in the presence of immune system is known as
   (a) Anergy (b) Opsonisation
   (c) Premunition (d) Atopy
2. An example of complement fixation test is
   (a) Weil-Felix reaction (b) Wasserman's reaction
   (c) Coomb's test (d) Rose-Waller test
3. Which cell causes phagocytosis?
   (a) B cell (b) T cell
   (c) Macrophage (d) None of the above
4. HLA typing is used in
   (a) Blood grouping (b) Assessing prognosis of disease
   (c) Cancer therapy (d) Cases of disputed paternity
5. MHC restriction applies to
   (a) Donor selection in tissue transplantation
   (b) Antigen presentation by macrophages to T cells
   (c) Feedback inhibition of antibody synthesis
   (d) Histocompatibility typing
6. Primary immune response is mediated by
   (a) IgA (b) IgD
   (c) IgG (d) IgM
7. Monoclonal antibodies are used in
   (a) Immunotherapy
   (b) Immunological identification of cell and tissues
   (c) Radioimmuno-imaging
   (d) All of the above

8. Anamnestic reaction is defined as
   (a) Production of heterologous but related antibody in response to antigenic stimulation
   (b) Selective proliferation of plasma cell produce antibodies
   (c) A kind of primary immunological reaction
   (d) None of the above
9. The function of an adjuvant in a vaccine is
   (a) Distribution (b) Absorption
   (c) Antigenicity (d) Metabolism
10. Anaphylaxis is mediated by
   (a) Cytotoxic antibodies (b) Chemotactic factors
   (c) Immune complexes (d) Incomplete antibodies
11. Which of the following is not a mediator of anaphylaxis?
   (a) 5-hydroxy tryptamine (b) Heparin
   (c) Platelet activating factors (d) Anaphylatoxins
12. Reaginic immunoglobulin is
   (a) IgG (b) IgD
   (c) IgA (d) IgE
13. The Prausnitz-Kustner (PK) reaction is used to demonstrate
   (a) Presence of secretory antibodies
   (b) Presence of Wasserman regain
   (c) Presence of skin sensitizing antibody
   (d) Atopic hypersensitivity
14. The most common complications following blood transfusion are
   (a) Allergic reaction (b) Volume overload
   (c) Infections (d) Hemolysis
15. Rh antibodies are detected by
   (a) Using a colloid medium such as 20% bovine serum albumin
   (b) Using red cells treated with enzymes such as trypsin
   (c) Indirect Coombs test
   (d) All of the above.
16. The most common complications following blood transfusion are
   (a) Allergic reaction (b) Volume overload
   (c) Infections (d) Hemolysis
17. Rh antibodies are detected by
   (a) Using a colloid medium such as 20% bovine serum albumin
   (b) Using red cells treated with enzymes such as trypsin
   (c) Indirect Coombs test
   (d) All of the above.

18. In typhoid, Widal test detects
   (a) O antigen *(b)* H antigen
   (c) Vi antigen *(d)* Both O and H antigen
19. All the following are true of Widal test EXCEPT
   (a) High titre in first sample is diagnostic
   (b) H antigen is specific for serotyping
   (c) Highly positive H titre is not diagnostic
   (d) Maximum titre is reached in the third week
20. Vibrio cholerae was discovered by
   (a) Robert Koch *(b)* John Snow
   (c) Louis Pasteur *(d)* Eberth and Gaffky

Answer Key

Question Number	Answer	Question Number	Answer
1	C	11	B
2	B	12	D
3	C	13	D
4	D	14	C
5	B	15	D
6	D	16	C
7	D	17	D
8	A	18	D
9	C	19	A
10	B	20	A

References

Akira, S., K. Takeda, and T. Kaisho. 2001. Toll-like receptors: Critical proteins linking innate and acquired immunity. Nature Immunol. 2:675.

Berke G. and Clark W. R. (2007) killer lymphocytes. Springer Dordrecst, The Netherlands.369pp.

Burnet, F. M. 1959. The Clonal Selection Theory of Acquired Immunity. Cambridge University Press, Cambridge.

Cohen, S. G., and M. Samter. 1992. Excerpts from Classics in Allergy. Symposia Foundation, Carlsbad, California.

Creagh E.M. and O'Neill L.A. (2006) TLRs, NLRs and RLRs: trinity of pathogen sensors that co-operate in Innate immunity. Trends In Immunology.8,352-357.

Delves P. J. and Roitt I.M (2000) The immune system: first of two parts. New England journal of medicine 343, 37-49.

Fritig, B., T. Heitz, and M. Legrand. 1998.Antimicrobial proteins in induced plant defence. Curr. Opin. Immunol. 10:12.

Janeway C.A. Jr and Medzhito R. (2002) Innate Immune Recognition. Annual Review of Immunology 20,197216.

Kimbrell, D. A., and B. Beutler. 2001. The evolution and genetics of innate immunity. Nature Rev. Genet. 2:256.

Kindt, T. J., and J. D. Capra. 1984. The Antibody Enigma. Plenum Press, New York.

Lawson, P. R., and K. B. Reid. 2000. The roles of surfactant proteins A and D in innate immunity. Immunologic Reviews173:66

Matzinger P. (2002) The Danger model: a renewed sense of self. Science. 296,301-305.

Medzhitov, R., and C. A. Janeway. 2000. Innate immunity. N. Eng. J. Med. 343:338.

Medzihitow R. (2008) origin and physiological rules of inflammation. Nature 454,428-35.

Metchnikoff, E. 1905. Immunity in the Infectious Diseases. MacMillan, New York'.

Metlan E., Tschoop J. and Karin M. (2006) Intra cellular pattern recognition receptors in the host response. Nature 424,39-44.

Otvos, L. 2000. Antibacterial peptides isolated from insects. J. Peptide Sci. 6:497

Palm N.W. and Medzhitov R. (2009) Pattern recognition receptors and control of adaptive Immunity. Immunological Review 227,221-233.

Paul, W., ed. 1999. Fundamental Immunology, 4th ed. Lippincott- Raven, Philadelphia

Steinman R.M. and Idoyaga J. (2010) features of the dendritic cell lineage. Immunological Reviews 234,5-17.

CHAPTER 2

Cells of Immune System

Introduction

The survival of a host, such as a human, depends upon an elaborate network of defenses that keeps harmful microorganisms and other foreign material away from infecting the body. We live in a potentially hostile world filled with a bewildering array of infectious agents of diverse shape, size, composition and subversive character that would very happily use us as rich sanctuaries for propagating their "selfish genes" had we not also developed a series of defense mechanisms at their equal in effectiveness and ingenuity. In these defense mechanisms that can establish a state of immunity against infection (Latin *immunitas,* freedom from) and whose operation provides the basis for the delightful subject called "Immunology".

Immune System

The immune system is remarkably versatile defense system that has evolved to protect animals from invading pathogenic microorganisms and cancer. It is able to generate an enormous variety of cells and molecules capable of specifically recognizing and eliminating an apparently limitless variety of foreign invaders. These cells and molecules act together in a dynamic network whose complexity rivals that of the nervous system. Functionally, an immune response can be divided into two related activities—recognition and response. Immune recognition is remarkable for its specificity. The immune system is able to recognize subtle chemical differences that distinguish one foreign pathogen from another. Furthermore, the system is able to discriminate between foreign molecules and the body's own cells and proteins. Immune system like any other system of the body is comprised of varieties of cells and organs, specified for a specific role. All the blood cells originate in the bone marrow having stem cells.

Stem Cells

The cells which develop into the blood cells are called stem cells. They are undifferentiated embryonic cells. They have the ability to develop into any type of blood cells. So, they are said to be pluripotent and totipotent. They are located in the bone marrow (figure 2.1). However, in the early embryo they originate in the yolk sac. Later they migrate into the liver. In the adult they reach the bone marrow. The stem cells develop into blood cells through a process called hemopoiesis. As the stem cells develop into blood cells they are also called haemocytoblasts or haemopoietic stem cells. Some of the stem cells develop into lymphocytes. The development of lymphocytes from stem cells is called lymphopoiesis. The stem cells proliferate and differentiate under the influence colony stimulating factors (CSF).

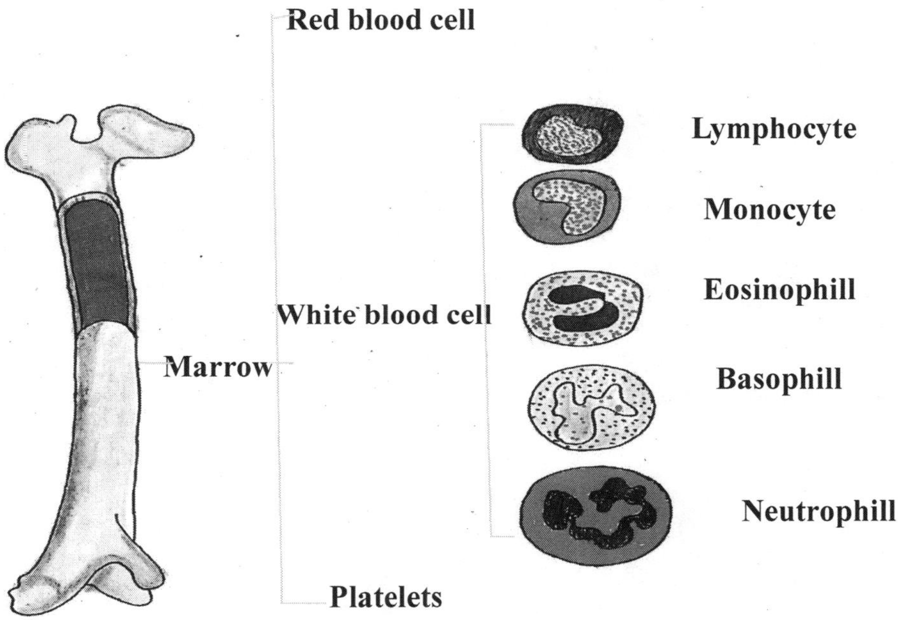

Fig. 2.1: Bone marrow, site of formation of blood cells

The stem cells develop in three lines namely lymphoid lineage, myeloid lineage and erythroid lineage (figure 2.2).

a) **Erythroid Lineage -** In erythroid lineage the stem cell develops into Red Blood Corpuscles (RBCs).

b) **Myeloid Lineage -** In myeloid lineage the stem cell develops into the myeloid progenitors. The myeloid progenitor develops into two groups namely monocytes and polymorphonuclear leucocytes. The monocytes differentiate into macrophages. The polymorphonuclear leucocytes include the eosinophils, basophils, neutrophils, mast cells, antigen presenting cells and megakaryocytes. The megakaryocyte differentiates into platelets.

c) **Lymphoid Lineage -** In lymphoid lineage the stem cells develop into lymphoid progenitor. The lymphoid progenitor cell develops into three groups of immune cells namely T lymphocytes, B lymphocytes and null cells. The null cells are of two types namely natural killer and killer cells.

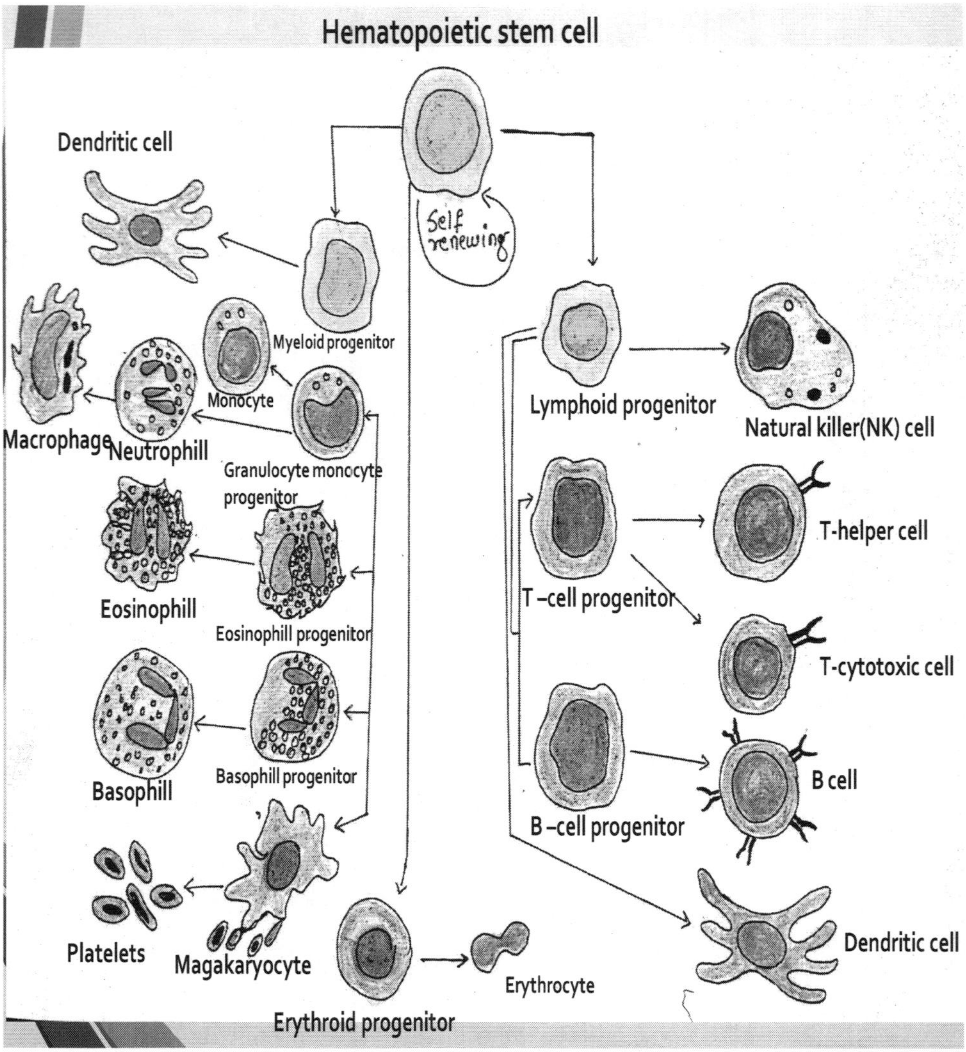

Fig. 2.2 – Various lineages of stem cells

(A) Immune Cells of Erythroid Lineage

Red Blood Corpuscles

Red Blood Corpuscles (RBCs) are derived from the erythroid lineage of bone marrow. Erythrocytes have surface complement receptors that bind to complement attached to small circulating immune complexes. They carry these complexes to the liver, where they are released to Kupffer cells which phagocytose them. Thus, erythrocytes play an important immunological role in clearing immune complexes from the circulation in persistent infections and in some autoimmune disease. Structure of RBCs is depicted in figure 2.3.

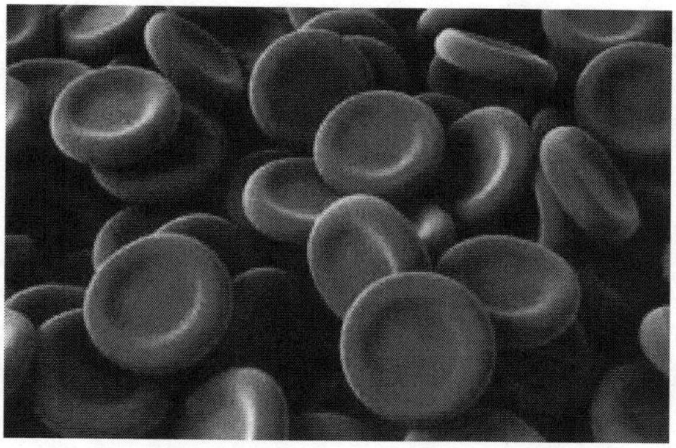

Fig. 2.3 : Structure of Red Blood Corpuscles

(B) Immune cells of myeloid lineage

1. The Monocytes

During hematopoiesis in the bone marrow, granulocyte-monocyte progenitor cells differentiate into promonocytes (figure 2.2), which leave the bone marrow and enter the blood, where they further differentiate into mature monocytes. Monocytes circulate in the bloodstream for about 8 h, during which they enlarge; they then migrate into the tissues and differentiate into specific tissue macrophages or, into dendritic cells.

Monocytes and macrophages are two mononuclear (i.e., a single large nucleus) cells. Both types are highly phagocytic and make up the monocyte-macrophage system. Monocytes circulate in the blood and macrophages are present in the tissues. Monocytes [Greek *monos,* single, and *cyte,* cell] are mononuclear phagocytic leukocytes with an ovoid or kidney-shaped nucleus (figure 2.4) and granules in the cytoplasm that stain gray-blue. Monocytes are present in the blood and settle in the tissues as macrophages [MO]. These phagocytes are attracted to sites of infection [chemotaxis], bind to the microbe [adhere], and ingest [phagocytose] and kill the microbe. Molecules coating a microbe, such as complement or antibody, enhance contact and ingestion [opsonization] of the microbe.

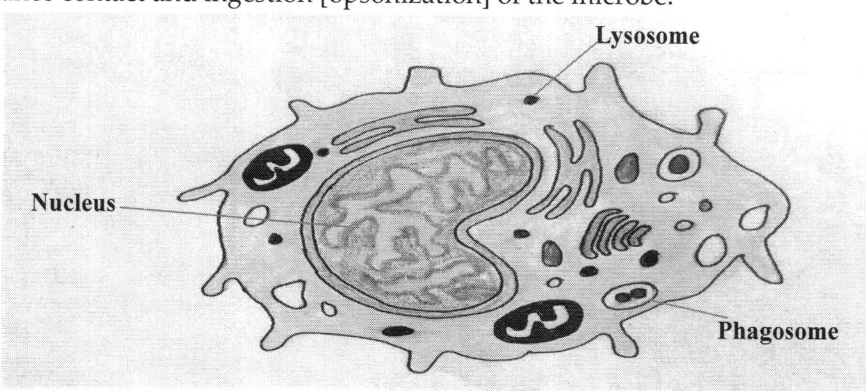

Fig. 2.4 : Structure of Monocyte

2. Macrophages

Macrophages originate from the stem cells of bone marrow. Some of the stem cells develop into myeloid progenitor cells and some of which turn into monoblasts. The monoblasts become promonocytes which change into monocytes. The monocytes develop into macrophages. The macrophages are derived from monocytes (figure 2.2). The monocytes circulate in the blood. They live only for 24 hours. Then they leave the blood and migrate into tissues where they enlarge and become macrophages. Differentiation of a monocyte into a tissue macrophage involves a number of changes: The cell enlarges five- to tenfold; its intracellular organelles increase in both number and complexity; and it acquires increased phagocytic ability, produces higher levels of hydrolytic enzymes, and begins to secrete a variety of soluble factors.

Macrophages are large mononuclear phagocytic cells derived from monocytes. Macrophages are components of the reticuloendothelial system. The macrophages are distributed throughout the body but they are concentrated in lymph nodes, spleen, bone marrow and liver. They are large lymphoid cells. They have a large nucleus. They contain a large number of lysosomes (figure 2.5). They are strongly phagocytic to a wide variety of particulate materials such as microorganisms, dead cells debris, immune complex etc. Usually macrophages are immobile but become actively mobile when stimulated by lymphokines secreted by T cells.

Macrophages may be larger than monocytes, contain more organelles (especially lysosomes and phagolysosomes), and have a plasma membrane covered with ruffles or microvilli (figure 2.5). Macrophages have receptors for antibodies and complement; these can coat microorganisms or foreign material and enhance phagocytosis. This enhancement is termed opsonization. Since macrophages are highly phagocytic, they provide nonspecific resistance. The macrophages are of two types namely resident macrophages and elicited macrophages. The resident macrophages are stationary and immobile. The elicited macrophages are wandering cells.

Macrophages are dispersed throughout the body. Some take up residence in particular tissues, becoming fixed macrophages, whereas others remain motile and are called free, or wandering, macrophages. Free macrophages travel by amoeboid movement throughout the tissues. Macrophages spread throughout the animal body and take up residence in specific tissues where they are given special names.

1. Kupffer cells - These are macrophages of liver.
2. Alveolar macrophages or Dust cells - These are the macrophages of lungs.
3. Peritoneal macrophages - They live in the peritoneal cavity.
4. Microglial cells - These cells live in the nervous system.
5. Giant cells - These are very large macrophages formed by the fusion of many macrophages. They are found in certain inflammatory processes.
6. Histiocytes in connective tissues
7. Mesangial cells in the kidney
8. Osteoclasts in bone

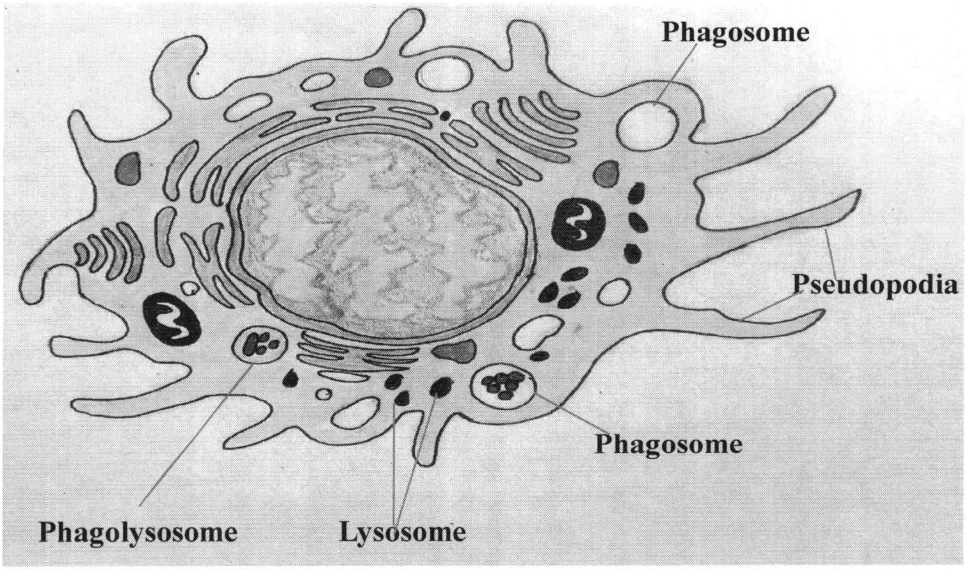

Fig. 2.5 : Structure of Macrophage

Although normally in a resting state, macrophages are activated by a variety of stimuli in the course of an immune response. Phagocytosis of particulate antigens serves as an initial activating stimulus. However, macrophage activity can be further enhanced by cytokines secreted by activated TH cells, by mediators of the inflammatory response, and by components of bacterial cell walls. One of the most potent activators of macrophages is interferon gamma (IFN-γ) secreted by activated TH cells. Activated macrophages are more effective than resting ones in eliminating potential pathogens, because they exhibit greater phagocytic activity, an increased ability to kill ingested microbes, increased secretion of inflammatory mediators, and an increased ability to activate T cells. In addition, activated macrophages, but not resting ones, secrete various cytotoxic proteins that help them eliminate a broad range of pathogens, including virus-infected cells, tumor cells, and intracellular bacteria. Activated macrophages also express higher levels of class II MHC molecules, allowing them to function more effectively as antigen-presenting cells. Thus, macrophages and TH cells facilitate each other's activation during the immune response.

3. The polymorphonuclear leucocytes (PMN)

Granulocytes are white blood corpuscles. They have irregular-shaped nuclei with two to five lobes, and the cytoplasmic matrix has granules that contain reactive substances that kill microorganisms and enhance inflammation. Because of the irregular-shaped nuclei, granulocytes are also called polymorphonuclear leukocytes or PMNs. Three types of granulocytes exist, viz. eosinophils, basophils and neutrophils.

3.1 Eosinophils

These are granular, motile, acidophilic leucocytes. Have a two lobed nucleus connected by a slender thread of chromatin, and the granules stain red with acidic dyes (eosin). An acid dye stains the granules of the cytoplasm of these cells intensely. The granules are rich in hydrolytic enzymes. The nucleus is usually bilobed or ellipsoid (figure 2.6). They can migrate from the bloodstream into tissue spaces.

Unlike basophils, eosinophils are mobile cells that their role is important only in the defense against protozoan and helminth parasites, mainly by releasing cationic proteins and reactive oxygen metabolites into the extracellular fluid to damage the parasite's plasma membranes. Increase in number of eosinophils [eosinophilia] is observed in allergic reactions especially during infection with intestinal parasites. They are present at low levels in the circulation [2-5% of blood leukocytes], have some phagocytic activity but are primarily responsible for extracellular killing of large parasites (e.g., schistosome worms) that cannot be phagocytosed. They usually bind to an antibody coated parasite through surface Fc receptors and release the contents of their granules (degranulate) onto the parasite surface. The granules contain peroxidase and toxin, major basic protein, which kill the parasite. Histamine is also present in the granules. The secreted contents of eosinophilic granules may damage the parasite membrane.

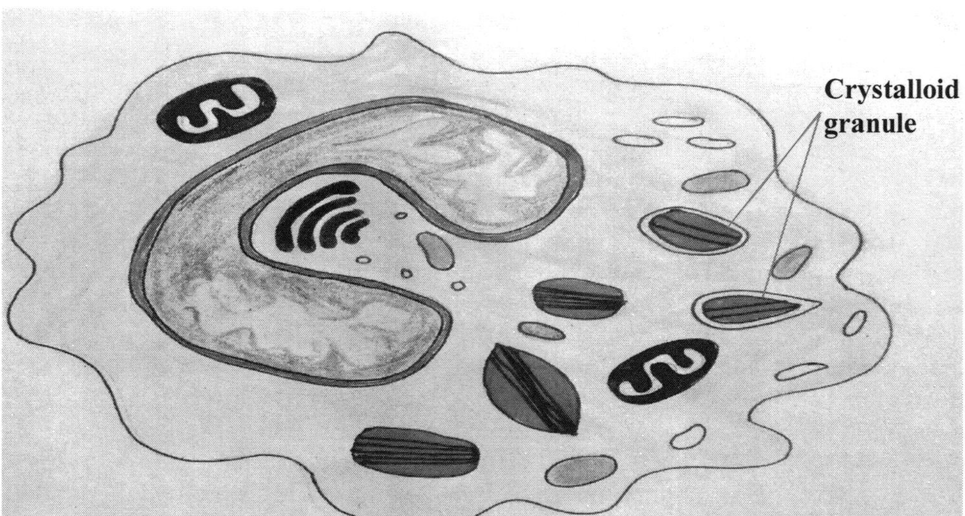

Fig. 2.6 : Structure of Eosinophil

3.2 Basophils

Basophils [Greek *basis,* base, and *philein,* to love] are non-phagocytic granulocytes that have an irregular-shaped nucleus with two lobes, and the granules stain bluish-black with basic dyes (figure 2.7). Basophils are non-phagocytic cells. The basophils granules are believed to contain heparin, histamine, serotonin, platelets, activating factor and other vasoactive amines that may be released at the site of inflammation or regions of immediate hypersensitivity reactions. Because these physiological mediators influence the tone and diameter of blood vessels, they are termed vasoactive agents. Basophils (and mast cells) possess high-affinity receptors for an immunoglobulin and thereby become coated with IgE antibodies. Once coated, antigens can trigger the cell to secrete vasoactive mediators. These inflammatory mediators play a major role in certain allergic responses such as eczema, hay fever, and asthma.

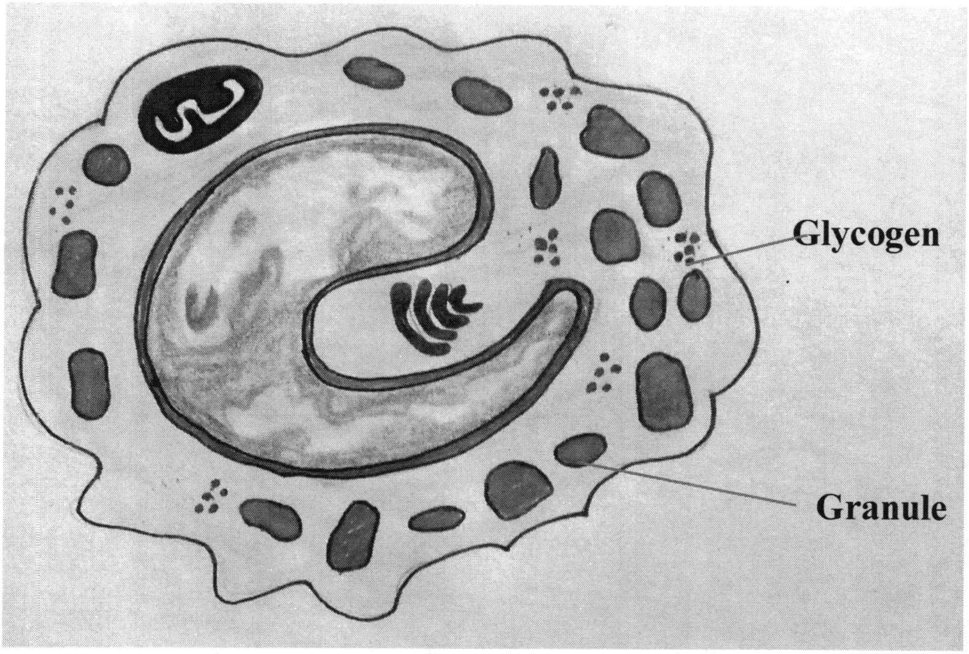

Fig. 2.7 : Structure of Basophil

3.2.1 Mast Cells

These are large tissue cells with basophilic granules in the cytoplasm. Mast cells are similar to basophils of the blood, in appearance and function. Basophils are circulating in the blood whereas the mast cells are sessile and present in the tissues throughout the body. These cells are about 10-30 μm in diameter and they have a polymorphous nucleus. When activated, these cells degranulate, releasing pharmacological mediators like serotonin, histamine, heparin, platelet activating factor, leukotrienes and prostaglandins which bring about the inflammatory and allergic reactions resulting in vasodilation, increased vascular permeability, and leukocyte migration (figure 2.8). Mast cells, along with basophils, play an important role in the development of allergies and hypersensitivities. The mast cells are of two types.

- Mucosal Mast Cells - The mast cells are found in the mucosa of the lung and gut. These cells are dependent on T lymphocytes for differentiation.
- Connective tissue Mast cells - These cells are not dependent on T lymphocytes and present at the sites of immediate hypersensitivity reactions.

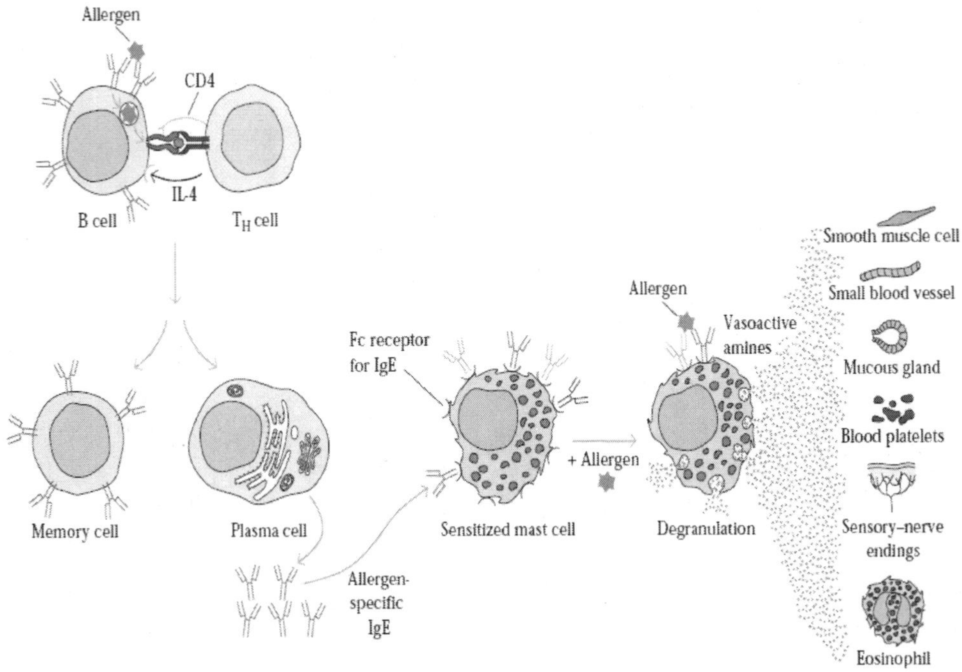

Fig. 2.8 : Degranulation of Mast cell, upon its sensitization with an allergen

3.3 Neutrophils

Neutrophils form the major part of the white blood corpuscles (40-75%). They are motile short-lived cells with multilobed nucleus (figure 2.9). Neutrophils [Latin *neuter*, neither, and *philien*] stain readily at a neutral pH, have a nucleus with three to five lobes connected by slender threads of chromatin, and contain fine primary and secondary inconspicuous granules. The cytoplasm contains granules which do not take up acidic or basic stains strongly and hence named neutrophils. The major function of the neutrophils is phagocytosis which is very similar to macrophages. Like macrophages, neutrophils have receptors for antibodies and complement proteins and are highly phagocytic cells. However, unlike the macrophage, neutrophils do not reside in healthy tissue but rapidly migrate to the site of tissue damage and infection where they are the principal phagocytic and microbicidal cells. The lytic enzymes and bactericidal substances in neutrophils are contained within large primary and smaller secondary granules. Primary granules contain peroxidase, lysozyme, and various hydrolytic enzymes, whereas secondary granules have collagenase, lactoferrin, and lysozyme. Both of these granules help accomplish intracellular digestion. Neutrophils also use oxygen-dependent and oxygen-independent pathways that generate antimicrobial substances and defensins to kill ingested microorganisms. Neutrophils can attack and destroy bacteria and viruses even in the circulating blood. When a tissue is damaged or inflamed the neutrophils reach that area along with macrophages and destroy the unwanted tissues by phagocytosis.

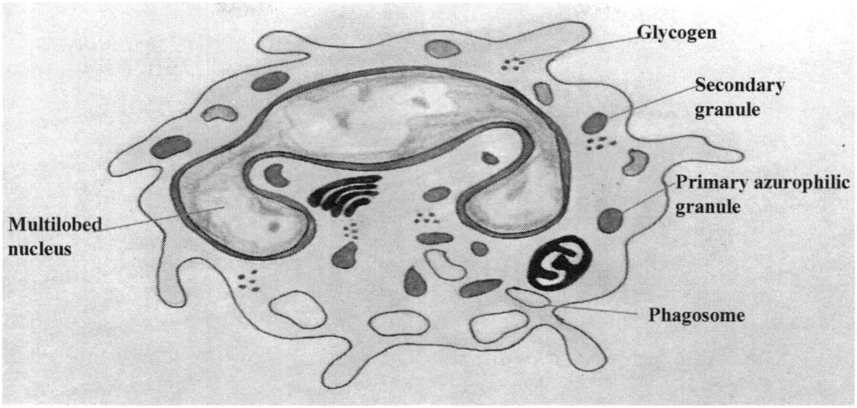

Fig. 2.9 : Structure of Neutrophil

4. Antigen presenting cells

Activation of both the humoral and cell-mediated branches of the immune system requires cytokines produced by TH cells. It is essential that activation of TH cells themselves be carefully regulated, because an inappropriate T-cell response to self-components can have fatal autoimmune consequences. To ensure carefully regulated activation of TH cells, they can recognize only antigen that is displayed together with class MHC II molecules on the surface of antigen-presenting cells (APCs). The cells which process and transfer the antigen to lymphocytes are called antigen presenting cells. These specialized cells, which include macrophages, B lymphocytes, Langerhans cells and dendritic cells, are distinguished by two properties: (1) they express class II MHC molecules on their membranes, and (2) they are able to deliver a co-stimulatory signal that is necessary for TH-cell activation. Antigen-presenting cells first internalize antigen, either by phagocytosis or by endocytosis, and then display a part of that antigen on their membrane bound to a class II MHC molecule (figure 2.10). The TH cell recognizes and interacts with the antigen–class II MHC molecule complex on the membrane of the antigen-presenting cell. An additional costimulatory signal is then produced by the antigen-presenting cell, leading to activation of the TH cell.

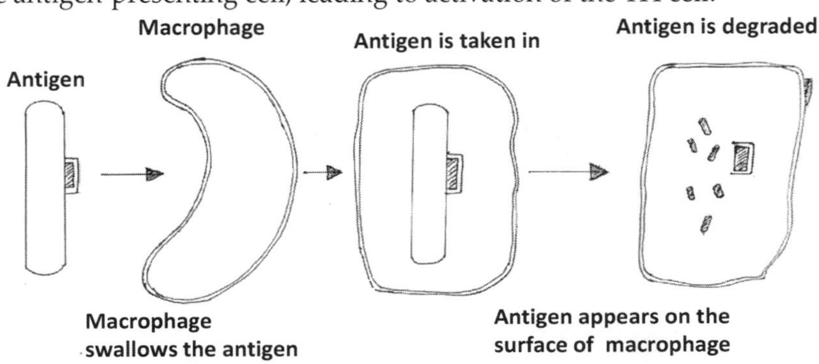

Fig. 2.10 : Processing of antigens by macrophages

Langerhans cells are present in the skin from the skin they can migrate into the spleen and lymph nodes. They contain Class 1 and 2 MHC molecules. Fc and C3 receptors. Dendritic cells (DCs) are present in the spleen and lymph nodes. They have long processes. They contain Fc receptors and class 2 MHC molecules. Dendritic cells can recognize specific pathogen associated molecular patterns on microorganisms and play an important role in nonspecific resistance. They can differentiate between potentially harmful microorganisms and "self" molecules. After the pathogen is recognized, it binds to the dendritic cell's pattern recognition receptors and then is phagocytosed. These cells are also stimulated by endogenous activators such as interferon α, heat-shock proteins, and tumor necrosis factor that are released in response to microbial infection. After stimulation, dendritic cells migrate to the bloodstream or lymphatic system and present antigens to T cells. Thus, dendritic cells also play an important role in the specific immune response. Table 2.1 depicts the types of dendritic cells, their characteristics and functions.

Table 2.1 : Types of Dendritic cells

Classification	Characteristics	Function
Myeloid	Localized in blood and tissues. Relatively short lived and replenished by bone marrow precursors.	Phagocytic when immature; migrate to lymphoid organs and tissues; main antigen presenting cells to prime CD4 T cells; regulate immune responses.
Plasmacytoid	Present in bone marrow and peripheral organs: usually long lived.	Produce large amounts of type 1 interferons following exposure to viruses; can present antigen to CD4 T cells and regulate immune responses.

5. Megakaryocytes

A megakaryocyte (mega- + karyo- + -cyte, "large-nucleus cell") is a large bone marrow cell with a lobated nucleus responsible for the production of blood thrombocytes (platelets), which are necessary for normal blood clotting. Megakaryocytes have two unique characteristics (1) They undergo a process known as endomitosis, in which the nucleus accumulates many times the normal number of chromosomes, and (2) they have specialized structures in the cytoplasm that permit fragments to be shed, as platelets, into the blood stream. Megakaryocytes have been identified in intravascular sites within the lung, leading to a theory that platelets are formed from their parent cell predominantly in the pulmonary circulation. Megakaryocytes are remarkably abundant in the lung and the pulmonary circulation, and some have estimated that 250,000 megakaryocytes reach the lung every hour. In addition, platelet counts are higher in the pulmonary vein than in the pulmonary artery, providing further evidence that the pulmonary bed contributes to platelet formation.

5.1 Platelets

Platelets are non-nucleated cells of blood usually spherical and colourless and are derived from the megakaryocytes of myeloid lineage of bone marrow. They have class 1 MHC products and receptors for IgG and low affinity receptors of IgE. Platelets, as well as having a major role in blood clotting, they play an important role in inflammation, as they contain important mediators that are released when they are activated at the site of a damaged blood vessel. Parasites coated with IgG and IgE antibodies are also thought to activate platelets through surface Fc receptors for these antibody classes. Released mediators activate also complement, which in turn attracts leukocytes to the site of tissue damage caused by trauma or infection by a parasite. They also contain granules which secrete histamine and serotonin and their release from the platelets contribute to immediate hypersensitivity reactions.

(C) Imm-une cells of Lymphoid Lineage

As mentioned earlier, in lymphoid lineage the stem cells develop into lymphoid progenitor. The lymphoid progenitor cell develops into three groups of immune cells namely T lymphocytes, B lymphocytes and null cells. The null cells are of two types namely natural killer and killer cells. The lymphocytes arise from pluripotential haemopoietic stem cells. Some of the haemopoietic stem cells turn into lymphoid stem cells which in turn develop into lymphocytes. Lymphocytes are one of many types of white blood cells produced in the bone marrow by the process of lymphopoiesis. Lymphocytes leave the bone marrow, circulate in the blood and lymphatic systems, and reside in various lymphoid organs.

Lymphocytes are mononucleate, nongranular leukocytes (WBC) of lymphoid tissue, participating in immunity. They are found in blood, lymph and lymphoid tissues such as spleen, lymph nodes, tonsils, Peyer's patches appendix etc. They are spherical or ovoid in shape. They have a diameter of 7 to 12 μm. They have a large nucleus and a rim of cytoplasm. They do not contain endoplasmic reticulum. The lymphocytes may be small or large. The surface membrane of lymphocytes contains certain unique proteins called surface markers. Because they produce and display antigen binding cell-surface receptors, lymphocytes mediate the defining immunologic attributes of specificity, diversity, memory, and self/non-self-recognition. The lymphocytes are of three types. They are T lymphocytes, B lymphocytes and null cells. The null cells constitute about 3% the B cells about 27% and the T cells about 70% of the total lymphocytes.

1. T- Lymphocytes

They are mononuclear, nonregular leucocyte. The T lymphocytes have a large nucleus and a rim of cytoplasm. They are highly concentrated in the blood and spleen. The T lymphocytes are derived from haemopoietic stem cells of bone marrow. Some of these cells turn into lymphopoietic progenitor. The lymphoid progenitor cells turn into pre-T lymphocytes. The pre t-cells leave the bone marrow and enter the thymus. Unlike B cells, which mature within the bone marrow, T cells migrate to the thymus gland to mature. The T lymphocytes are thymus dependent cells. The T lymphocytes mature in the thymus under the influence of thymic hormones. The T lymphocytes bring about cell mediated immunity. The T cells are responsible for the killing of cancer cells, killing viral infected cells, allograft rejection etc.

During its maturation within the thymus, the T cell comes to express a unique antigen-binding molecule, called the T-cell receptor (TCR), on its membrane. Unlike membrane-bound antibodies on B cells, which can recognize antigen alone, T-cell receptors can recognize only antigen that is bound to cell-membrane proteins called major histocompatibility complex (MHC) molecules. MHC molecules that function in this recognition event, which is termed "antigen presentation," are polymorphic (genetically diverse) glycoproteins found on cell membranes. There are two major types of MHC molecules: Class I MHC molecules, which are expressed by nearly all nucleated cells of vertebrate species, consist of a heavy chain linked to a small invariant protein called β2-microglobulin. Class II MHC molecules, which consist of an alpha and a beta glycoprotein chain, are expressed only by antigen-presenting cells. When a naive T cell (one that has not previously encountered antigen) encounters antigen combined with a MHC molecule on a cell, the T cell proliferates and differentiates into memory T cells and various effector T cells.

All the T cells are not similar. There are two well-defined subpopulations of T cells: T helper (TH) and T cytotoxic (TC) cells. Although a third type of T cell, called a T suppressor (TS) cell, has been postulated, recent evidence suggests that it may not be distinct from TH and TC subpopulations. T helper and T cytotoxic cells can be distinguished from one another by the presence of either CD4 or CD8 membrane glycoproteins on their surfaces. T cells displaying CD4 generally function as TH cells, whereas those displaying CD8 generally function as TC cells. T cells are functionally classified into 2 types namely regulator cells and effectors cells. The T helper cells and T suppressor cells are regulator cells, whereas the T cytotoxic cells are effector cells.

1.1 T Helper Cells [Th cells]

T helper cells are a sub population of T lymphocytes that help B cells and other T cells in immune response. They are the regulator cells. The T helper cells are activated even by very small quantities of antigens which cannot activate other cells. After a TH cell recognizes and interacts with an antigen–MHC class II molecule complex, the cell is activated—it becomes an effector cell that secretes various growth factors known collectively as cytokines. The secreted cytokines play an important role in activating B cells, TC cells, macrophages, and various other cells that participate in the immune response. The B cells are activated to produce antibodies. Differences in the pattern of cytokines produced by activated TH cells result in different types of immuneresponse. The T helper cells secrete another lymphokine called macrophage migration inhibition factor which causes the accumulation of macrophages around the antigen and the activation of macrophages to perform phagocytosis.

1.2 T Suppressor Cells [Ts cells]

T suppressor cells are a subpopulation of T cells that suppress the activity of B cells and other T cells. They are the regulatory T cells. They inhibit antibody production by B cells. They suppress the functions of the T killer cells and T helper cells. Suppressor T cells are responsible for immune tolerance by limiting the ability of the immune system to attack a person's own body tissues.

1.3 T Cytotoxic Cells [Tc] or T killer Cells [Tk]

The killer cells are a sub population of T lymphocytes that kills microorganisms or body's own cells. The cytotoxic T cell can directly attack a cell thereby capable of killing microorganisms and at times even some of the body's own cells. The receptor proteins on the surface of the cytotoxic cells help them in binding to the microorganisms or cells. The immediate effect of binding is the swelling of the Tc cells and release of cytotoxic substances directly into the attacked cell. The cytotoxic substances are probably lysosomal enzymes manufactured in the Tc cells. It is remarkable to see that each killer cell can attack many microorganisms one after another thereby killing many without the killer cells being harmed. The cytotoxic T cells (Tc) are lethal to tissue cells that have been invaded by viruses. The virus particles are entrapped in the membranes of these cells which attract the Tc cells because of the viral antigenicity and the Tc cells ultimately damage the virus infected tissue cells. The cytotoxic cells also play an important role in destroying cancer cells, heart transplant cells or other types of cells that are foreign to the person's own body.

Under the influence of TH-derived cytokines, a TC cell that recognizes an antigen–MHC class I molecule complex proliferates and differentiates into an effector cell called a cytotoxic T lymphocyte (CTL). In contrast to the TC cell, the CTL generally does not secrete many cytokines and instead exhibits cell-killing or cytotoxic activity. The CTL has a vital function in monitoring the cells of the body and eliminating any that display antigen, such as virus-infected cells, tumor cells, and cells of a foreign tissue graft. Cells that display foreign antigen complexed with a class I MHC molecule are called altered self-cells; these are targets of CTLs.

2. B-Lymphocytes

The B cells are derived from haemopoietic stem cells. Some of the haemopoietic stem cells turn into lymphoid progenitor. The lymphopoietic progenitor differentiates into pre-B cells (figure 2.2). Pre–B cells enter the bursa of Fabricius and develop into B lymphoblasts. In mammals this change occurs in the bone marrow itself. The B lymphoblast changes into immature B cell which has IgM molecules on the surface. The immature B cell changes into mature B cell which has IgD molecules on the surface in addition to IgM.

The B lymphocytes mature in bursa of fabricius (in Aves) or in bone marrow (in mammals), hence the B lymphocytes are bursa or bone marrow dependent cells. The B lymphocytes produce antibodies and hence they are responsible for humoral immunity. The B lymphocytes are mononucleate nongranular leucocytes. They have a large nucleus and a rim of cytoplasm. They are found in the blood and lymph but they are highly concentrated in the lymph nodes and spleen. The B lymphocytes contain immunoglobulins on their surface. These are called surface immunoglobulins. The B cells kill bacteria virus etc.

The mature B lymphocytes move into the lymph nodes and spleen from the bursa or bone marrow. Here the B lymphocyte is put into action when it is exposed to antigen. When a naive B cell (one that has not previously encountered antigen) first encounters the antigenic stimulations (viruses, bacterial infection and toxins) that matches its membrane bound antibody, the binding of the antigen to the antibody causes the cell to divide rapidly; its progeny differentiate into memory B cells (secondary B cells) and effector B cells called plasma cells (figure 2.11). Memory B cells have a longer life span than naive cells, and they express the same membrane-bound antibody as their parent B cell. The memory cells move more actively from blood to lymph. They survive for a longer time and they respond quickly and effectively during the subsequent similar antigenic stimulation. They produce antibodies and thus bring about secondary immune response. The plasma cells secrete antibodies in response to specific antigen (figure 2.11). Plasma cells produce the antibody in a form that can be secreted and have little or no membrane-bound antibody. Although plasma cells live for only a few days, they secrete enormous amounts of antibody during this time. It has been estimated that a single plasma cell can secrete more than 2000 molecules of antibody per second. Secreted antibodies are the major effector molecules of humoral immunity.

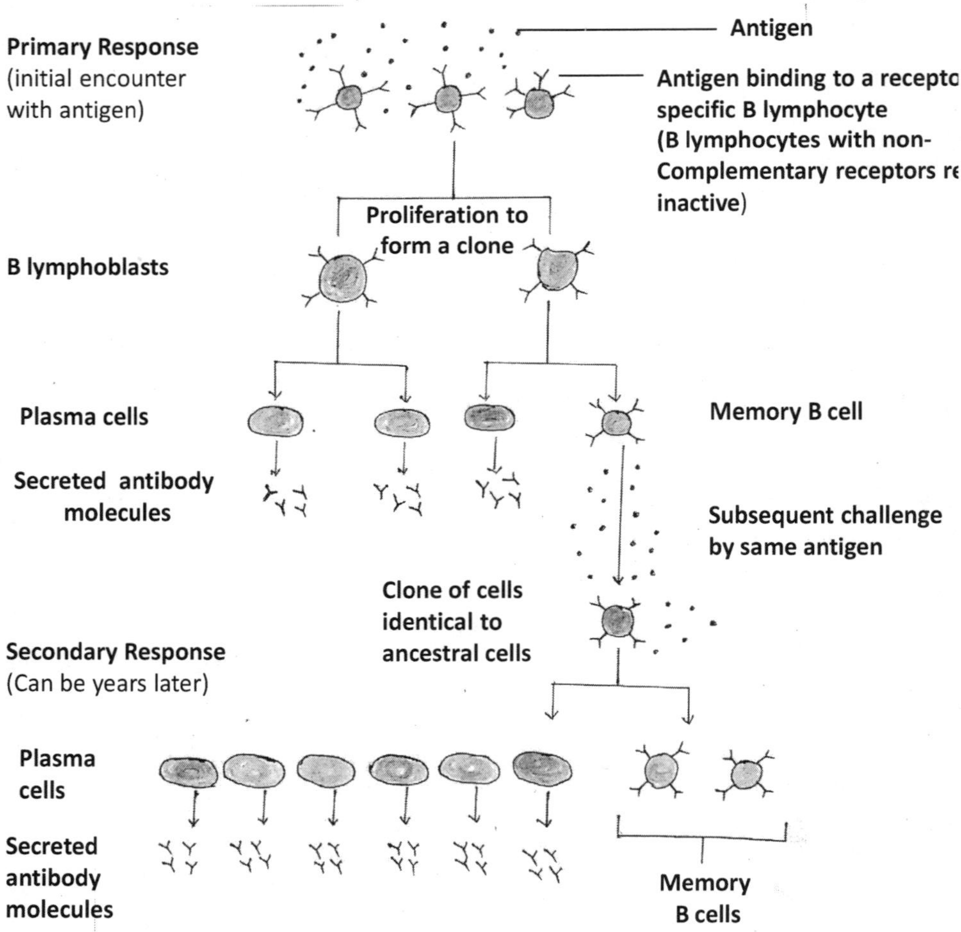

Fig. 2.11 : Production of antibodies by B lymphocytes upon antigenic stimulation

2.1 Plasma Cells

These are the end cells of the B lymphocytes. They secrete immunoglobulins. Despite their name plasma cells, they are very rarely seen in the plasma of blood but are found mainly in the secondary lymphoid organs namely lymph node and spleen. They have an eccentrically placed nucleus and the sparse cytoplasm is often gathered on one side. The nucleus gives a cartwheel appearance.

The protein synthesizing machinery is well formed. The cytoplasm is filled completely with rough endoplasmic reticulum which are heavily laden with ribosome. This is the site of protein synthesis namely synthesis of immunoglobulins. Two types of polysomes are found- one engaged in the synthesis of light chains and other in the synthesis of heavy chains. The Golgi body is also well developed. The plasma cell is devoid of surface receptors but rich in immunoglobulins in the cytoplasm. The immunoglobulin is localized in the spaces of the endoplasmic reticulum, where it sometimes forms distinct aggregates termed Russel's bodies. Plasma cells do not divide and have a half-life of about two to four days.

2.2 Memory Cells

These cells are also produced along with plasma cells when B lymphocytes are stimulated by an antigen attached on its surface. Memory cells forms the basis of vaccination, as on secondary exposure to the same antigen, they manifest the formation of antibodies very speedily.

3 Null Cells

The null cells form a third population of lymphocytes. They are intermediate between T and B cells. They have cytotoxic property. Null cells are lymphocytes with cytotoxic properties. They are neither B cells nor T cell. There are two types of null cells namely, natural killer cells and killer cells.

3.1 Natural Killer Cells [NK Cells]

The natural killer cell was first described in 1976, and constitute 5%–10% of lymphocytes in human peripheral blood. NK cells are a group of null cells. They form the third population of lymphocytes. They are the small population of large, granular lymphocytes. The Nk cells are have 2 or 3 large granules in the cytoplasm. Hence, they are also called large granular lymphocytes (LGL). They have a kidney shaped nucleus. They do not need antibody for activity. They are activated by interferons and interleukin-2. NK cells are found throughout the tissues of the body but mainly in the circulation. These cells do not express the membrane molecules and receptors that distinguish T- and B-cell lineages. Cell surface possesses FC receptors for Ig and CR3 receptor for complement. As they kill the target cells without the aid of antibody or complement, so they are antibody independent.

NK cells were subsequently shown to play an important role in host defense both against tumor cells and against cells infected with some, though not all, viruses. They recognize altered cell surface and bring about cytolysis and cytotoxicity against a wide range of tumor cells. Changes in the surface molecules of cells as the result of virus infection allow NK cells to bind to and kill infected cells by releasing perforins and inducing apoptosis. In addition, on binding to virus infected cells, NK cells secrete interferon gamma (IFNy), which protects adjacent cells from infection by viruses (herpes and mumps virus) and helps to activate T-cell mediated immunity.

Although NK cells do not have T-cell receptors or immunoglobulin incorporated in their plasma membranes, they can recognize potential target cells in two different ways. In some cases, an NK cell employs NK cell receptors to distinguish abnormalities, notably a reduction in the display of class I MHC molecules and the unusual profile of surface antigens displayed by some tumor cells and cells infected by some viruses. Another way in which NK cells recognize potential target cells depends upon the fact that some tumor cells and cells infected by certain viruses display antigens against which the immune system has made an antibody response, so that antitumor or antiviral antibodies are bound to their surfaces. Because NK cells express CD16, a membrane receptor for the carboxyl-terminal end of the IgG molecule, called the Fc region, they can attach to these antibodies and subsequently destroy the targeted cells. This is an example of a process known as antibody-dependent cell mediated cytotoxicity (ADCC).

Several observations suggest that NK cells play an important role in host defense against tumors. For example, in humans the Chediak-Higashi syndrome - an autosomal recessive disorder—is associated with impairment in neutrophils, macrophages, and NK cells and an increased incidence of lymphomas. Likewise, mice with an autosomal mutation called *beige* lack NK cells; these mutants are more susceptible than normal mice to tumor growth following injection with live tumor cells.

3.2 Killer Cells [K cells]

Killer cells are a group of null cells. They form the third population of lymphocytes. They are antibody dependent. These cells possess Fc receptors for binding with IgG antibodies. Hence, they can bind with cells coated with IgG antibodies and kill them. As the reaction is dependent on the presence of bound antibody, it is termed as antibody-dependent cell-mediated cytotoxic reaction (ADCC). These cells can combine with specific antibody when it is in complex with antigen. If the complex is on the surface of a target cell, these lymphocytes become activated destroying the target cell. By this cytotoxic property, the K cells can kill a variety of cells such as tumor cells, bacteria, viruses, fungi and parasites.

Question Bank

1. Very short answer type questions

   (a) Where does B cell mature?

   (b) Where does T cell mature?

   (c) Name the macrophages found in liver.

   (d) Name the chemicals found in mast cells.

   (e) How many lobes are found in nucleus of neutrophils?

   (f) Name one primary lymphoid organ.

   (g) Name one secondary lymphoid organ.

(h) Name one well organized secondary lymphoid organ.
(i) Which cell is responsible for humoral immunity?
(j) Which cell is responsible for CMI?
(k) Name one granulocytes.
(l) Name one agranulocytes.

2. Short answer type questions
(a) Write short note on macrophages.
(b) Write short note on lymphocytes.
(c) Write short note on thymus.
(d) Write short note on bone marrow.
(e) Write short note on granulocytes.
(f) Write short note on mast cells.
(g) Write short note on lymph node.
(h) Write short note on spleen.
(i) Write short note on T cell & B cell.

3. Very long answer type questions
(a) Describe in detail various lineages of stem cells.
(b) Describe in detail of lymphoid lineage.
(c) Describe in detail of myeloid lineage.
(d) Describe in detail structure and function of bone marrow.
(e) Describe in detail structure and function of thymus.
(f) Describe in detail structure and function of spleen.
(g) Describe in detail structure and function of lymph node.
(h) Describe in detail structure and function of unorganised secondary lymphoid organ.
(i) Describe in detail the types and functions of lymphocytes.
(j) Describe in detail the type and functions of granulocytes

Multiple Choice Questions

1. Which sentence is true about stem cells?
(a) They are undifferentiated embryonic cells
(b) Can develop into any type of blood cells
(c) They are said to be pluripotent
(d) All of the above

2. In adult stem cell are found in
(a) Spleen (b) Liver
(c) Bone marrow (d) Thymus

3. Haemopoesis the process of formation of
(a) R.B.C (b) W.B.C
(c) Platelets (d) Blood cells

4. B-Cells are formed by
   (a) Lymphoid lineage (b) Myeloid lineage
   (c) Erythroid lineage (d) None of the above
5. T - cells originate from
   (a) Lymphoid lineage (b) Myeloid lineage
   (c) Erythroid lineage (d) All of above
6. Mast cell originate from
   (a) Lymphoid lineage (b) Myeloid lineage
   (c) Lymphoid lineage (d) None of above
7. Which cells originate from myeloid lineage?
   (a) Eosinophil (b) Basophils
   (c) Neutrophils (d) All of the above
8. Which cells does not originate from myeloid lineage?
   (a) T - Cells (b) B-Cells
   (c) R.B.C (d) All of the above
9. Macrophages originates from
   (a) Basophils (b) Monocytes
   (c) Platelets (d) Neutrophils
10. Platelets originates from
    (a) Basophils (b) Megakaryocytes
    (c) Monocytes (d) T -cells
11. Polymorphonuclear leucocytes are found in
    (a) Lymphoid lineage (b) Myeloid lineage
    (c) Erythroid lineage (d) All of the above
12. B- lymphocytes matures in
    (a) Thymus (b) Bone marrow
    (c) Bursa of fabricus (d) Both b and c
13. Immunoglobulins are produced by
    (a) B- Cells (b) T- cells
    (c) Plasma cells (d) Null cells
14. Lymphocytes are
    (a) Granular (b) Non granular
    (c) Sometimes granular (d) Sometimes non granular
15. Plasma cells are rich in
    (a) Rough ER (b) Smooth ER
    (c) Mitochondria (d) Cytoplasm
16. Alveolar macrophages are found in
    (a) Liver (b) Brain
    (c) peritoneal cavity (d) lungs

17. Kupffer cells are found in
    (a) Liver
    (b) Brain
    (c) Lungs
    (d) Peritoneal cavity
18. Eosinophils are
    (a) Acidophilic leucocytes
    (b) Basophilic leucocytes
    (c) Neutrophilic leucocytes
    (d) Mast cells
19. Eosinophilia is
    (a) decrease in number of eosinophils
    (b) increase in number of eosinophils
    (c) decrease in size of eosinophils
    (d) increase in size of eosinophils
20. Basophils contain
    (a) Heparin
    (b) Serotonin
    (c) PAF
    (d) All of the above

Answer Key

Question Number	Answer	Question Number	Answer
1	D	11	B
2	C	12	D
3	D	13	C
4	A	14	B
5	A	15	B
6	B	16	D
7	D	17	A
8	D	18	A
9	B	19	B
10	B	20	D

References

Agace W.W. (2008) T- Cell recruitment to the intestinal mucosa. Trends in Immunology 29, 514-522.

Banchereau J., F. Briere, C. Caux, J. Davoust, S. Lebecque, Y. J. Liu, B. Pulendran, and K. Palucka. 2000. Immunobiology of dendritic cells. Annu. Rev. Immunology. 18:767.

Bencherau J. & Steinman R.M. (1998) Dendritic cells and the control of immunity. Nature 392, 245-252.

Bendelac, A., M. N. Rivera, S-H. Park, and J. H. Roark. 1997. Mouse CD1-specific NK1 T cells: Development, specificity and function. Annu. Rev. Immunol. 15:535.

Berke G. & Clark W.R. (2007) Killer lymphocytes. Springer, Dordrecht, The Netherlands. 369 pp.

Bos J.D.(ed.) (2004) skin immune system (SIS): Cutaneous immunology and clinical Immunodermatology, 3rd edn. Boca Raton. CRC Press.

Clevers, H. C., and R. Grosschedl. 1996. Transcriptional control of lymphoid development: lessons from gene targeting. Immunol. Today 17:336.

Cory, S. 1995. Regulation of lymphocyte survival by the BCL-2 gene family. Annu. Rev. Immunol. 12:513. Ganz, T., and R. I. Lehrer. 1998.Antimicrobial peptides of vertebrates. Curr. Opin. Immunol. 10:41.

Coss S.C., Gahan C.C.& Hill c. (2008) M- cells: origin, morphology and role in mucosal immunity and microbial pathogenesis. FEMS Immunology and medical microbiology 52, 2-12.

Crispe N. (2009) The liver as a lymphoid organ. Annual Review of Immunology 27, 147-163.

Cullen S.P. & Martin S.J. (2008) Mechanisms of granule-dependent killing. Cell death & differentiation 15, 215-262.

Junt T., Scandella E. & Ludewig B. (2008) from follows function: Lymphoid tissue micro architecture in antimicrobial immune defence. Nature Review Immunology 8, 764-775.

Liu,Y. J. 2001. Dendritic cell subsets and lineages, and their functions in innate and adaptive immunity. Cell 106:259.

Medzhitov R. (2008) orIgin and physiological role of inflammation. Nature 454, 428-35

Melchers, F., and A. Rolink. 1999. B-lymphocyte development and biology. In Fundamental Immunology, 4th ed., W. E. Paul, ed., p. 183. Lippincott-Raven, Philadelphia.

Melchers, F., and A. Rolink. 1999. B-lymphocyte development and biology. In Fundamental Immunology, 4th ed.,W. E. Paul, ed., p. 183. Lippincott-Raven, Philadelphia.

Ohtani O. & Ohtani Y. (2008) structure and function of rat lymph nodes. Archives of histology and cytology 71,69-76.

Osborne, B. A. 1996. Apoptosis and the maintenance of homeostasis in the immune system. Curr. Opin. Immunol. 8:245.

Picker, L. J., and M. H. Siegelman. 1999. Lymphoid tissues and organs. In Fundamental Immunology, 4th ed., W. E. Paul, ed., p. 145. Lippincott-Raven, Philadelphia.

Pribila J.T., Quale A.C., Mueller K.L. & Shimizu Y. (2004) Integrins and T cell-mediated immunity. Annual Reviews of immunology 22, 157-180.

Sayed B.A., Christy A., Quirion M.R. &Brown M.A. (2008) The master switch: the role of mast cells in autoimmunity and tolerance. Annual Review of Immunology 26, 705-739

Steinman R.M Idoyaga J (2010) features of the dendritic cell lineage. Immunological Reviews 234.

Ward,A. C.,D. M. Loeb, A.A. Soede-Bobok, I. P. Touw, and A.D. Friedman. 2000. Regulation of granulopoiesis by transcription factors and cytokine signals. Leukemia 14:973.

Weissman, I. L. 2000. Translating stem and progenitor cell biology to the clinic: barriers and opportunities. Science 287:1442.

CHAPTER 3

Organs of Immune System

A number of morphologically and functionally diverse organs and tissues have various functions in the development of immune responses. These can be distinguished by function as the primary and secondary lymphoid organs. The thymus and bone marrow are the primary (or central) lymphoid organs, where maturation of lymphocytes takes place. The lymph nodes, spleen, and various mucosal associated lymphoid tissues (MALT) such as gut-associated lymphoid tissue (GALT) are the secondary (or peripheral) lymphoid organs, which trap antigen and provide sites for mature lymphocytes to interact with that antigen. In addition, tertiary lymphoid tissues, which normally contain fewer lymphoid cells than secondary lymphoid organs, can import lymphoid cells during an inflammatory response. Most prominent of these are cutaneous-associated lymphoid tissues. Once mature lymphocytes have been generated in the primary lymphoid organs, they circulate in the blood and lymphatic system, a network of vessels that collect fluid that has escaped into the tissues from capillaries of the circulatory system and ultimately return it to the blood.

(A) Primary (Central) Lymphoid Organs

Based on function, the organs and tissues of the immune system can be divided into primary or secondary lymphoid organs or tissues. The primary organs or tissues are where immature lymphocytes mature and differentiate into antigen-sensitive mature B and T cells. The thymus and bone marrow are the primary lymphoid tissue.

1. Bone Marrow

The bone marrow contains two types of stem cells, mesenchymal and hematopoietic. Red bone marrow consists of a delicate, highly vascular fibrous tissue containing hematopoietic stem cells. These are blood-forming stem cells. Yellow bone marrow contains mesenchymal stem cells, also known as marrow stromal cells. These produce fat, cartilage, and bone. Stem cells are immature cells that can turn into a number of different types of cell. Hematopoietic stem cells in the bone marrow give rise to two main types of cells: myeloid and lymphoid lineages (chapter 2). These include monocytes, macrophages, neutrophils, basophils, eosinophils, erythrocytes, dendritic cells, and megakaryocytes or platelets, as well as T cells, B cells, and natural killer cells (figure 3.1). The different types of hematopoietic stem cells vary in their regenerative capacity and potency. Some are multipotent, oligopotent or unipotent as determined by how many types of cell they can create. Pluripotent hematopoietic stem cells have the following properties:

- Renewal: They can reproduce another cell identical to themselves.
- Differentiation: They can generate one or more subsets of more mature cells.

The process of development of different blood cells from these pluripotent stem cells is known as hematopoiesis. It is these stem cells that are needed in bone marrow transplant. Stem cells constantly divide and produce new cells. Some new cells remain as stem cells and others go through a series of maturing stages, as precursor or blast cells, before becoming formed, or mature, blood cells. Stem cells rapidly multiply to make millions of blood cells each day. Blood cells have a limited life span. This is around 100-120 days for red blood cells. They are constantly being replaced. The production of healthy stem cells is vital. The blood vessels act as a barrier to prevent immature blood cells from leaving the bone marrow. Only mature blood cells contain the membrane proteins required to attach to and pass through the blood vessel endothelium. Hematopoietic stem cells can cross the bone marrow barrier, however. These may be harvested from peripheral, or circulating, blood.

Once mature, these blood cells move from the marrow into the bloodstream, where they perform important functions required to keep the body alive and healthy. Mesenchymal stem cells are found in the bone marrow cavity. They differentiate into a number of stromal lineages, such as: chondrocytes (cartilage generation), osteoblasts (bone formation), osteoclasts, adipocytes (adipose tissue), myocytes (muscle), macrophages, endothelial cells and fibroblasts.

Red bone marrow

Red bone marrow produces all red blood cells and platelets in human adults and around 60 to 70 percent of lymphocytes. Other lymphocytes begin life in the red bone marrow and become fully formed in the lymphatic tissues, including the thymus, spleen, and lymph nodes. Together with the liver and spleen, red bone marrow also plays a role in getting rid of old red blood cells.

Yellow bone marrow

Yellow bone marrow mainly acts as a store for fats. It helps to provide sustenance and maintain the correct environment for the bone to function. However, under particular conditions, such as severe blood loss or fever, the yellow marrow may revert to red marrow. Yellow marrow tends to be located in the central cavities of long bones, and is generally surrounded by a layer of red marrow with long trabeculae (beam-like structures) within a sponge-like reticular framework.

Bone marrow timeline

Before birth, bone marrow first develops in the clavicle toward the end of fetal development. It becomes active about 3 weeks later. Bone marrow takes over from the liver as the major hematopoietic organ at 32 to 36 weeks' gestation. Bone marrow remains red until around the age of 7 years, as the need for new continuous blood formation is high. As the body ages, the red marrow is gradually replaced by yellow fat tissue. Adults have an average of about 2.6 kg (5.7 lbs) of bone marrow, about half of which is red. In adults, the highest concentration of red marrow is in the bones of the vertebrae, hips (ilium), breastbone (sternum), ribs, skull and at the metaphyseal and epiphyseal ends of the long bones of the arm (humerus) and leg (femur and tibia). All other cancellous, or spongy, bones and central cavities of the long bones are filled with yellow marrow.

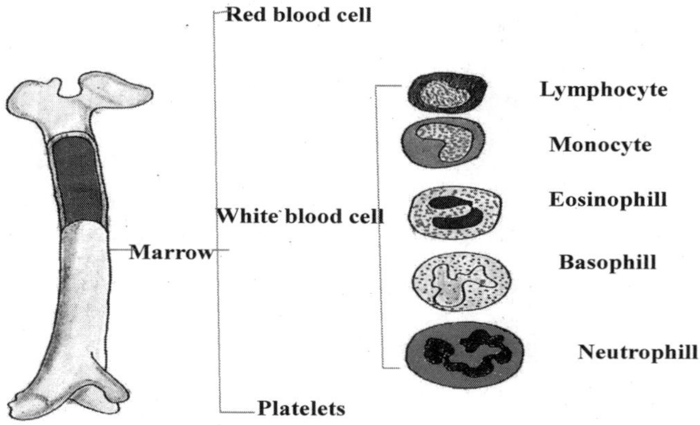

Fig. 3.1 : Various cells produced in Bone Marrow

2. Bursa of Fabricus

In birds, the bursa of Fabricius (Latin: Bursa cloacalis or Bursa fabricii) is the site of hematopoiesis, a specialized organ that, as first demonstrated by Bruce Glick and later by Max Cooper and Robert Good, is necessary for B cell (part of the immune system) development in birds.

The bursa of Fabricius functions as a central lymphoid organ, required for development of the antigen-specific B cell repertoire. The bursa of Fabricius is a saclike structure (figure 3.2) arising as an evagination of the dorsal wall of the cloaca on the fifth day of embryonation. Hematopoietic stem cells originating in the yolk sac first enter the bursal structure via the blood stream at around the twelfth or thirteenth day of incubation.

The bursa of Fabricius is critical to the normal development of B lymphocytes and the antibodies they go on to produce. While antibody production and B cells are common to all vertebrates, the bursa as an organ of primary B cell lymphopoiesis is unique to birds and was first implicated in the development or generation of antibody responses nearly 60 years ago. At that time, Glick and colleagues demonstrated that surgical removal of the bursa from neonatal chicks impaired subsequent antibody responses to *Salmonella typhimurium* type O antigen. Since then, it has become clear that the bursa is indeed the primary site of B cell lymphopoiesis in birds and that avian B cell lymphopoiesis has several characteristics that distinguish it from pathways of B cell development in human or rodent models. The bursa itself is colonized during embryonic development by lymphoid precursors that expand and mature in the bursa before emigrating from the bursa to the periphery, where they have the potential to take part in immune responses. As a consequence, we can consider B cell development as occurring in three distinct stages, pre-bursal, bursal and post-bursal. The bursa of Fabricius is necessary for the development of the postbursal B cell population, including the mature antigen-specific B cells and the self-renewing postbursal stem cells. It is necessary for the differentiation of prebursal stem cells into bursal stem cells present in the bursa until the 5th week after hatching. These cells are capable of reconstituting the bursal morphology and specific antibody production when transferred into birds with the bursal lymphoid structures destroyed with cyclophosphamide in the newly hatched period. They comprise a clearly defined stage in the stepwise maturation of the avian antibody-producing cells.

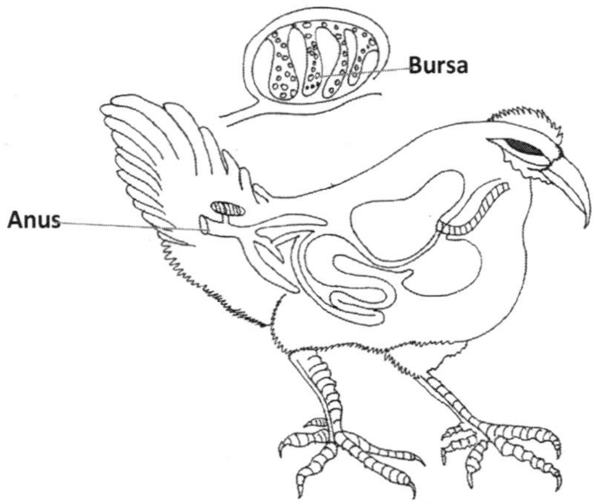

Fig. 3.2 : Bursa of Fabricius

3. Thymus

The thymus gland is a small organ behind the breastbone that plays an important function both in the immune system and endocrine system. Though the thymus begins to atrophy (decay) during puberty, its effect in "training" T lymphocytes to fight infections and even cancer lasts for a lifetime. The thymus gland lies in the chest, directly behind the breastbone (sternum), and in front of the heart in the area between the lungs called the anterior mediastinum. Sometimes, however, the thymus gland is found in another (ectopic) location, such as in the neck, the thyroid gland, or on the surface of the lungs (the pleura) near the area where the blood vessels and bronchi enter the lungs.

It is named the thymus due to its shape being similar to that of a thyme leaf—pyramid shaped with two lobes. The two lobes of the thymus are broken down into lobules. These lobules have an outer cortex occupied by immature T lymphocytes, and an inner medulla occupied by mature T lymphocytes (figure 3.3). It is considered a lymphoid organ (an organ of the immune system) similar to the tonsils, adenoids, and spleen.

A number of different cell types are present within the thymus gland.

- **Epithelial cells:** cells that line body surfaces and cavities
- **Kulchitsky cells:** cells that are the hormone-producing cells of the thymus or neuroendocrine cells

- **Thymocytes:** cells that become mature T lymphocytes

The thymus gland is also home to some macrophages. Macrophages are known as the "garbage trucks" of the immune system because they eat foreign matter. Dendritic cells, and a few B lymphocytes (the types of lymphocytes that produce antibodies) also reside in the thymus. Interestingly, the thymus gland also contains some myoid (muscle-like) cells. The thymus gland is large in infants, but after infancy, it grows and reaches its maximum size during puberty. The gland is very small in elderly people, but can sometimes atrophy prematurely in response to severe stress. The term used to describe the atrophy of the thymus gland with age is "thymic involution."[1]

The thymus gland is very active from before birth until puberty, and it functions as both a lymphatic organ and an endocrine organ (an organ of the endocrine system that produces hormones). In order to understand the role, the thymus gland plays in immunity, it's helpful to first distinguish between T lymphocytes and B lymphocytes. T cells (also known as T lymphocytes or thymus derived lymphocytes) mature in the thymus gland and play a central role in cell-mediated immunity, meaning that the cells themselves are active in fighting off foreign invaders such as bacteria, viruses, cancer cells, and more. In contrast, B lymphocytes are part of the humoral immune system and produce antibodies directed at specific invaders.

As part of the adaptive immune system, the thymus can be thought of as the training ground for T lymphocytes. During childhood, immature T cells (called progenitor cells) that originate in the bone marrow travel via the bloodstream to the thymus gland where they mature and differentiate into specialized T cells.

The immature T cells that leave the bone marrow enter the thymus in the cortex (known as the classroom of the thymus) (figure 3.3). During "training," these cells are taught to recognize antigens associated with foreign cells and matter in a process called positive selection. Cells are positively selected for usefulness. Once the T cells have learned to recognize specific pathogens, they travel to the medulla to undergo "negative selection." In the medulla, the mature T cells are introduced to the body's own antigens. Since T cells that would react with the body's antigens could attack a person's own cells, these cells are eliminated. T cells are negatively selected for autoimmunity, and these self-attacking cells either die or are turned into regulatory cells. The survivors are then exposed to hormones produced by the thymus gland to complete their maturation before being released to do their job (circulating in the bloodstream or waiting in the lymph nodes for foreign invaders).

Within each lobule, the cells are arranged into an outer cortex and an inner medulla (figure 3.3). The cortex tightly packed with proliferating immature lymphocytes while the medulla contains more mature cells. As the cells mature, they move from the cortex to the medulla. The cortex consists of lymphocytes (thymocytes) and reticular cells. The reticular cells are larger than lymphocytes and they form a three-dimensional network and in the meshes of which the lymphocytes are found. The lymphocytes multiply rapidly and form thymic lymphocytes (T lymphocytes) which cause the cell mediated immunity. The medulla consists of vascular structure reticular epithelial cells and scattered lymphocytes. The reticular cells are relatively more in number than the lymphocytes. There are also some interdigitating cells associated with the epithelial network and these cells are rich in MHC class 2 antigens.

In addition, there are some peculiar structure in the medulla called Hassall's corpuscles. These are small masses or wholes of epithelial cells around a central core of degenerating epithelial cells. Their functions are not known inside the thymus as they do not come in contact with the antigens. The non-execution of the immune response is due to the epithelial barrier which prevents the antigens of the blood to contact the lymphocytes of the thymus. These non-functional T lymphocytes travel through the blood and lymph circulation and ultimately reach the thymus dependent areas of the peripheral lymphoid organs and get colonized there. In these organs these T lymphocytes become functional by antigenic stimulation.

The thymus gland produces several hormones including:

- thymopoietin and thymulin, which are hormones that assist in the process where T cells differentiate into different types
- thymosin, which accentuates the immune response as well as stimulating pituitary hormones such as growth hormone
- thymic humoral factor, which acts similarly to thymosin, but increases the immune response to viruses in particular

Surgery to remove the thymus gland (thymectomy) may be done for a number of reasons. One is for congenital heart surgery. A congenital heart condition is a birth defect of the heart. Due to the location of the thymus gland, it must be removed for surgeons to gain access to the heart in infants. Another common reason for this surgery is for a person with thymic cancer. In addition, myasthenia gravis (MG) is another condition treated with a thymectomy. When the thymus gland is removed, roughly 60 percent of people with myasthenia gravis achieved remission. However, it can take months to years for these effects to be apparent with myasthenia gravis. When used for MG, surgery is usually done between puberty and middle age to avoid the potential consequences of removing the thymus gland earlier in life.

The thymus gland provides a critical role in cell-mediated immunity, but fortunately, a significant part of this benefit occurs before birth (the T cells formed during development in the uterus are long-lasting). However, there are potential consequences of removal early in life, such as when the thymus is removed during heart surgery in infants. It appears that early removal may increase the risk of developing infections, the development of autoimmune diseases (such as autoimmune thyroid disease), the risk of atopic disease (allergies, asthma, and eczema), and possibly the risk of cancer, as T cells perform a vital role in cancer. There is also some evidence that thymus removal may be associated with premature aging of the immune system.

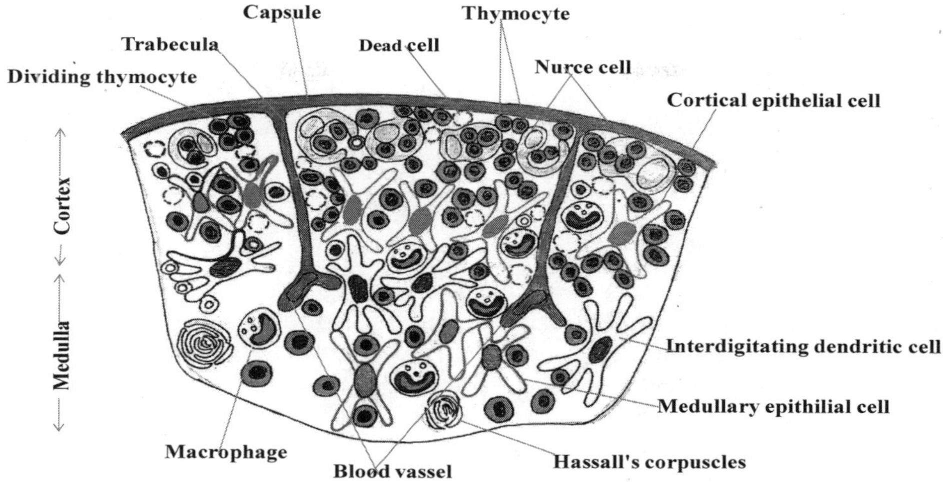

Fig. 3.3 : Structure of Thymus

(B) Secondary (Peripheral) Lymphoid Organs

The Secondary lymphoid organs are concerned with immune reactions. In the secondary lymphoid organs, the lymphocytes are made functional. Here the cells are exposed to antigen and they produce antibodies or sensitized cells. The secondary lymphoid organs are small and poorly developed at birth and they grow progressively with age. The secondary organs and tissues serve as areas where lymphocytes may encounter and bind antigen, where upon they proliferate and differentiate into fully mature, antigen-specific effector cells. The spleen is a secondary lymphoid organ and the lymph nodes and mucosal-associated tissues (GALT, gut-associated lymphoid tissue and SALT, skin associated lymphoid tissues) are the secondary lymphoid tissues.

1. Spleen

The spleen is the large secondary lymphoid organ located in the abdominal cavity. Whereas lymph nodes are specialized for trapping microorganisms and antigens from local tissues, the spleen specializes in filtering the blood and trapping blood-borne microorganisms and antigens. Once trapped by macrophages and dendritic cells, the pathogen is phagocytosed and antigens are presented to B and T cells, which become activated to carry out their immune functions.

Although it varies in size between individuals, a spleen is typically around 3–5.5 inches long and weighs 5.3–7.1 ounces (oz). The spleen is a soft organ with a thin outer covering of tough connective tissue, called a capsule (figure 3.4). Anything that relates to the spleen is referred to as splenic; the spleen receives blood through the splenic artery, and blood leaves the spleen through the splenic vein. Although the spleen is connected to the blood vessels of the stomach and pancreas, it is not involved in digestion. The spleen contains two main regions of tissue called white pulp and red pulp. Red pulp contains venous sinuses (cavities filled with blood), and splenic cords (connective tissues containing red blood cells and white blood cells). White pulp mostly consists of immune cells (T cells and B cells). The major part of the lymphoid tissue is arranged around a central arteriole it is known as periarteriolar lymphatic sheath (PALS) consist of B lymphocytes grouped in small masses called follicles. In between the follicles are distributed the T lymphocytes. The B lymphocytes follicles may also contain germinal centre when it is known as secondary follicle. Surrounding the germinal centre is a layer of lymphocytes known as mantle layer. The PALS is separated from the red pulp by the marginal zone consisting of both T and B lymphocytes.

The spleen's primary job is to filter the blood. As blood flows into the spleen, it performs a quality control service, detecting any red blood cells that are old or damaged. Blood flows through a maze of passages in the spleen. Healthy cells flow straight through, but those considered to be unhealthy are broken down by large white blood cells called macrophages. Once the red blood cells are broken down, the spleen stores useful leftover products, such as iron, which it eventually returns to the bone marrow, which makes hemoglobin (the iron-containing part of blood). The spleen also stores blood, the blood vessels of the spleen can expand significantly. In humans, around 1 cup of blood is kept in the spleen, ready to be released if there is a significant loss of blood, after an accident, for instance. The spleen also plays a role in the immune response by detecting pathogens (bacteria, for instance), and producing white blood cells in response. Around one-quarter of our lymphocytes are stored in the spleen at any one time. The spleen clears out old platelets from the blood; it also acts as a reservoir for platelets. As a fetus is developing, the spleen makes red blood cells, but after the fifth month of gestation, it stops. The spleen also produces compounds called opsonins, such as properdin and tuftsin, that help the immune system.

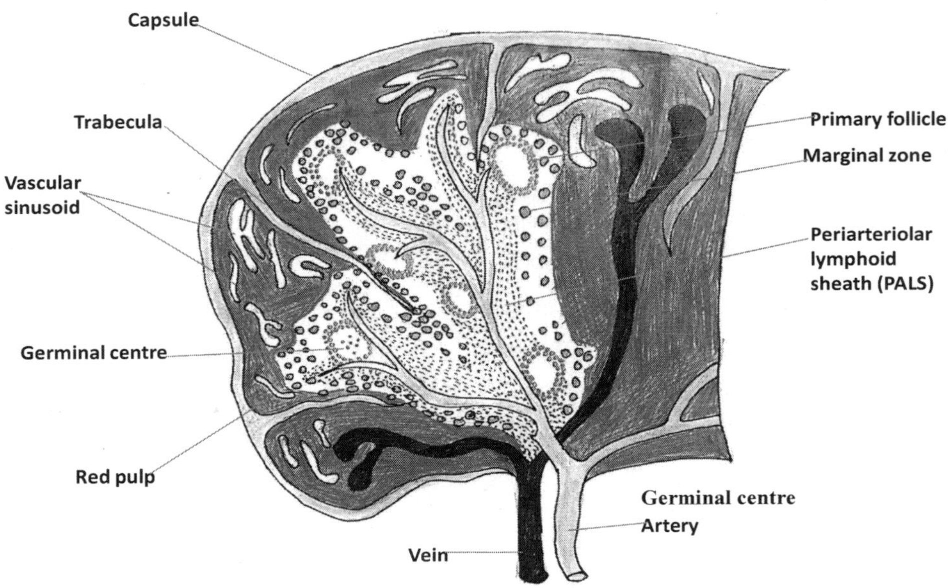

Fig. 3.4 : Structure of Spleen

2. Lymph Node

Lymph nodes are kidney or oval shaped and range in size from 0.1 to 2.5 cm long. Each lymph node is surrounded by a fibrous capsule, which extends inside a lymph node to form trabeculae (figure 3.5). The substance of a lymph node is divided into the outer cortex and the inner medulla. These are rich with cells. Lymph nodes or lymph glands are an important part of the immune system, acting as «nodes» between the lymphatic vessels that span the body. Immune cells that are «parked» in these nodes stand ready to attack any bacteria, viruses, or other foreign substances that enter the body. Like other parts of the body, lymph nodes are also susceptible to diseases, such as infections, cancer, and trauma.

Lymph nodes are small, bean-shaped glands that are located along the lymphatic system (a system of vessels similar to arteries and veins through which lymph fluid travels).

The structure of a lymph node is actually quite complex. Lymph nodes are divided into lobules, each of which contains an outer cortex, followed by a paracortex, with the medulla (core) on the inside. Simplistically, B lymphocytes (B cells) are found in the cortex, with T lymphocytes (T cells) and dendritic cells in the paracortex. Plasma cells and macrophages are present in the medulla. The entire lymph node is enclosed by a tough fibrous capsule. The lymph node is covered by a capsule. The capsule penetrates into the lymph node to form septa called trabeculae (figure 3.5).

Lymph nodes lie at the junctions of lymphatic vessels where they filter out harmful microorganisms and antigens from the lymph; pathogens and antigens are trapped by phagocytic and dendritic cells. Fixed macrophages then phagocytose the foreign material. It is within the lymph nodes that B cells proliferate into antibody-secreting plasma cells. Dendritic and T cells are also found here; dendritic cells serve as antigen-presenting cells and T helper cells promote the B-cell immune response. Lymph nodes work like filters, or in our analogy security guards to filter bacteria, viruses, parasites, other foreign material (even cancer cells) that are brought to the nodes via lymphatic vessels. This is the reason that lymph nodes are evaluated in people with cancer, as this is the first place where cancer cells may be "caught" on their journey to explore and set up home elsewhere in the body. Lymph nodes play an important role in fighting infections in a few ways. Not only do they "trap" viruses and bacteria so that T cells can attack, but one type of T cells presents the invader (or an antigen from the invader) to B cells so the B cells can make antibodies against the invader. In this way, lymph nodes are a place where immune cells can communicate and work together. Lymph nodes are well-known as the "swollen glands" people may note in their neck when they are fighting a cold or sore throat, but these nodes are actually located in many regions of the body.

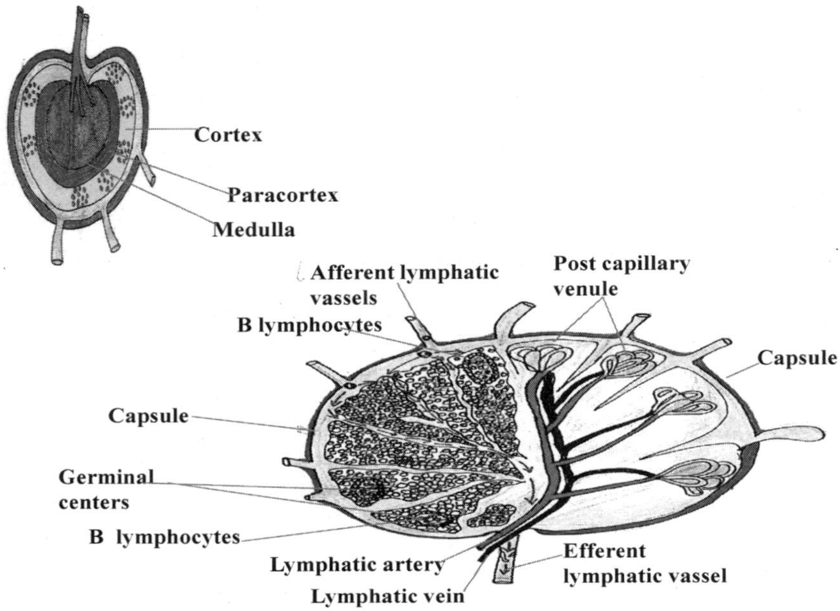

Fig. 3.5 : Structure of Lymph node

3. Mucosa Associated Lymphoid Tissues

Mucous membranes have a specialized immune barrier called *m*ucosal-*a*ssociated *l*ymphoid *t*issue (MALT). The mucosal layer of the alimentary canal, respiratory and urinogenital tracts is provided with dispersed groups of lymphoid tissues known as MALT. These tissues are usually without a capsule (uncapsulated). There are several types of MALT. The system most studied is the *g*ut-*a*ssociated *l*ymphoid *t*issue (GALT). In human beings the Peyer's patches, the tonsils and appendix are good examples of lymphoid tissues found in the mucosal layer of the alimentary canal. Hence these tissues are also referred to as GALT (Gut Associated Lymphoid Tissue).

Less well-organized mucosal-associated lymphoid tissue also occurs in the respiratory system and is called *b*ronchial *a*ssociated *l*ymphoid *t*issue (BALT); the diffuse MALT in the urogenital system does not have a specific name. MALT can operate by two basic mechanisms. First, when an antigen arrives at the mucosal surface, it contacts a type of cell called the M cell (figure 3.6). The M cell does not have the brush border or microvilli found on adjacent columnar epithelial cells but does have a large pocket containing B cells, T cells, and macrophages. When an antigen contacts the M cell, it is phagocytosed and released into the pocket. Macrophages engulf the antigen or pathogen and try to destroy it. An M cell also can phagocytose an antigen and transport it to a cluster of cells called an organized lymphoid follicle. The B cells within this follicle recognize the antigen and mature into plasma cells. The plasma cells leave the follicle and secrete a class of antibody called secretory IgA (sIgA). Secretory IgA is then transported into the lumen of the gut where it interacts with the antigen that caused its production.

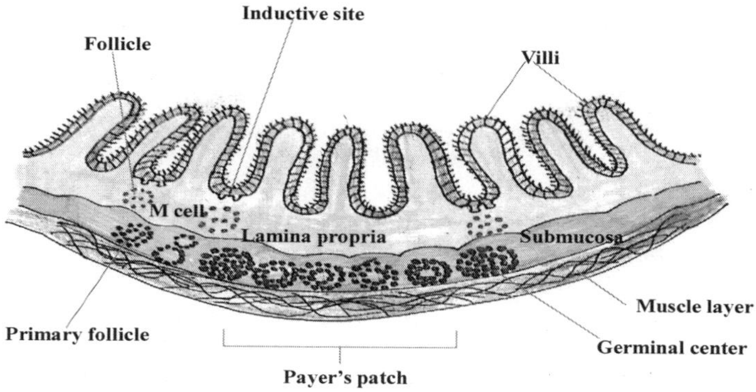

Fig. 3.6 : Mucosa Associated Lymphoid Tissue (MALT)

Peyer's patches are secondary lymphoid tissues. They are Mucosa Associated Lymphoid Tissue. They are collection of lymphoid nodules packed together to form oblong elevations of the mucous membrane of the small intestine. They consist of a mixture of T and B lymphocytes where the T cells predominate. The Peyer's patches are covered by specialized epithelial cells which have no microvilli but the surface seems wrinkled or folded under the scanning electron microscope (figure 3.7) This is called microfold. The cells of the microfold the M cells contain vesicles which actively transport particulate antigens from the lumen of the gut into the "dome" area (area below the folded area). Here the priming of both T and B lymphocytes occurs as a result of antigenic stimulation. The primed B lymphoblasts migrate via efferent lymphatics and the mensenteric lymph nodes to the thoracic duct and thus enter the blood. These cells very soon recenter the lamina propria of the gut where they mature into IgA plasma cells. These IgA plasma cells later form into secretory IgA molecules. The secretory IgA gets transported across the mucosa into the intestinal lumen where it neutralizes viruses, bacteria and toxins and blocks the entry of these antigens into circulation by acting as an antiseptic paint.

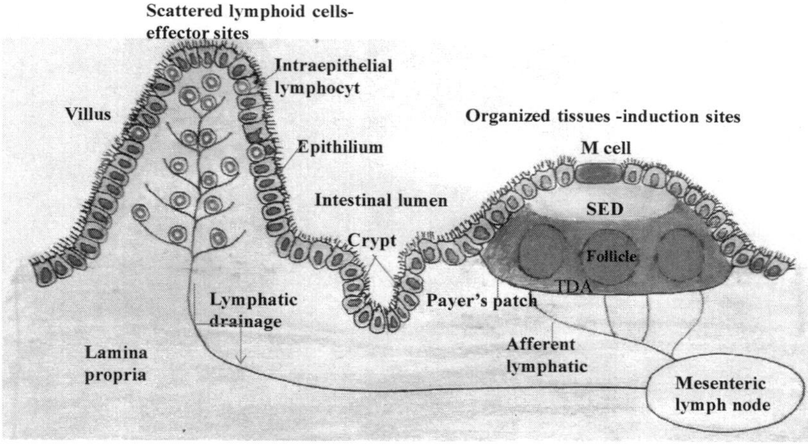

Fig. 3.7 : Payer's patch

Tonsils are lymphoid tissues encircling the pharynx. They are secondary lymphoid tissues. They also form MALT. They are very similar to thymus in the internal structure. They are rather larger in childhood and tend to diminish with age. The tonsils contain a considerable amount of lymphoid tissue and composed mostly of B lymphocytes. The lymphocytes are compactly arranged in follicles which usually contain large germinal centers. There are 3 types of tonsils, viz. palatine tonsils, lingual tonsils and pharyngeal tonsils (figure 3.8). The tonsils (palatine tonsils) are a pair of soft tissue masses located at the rear of the throat (pharynx). Each tonsil is composed of tissue similar to lymph nodes, covered by pink mucosa (like on the adjacent mouth lining). Running through the mucosa of each tonsil are pits, called crypts. The lingual tonsils are at the base of the tongue and the pharyngeal tonsils also called stenoids are at the back of the pharynx. Like the spleen and lymph nodes the tonsils also setup resistance to infecting to infecting microbes. It is said that the tonsils sample the microbes in the inhaled air and form suitable antibodies.

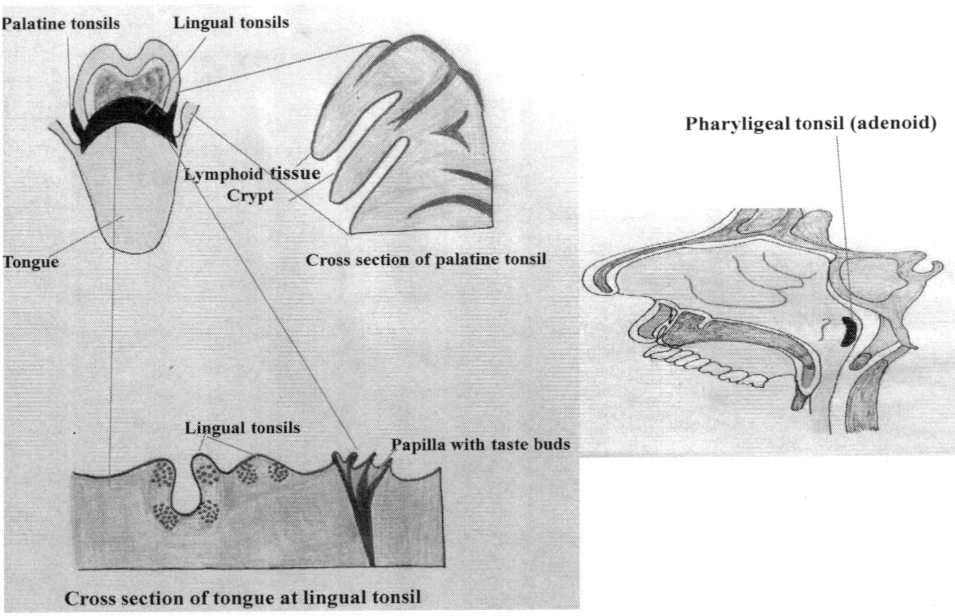

Fig. 3.8 – Types of Tonsils

Multiple Choice Questions

1. Which of the following is lymphoid organ?

   (a) Liver *(b)* Pancreas

   (c) Tonsils *(d)* Gall bladder

2. T-Cells becomes immune-competent in

   (a) Stomach *(b)* Thyroid

   (c) Tonsils *(d)* Thymus

3. Which organs filters blood?
   (a) Heart (b) Spleen
   (c) Liver (d) Payer patches
4. Spleen is a
   (a) Primary lymphoid organ (b) Secondary lymphoid organ
   (c) MALT (d) GALT
5. Mature B lymphocytes are present in which part of spleen?
   (a) Cortex (b) Paracortex
   (c) Medula (d) Both a and c
6. Bursa of fibricus is found in
   (a) Hind gut (b) Mid gut
   (c) Upper gut (d) Can be found any where
7. Lymph gets filtered in
   (a) Spleen (b) Lymph node
   (c) Heart (d) Lymphatic ducts
8. Immature T-cells are found in which part of thymus?
   (a) Medulla (b) Cortex
   (c) Paracortex (d) None of the above
9. Cell mediated immunity gets affected by the removal of
   (a) Bone marrow (b) Spleen
   (c) Lymph node (d) Thymus
10. Thymectomy is the surgical removal of
   (a) Spleen (b) Thymus
   (c) Thyroid gland (d) T- cells
11. Which organ is involved in graft rejection?
   (a) Tonsils (b) Bone marrow
   (c) Thymus (d) spleen
12. Weight of bone marrow is about
   (a) 2 Kg (b) 3 Kg
   (c) 5 Kg (d) 7 Kg
13. Stems cells are found in
   (a) Red marrow (b) Yellow marrow
   (c) Adipose part (d) None of the above
14. Which organ is the source of antibody synthesis?
   (a) Spleen (b) Thymus
   (c) Bone marrow (d) Both c and a
15. Which organ gets atrophy by age?
   (a) Thymus (b) Bursa of fabricus
   (c) Both a and b (d) Bone marrow

16. Which are primary lymphoid organs?
    (a) Thymus *(b)* Spleen
    (c) Lymph node *(d)* Tonsils
17. Which of the following is secondary lymphoid organ?
    (a) Thymus *(b)* Bone marrow
    (c) Bursa of fabricus *(d)* Lymph node
18. Medulla of spleen and lymph node contain
    (a) B- cells *(b)* T- Cells
    (c) Both B and T cells *(d)* None of the above
19. Which organ is the largest secondary lymphoid organ?
    (a) Lymph node *(b)* Spleen
    (c) Peyer's patches *(d)* tonsils
20. Humoral and cell mediated immunity is mediated by
    (a) Spleen *(b)* Lymph node
    (c) Both a and b *(d)* Thymus

Answer Key

Question Number	Answer	Question Number	Answer
1	C	11	C
2	D	12	B
3	B	13	A
4	B	14	D
5	D	15	C
6	A	16	A
7	B	17	D
8	B	18	C
9	D	19	B
10	B	20	C

References

Agace W.W. (2008) T- Cell recruitment to the intestinal mucosa. Trends in Immunology 29, 514-522.

Banchereau J., F. Briere, C. Caux, J. Davoust, S. Lebecque, Y. J. Liu, B. Pulendran, and K. Palucka. 2000. Immunobiology of dendritic cells. Annu. Rev. Immunology. 18:767.

Bencherau J. & Steinman R.M. (1998) Dendritic cells and and the control of immunity. Nature 392, 245-252.

Bendelac, A., M. N. Rivera, S-H. Park, and J. H. Roark. 1997. Mouse CD1-specific

NK1 T cells: Development, specificity and function. Annu. Rev. Immunol. 15:535.

Berke G. & Clark W.R. (2007) Killer lymphocytes. Springer, Dordrecht, The Netherlands. 369 pp.

Bos J.D. (ed.) (2004) skin immune system (SIS): Cutaneous immunology and clinical Immunodermatology, 3rd edn. Boca Raton. CRC Press.

Clevers, H. C., and R. Grosschedl. 1996. Transcriptional control of lymphoid development: lessons from gene targeting. Immunol. Today 17:336.

Cory, S. 1995. Regulation of lymphocyte survival by the BCL-2 gene family. Annu. Rev. Immunol. 12:513. Ganz, T., and R. I. Lehrer. 1998.Antimicrobial peptides of vertebrates. Curr. Opin. Immunol. 10:41.

Coss S.C., Gahan C.C.& Hill. (2008) M- cells: origin, morphology and role in mucosal immunity and microbial pathogenesis. FEMS Immunology and medical microbiology 52, 2-12.

Crispe N. (2009) The liver as a lymphoid organ. Annual Review of Immunology 27, 147-163.

Cullen S.P. & Martin S.J. (2008) Mechanisms of granule-dependent killing. Cell death & differentiation 15, 215-262.

Junt T., Scandella E. & Ludewig B. (2008) from follows function: Lymphoid tissue micro archetecture in antimicrobial immune defence. Nature Review Immunology 8, 764-775.

Liu,Y. J. 2001. Dendritic cell subsets and lineages, and their functions in innate and adaptive immunity. Cell 106:259.

Medzhitov R. (2008) Origin and physiological role of inflammation. Nature 454, 428-35

Melchers, F., and A. Rolink. 1999. B-lymphocyte development and biology. In Fundamental Immunology, 4th ed.,W. E. Paul, ed., p. 183. Lippincott-Raven, Philadelphia.

Melchers, F., and A. Rolink. 1999. B-lymphocyte development and biology. In Fundamental Immunology, 4th ed.,W. E. Paul, ed., p. 183. Lippincott-Raven, Philadelphia.

Ohtani O. & Ohtani Y. (2008) structure and function of rat lymph nodes. Archives of histology and cytology 71,69-76.

Osborne, B. A. 1996. Apoptosis and the maintenance of homeostasis in the immune system. Curr. Opin. Immunol. 8:245.

Picker, L. J., and M. H. Siegelman. 1999. Lymphoid tissues and organs. In Fundamental Immunology, 4th ed.,W. E. Paul, ed., p. 145. Lippincott-Raven, Philadelphia.

Pribila J.T., Quale A.C., Mueller K.L. & Shimizu Y. (2004) Integrins and T cell-mediated immunity. Annual Reviews of immunology 22, 157-180.

Sayed B.A Christy A., Quirion M.R. &Brown M.A. (2008) The master switch:

the role of mast cells in autoimmunity and tolerance. Annual Review of Immunology 26, 705-739

Steinman R.M Idoyaga J. (2010) features of the dendritic cell lineage. Immunological Reviews 234.

Ward, A. C., D. M. Loeb, A.A. Soede-Bobok, I. P. Touw, and A.D. Friedman. 2000. Regulation of granulopoiesis by transcription factors and cytokine signals. Leukemia 14:973.

Weissman, I. L. 2000. Translating stem and progenitor cell biology to the clinic: barriers and opportunities. Science 287:1442.

CHAPTER 4

Antigens

Introduction

The first stage of removing an invading organism is to recognize it as being foreign, that is not "self". The immune system distinguishes between "self" and "nonself" through an elaborate recognition process. Prior to birth, the body inventories the proteins and various other large molecules present (self) and removes most T cells specific for self-determinants. Subsequently self-substances can be distinguished from nonself substances, and lymphocytes can produce specific immunologic reactions against the latter, leading to their removal. The immune system sees the invader as having a number of antigens. A substance that can produce a specific immune response when it is introduced into the tissues of an animal that can react specifically with antibodies or sensitized cells is known as an antigen. Antigens are defined as substances which induce an immune response. They include proteins, carbohydrate, lipids, and nucleic acids.

Microbes have many different components which can be recognized by innate and adaptive immune systems. Antigens recognized by cells of the innate immune system are called "pathogen- associated molecular patterns" (PAMPs) and initiate production of cytokines, chemokines, and antimicrobial peptides by these cells. The ability of an antigen to produce an immune response and to react with the product is known as antigenicity. The ability of a material to induce an immune response is referred to as immunogenicity and such materials are known as immunogens. Hence, immunogen is any substance which elicits an immune response. Whilst all immunogens are antigens, not all antigens are immunogens. Very small molecules, which can be viewed as single antigenic determinants, are incapable of eliciting an antibody response by themselves.

Certain antigens provoke such a drastic immune response that they are termed superantigens. Superantigens are bacterial proteins. These superantigens nonspecifically stimulate T cells to proliferate by interacting with both class II major histocompatibility complex products on antigen-presenting cells and the T-cell receptor. Good examples of superantigens are the staphylococcal enterotoxins that cause food poisoning and the toxin that causes toxic shock syndrome. Superantigens cause symptoms by stimulating the release of massive quantities of cytokines from T cells and should be considered possible chronic associates in such diseases as rheumatic fever, arthritis, Kawasaki syndrome, atopic dermatitis, and one type of psoriasis.

Hapten is low molecular weight molecule that is recognized by preformed antibody, but is not itself immunogenic unless conjugated to a carrier molecule which provides epitopes recognized by helper T-cells. These haptens, as they are called, can be attached to larger molecules and in this physical form can with the help of T cells, induce the formation of antibodies. Therefore, one can distinguish between molecules which can stimulate an immune response (immunogens) and those which react with antibodies but cannot initiate an immune response (haptens or individual antigenic determinants). It is logical to refer a hapten as the antigen and hapten- protein complex as the immunogen, although strictly the word "antigen" is derived from "*a*ntibody *g*enerating" substance.

Antigen is any molecule capable of being recognized by an antibody or T-cell receptor; the antigen is not necessarily immunogenic in its own right. An extreme example of the distinction between the ability to be recognized by an antibody and the ability to elicit antibodies when used to immunize an animal is provided by experimentations using small molecules known as haptens such as *m*-aminobenzene sulphonate. Immunization with free hapten produces no antibodies to the hapten. However immunization with hapten groups linked to a protein carrier generates antibodies that react with high affinity to hapten alone or linked to a molecule other than a carrier.

When lymphocytes are stimulated by the combined molecule, they can react to either the hapten or the larger carrier molecule. Conjugation of a hapten to a carrier protein makes the hapten immunogenic because the carrier protein can be processed and presented to specific T cells. As a result, both hapten-specific and carrier-specific antibodies can be made. Many biologically important substances, including drugs, peptide hormones, and steroid hormones, can function as haptens. One example of a hapten is penicillin. By itself penicillin is not antigenic. However, when it combines with certain serum proteins of sensitive individuals, the resulting molecule does initiate a severe and sometimes fatal allergic immune reaction. In these instances, the hapten is acting as an antigenic determinant on the carrier molecule. Conjugates of these haptens with large protein carriers can be used to produce hapten-specific antibodies. These antibodies are useful for measuring the presence of various substances in the body. For instance, the original home pregnancy test kit employed anti-hapten antibodies to determine whether a woman's urine contained human chorionic gonadotropin (HCG), which is a sign of pregnancy.

The most potent immunogens are proteins and polysaccharides but lipids, nucleic acids and synthetic polypeptides can also be immunogenic. Immunogenicity appears to be enhanced by large molecular size and molecular complexity. Although the linear sequences of the residues in a molecules has been equated with an antigenic determinant, the physical structures to which antibodies bind are primarily the result of the conformation of the molecule. As a result of folding, residues are different parts of the molecule may be close together and may be recognized by B-cell receptor or an antibody as part of the same determinant. Thus antibodies made against the native [natural] conformation of a molecule will not, in most instances react with the denatured molecule even though the primary sequence has not changed. This is in contrast to the way in which T-cell receptors recognize antigenic determinants- in the form of linear amino acid sequences, which have to be presented by major histocompatibility complex (MHC) molecules. The anchor amino acid residues of the linear peptide are important for attachment to the MHC molecules.

Epitopes and Paratopes

The part of the antigen with which the antibody reacts is known as the epitope or antigenic determinant (figure 4.1). Antigenic determinants or "epitopes" are the smallest unit of an antigen to which an antibody or cell can bind. These antigenic determinants are usually expressed in multiple copies on the foreign material, e.g. proteins or carbohydrates on a bacterial cell surface of a virus. For a protein, an antibody binds to a unit which is about three to six amino acids while for a carbohydrate it is about five to six sugar residues. Therefore, most large molecules possesses many antigenic determinants per molecule, that is they are "multideterminant". However, these determinants may be identical or different from each other on the same molecule. For example a carbohydrate with repeating sugar units will have repeating 3-5 amino acid sequences, and will thus have many different antigenic determinants.

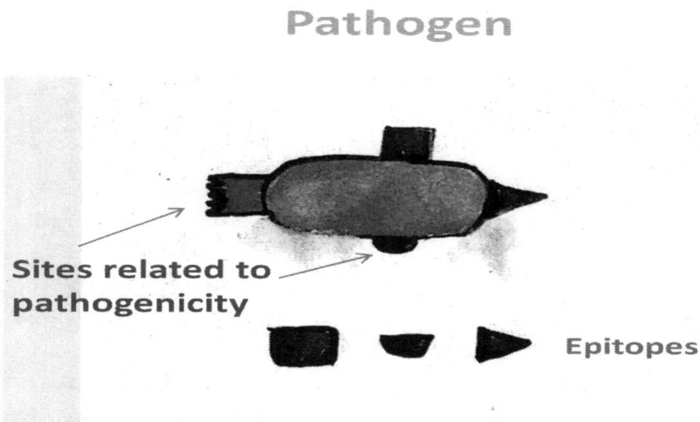

Fig. 4.1 : Presence of epitopes on a pathogen (antigen)

It is usual that an antigen, a molecule which is capable of initiating an adaptive immune response, possesses several unique molecular structures, each of which can elicit an adaptive immune response. Thus antibodies or cells recognizing an antigen are not directed against the whole molecules but against different parts of the molecule. The portion of the antibody molecule that binds to the epitope is called the paratope (figure 4.2). The epitope determinant is bound to the specific antibody by non-covalent bonds and their binding is more or less three dimensional and may be similar to a lock and key fit. An epitope on an antigen may bind very tightly to a given antibody but it may elicit such antibodies infrequently when the antigen is used to immunize an animal. In other words, there may be a perfectly good site on a pathogen for antibody binding but the antibody response to that site is so poor it cannot contribute to antibody protection against the pathogen. We say that the site has low immunogenicity and the consequences can clearly be great.

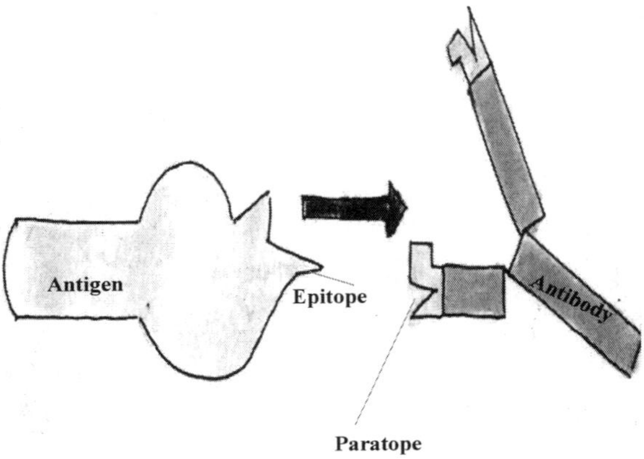

Fig. 4.2 : Epitope (antigen) and paratope (antibody)

Each antigen usually contains more than one epitope. Usually, the epitopes are found on the surface of the antigen, but denaturation and unfolding of the antigens have revealed that the antigens has some hidden epitopes in addition to the functional surface epitopes. In practical terms, microbes have a large number of different molecules and therefore potentially many different antigenic determinants, all of which could stimulate an immune response. However, all antigenic determinants are not equal- some may elicit strong and others weak responses. This is determined by the health, age and genetics of the individual. The number of epitopes per molecule of antigen is referred to as the valency. The functional valency of an antigen is different from the total valency of an antigen. The functional valency sites are all on the outer surface of the antigenic molecule and can be measured by determining the number of antibody molecules that attach to the antigen (figure 4.3). The valence determines the number of antibody molecules that can combine with the antigen at one time. If one determinant site is present, the antigen is monovalent. Most antigens, however, have more than one determinant site or more than one copy of the same epitope, and are termed multivalent. Multivalent antigens generally elicit a stronger immune response than do monovalent antigens (figure 4.4).

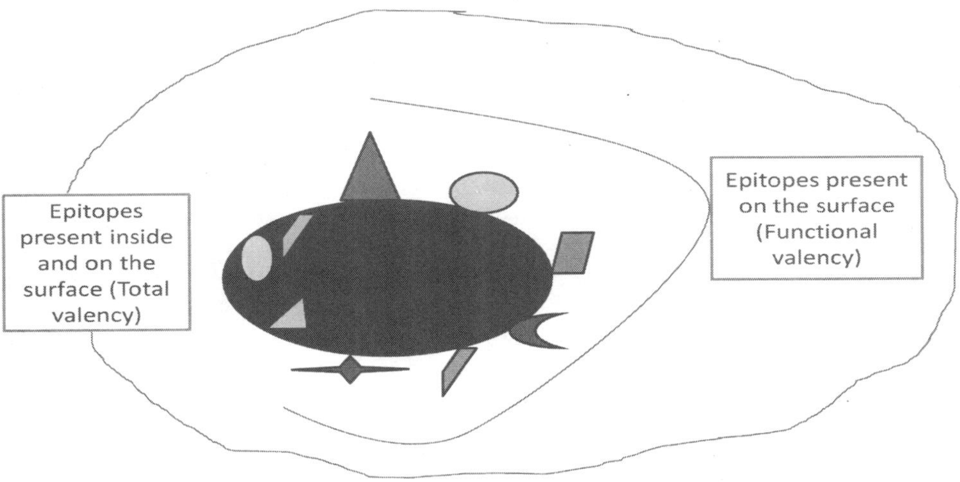

Fig. 4.3 : Concept of total valency and functional valency.

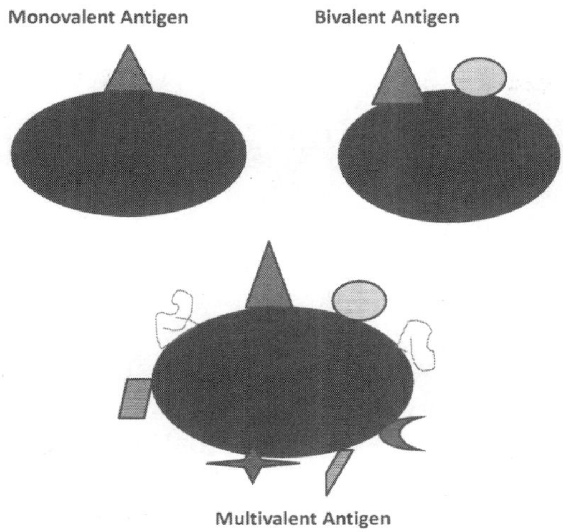

Fig. 4.4 : Types of antigens based on their valency

Antigens can be separated on the basis of molecular mass upon electrophoresis through polyacrylamide gels. Antigens separated in this way can be blotted onto nitrocellulose membranes and their presence detected by probing with suitable antibodies. Higher concentrations of antigens are frequently estimated by nephelometry. Protein microarrays, containing thousands of protein immobilized on solid support, can be probed with antibody for the simultaneous screening of many antigens. Similarly, antibody microarrays can be used to screen for the presence of multiple antigens in a single sample.

Essential Factors for Antigenicity

1. **Size:** The molecular size of an antigen has a direct relation to antigenicity. The most active immunogens tend to have a molecular mass of 100,000 daltons (Da). Generally, substances with a molecular mass less than 5000–10,000 Da are poor immunogens, although a few substances with a molecular mass less than 1000 Da have proven to be immunogenic (figure 4.5). Very large molecules such as hemocyanin (6000000 mol wt), thyroglobulin (669000 mol wt) and tetanus toxin (55000 mol wt) are excellent antigens. Whereas, molecules of low molecular size are poor antigens. For example protein like insulin (5700 mol wt) and histones (6000 mol wt) are poor antigens.

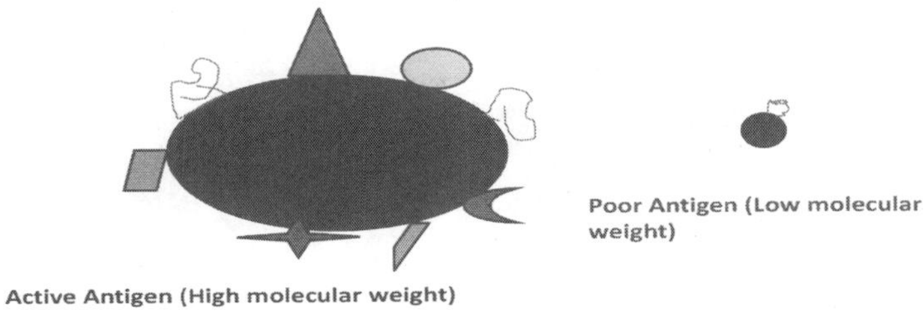

Fig. 4.5 : Effect of molecular weight on immunogenicity

2. **Solubility:** The non-antigenicity of synthetic polymer is attributed to their insolubility in body fluids and any substance which is not converted to soluble forms by tissue enzymes are also not antigenic.
3. **Chemical nature:** Most of the naturally occurring antigens are proteins and polysaccharides and these antigens are found to be comparatively more antigenic than lipid and nucleic acids. Proteins are better antigenic when compared to polysaccharides of the same size. Synthetic homopolymers (polymers composed of a single amino acid or sugar) tend to lack immunogenicity regardless of their size. Studies have shown that copolymers composed of different amino acids or sugars are usually more immunogenic than homopolymers of their constituents. These studies show that chemical complexity contributes to immunogenicity. In this regard it is notable that all four levels of protein organization- primary, secondary, tertiary, and quaternary-contribute to the structural complexity of a protein and hence affect its immunogenicity. Synthetic polymers are macromolecular in size, but not antigenic as they lack higher internal molecular complexity, that is usually possessed by polypeptide. Presence of aromatic amino acids in a polypeptide contributes to enhancement of its antigenicity.
4. **Foreignness:** This property allows a macromolecule to be antigenic. To be antigenic the macromolecule must come from a foreign source. Antigens from related species are less antigenic than that of unrelated species and antigens from members of the same species are less antigenic than that of other species. The more distant or foreign the antigen source the better the antigenicity will be. In order to elicit an immune response, a molecule must be recognized as nonself by the biological system. The capacity to recognize nonself is accompanied by tolerance of self, a specific unresponsiveness to self antigens. Much of the ability to tolerate self antigens arises during lymphocyte development, during which immature lymphocytes are exposed to self-components. Antigens that have not been exposed to immature lymphocytes during this critical period may be later recognized as nonself, or foreign, by the immune system. When an antigen is introduced into an organism, the degree of its immunogenicity depends on the degree of its foreignness. Generally, the greater the phylogenetic distance between two species, the greater the structural (and therefore the antigenic) disparity between them. For example, plant proteins are good antigens in animals whereas duck serum proteins are not good antigens for chick. For example, the common experimental antigen bovine serum albumin (BSA) is not immunogenic when injected into a cow but is strongly immunogenic when injected into a rabbit. Moreover, BSA would be expected to exhibit greater immunogenicity in a chicken than in a goat, which is more closely related to bovines. There are some exceptions to this rule. Some macromolecules (e.g., collagen and cytochrome *c*) have been highly conserved throughout evolution and therefore display very little immunogenicity across diverse species lines.

Conversely, some self-components (e.g., corneal tissue and sperm) are effectively sequestered from the immune system, so that if these tissues are injected even into the animal from which they originated, they will function as immunogens.

5. **Susceptibility to antigen processing and presentation-** The development of both humoral and cell-mediated immune responses requires interaction of T cells with antigen that has been processed and presented together with MHC molecules. Large, insoluble macromolecules generally are more immunogenic than small, soluble ones because the larger molecules are more readily phagocytosed and processed. Macromolecules that cannot be degraded and presented with MHC molecules are poor immunogens. This can be illustrated with polymers of D-amino acids, which are stereoisomers of the naturally occurring L-amino acids. Because the degradative enzymes within antigen-presenting cells can degrade only proteins containing L-amino acids, polymers of D-amino acids cannot be processed and thus are poor immunogens.

Cross Reactive Antigens

Antigen antibody reaction is specific and the specificity is determined by spatial configuration of the antigenic determinant group. But the antigen specificity is not absolute. Cross reactions can occur between the antigens which bear stereochemical similarities. Cross reacting antigen is one which is capable of binding to antibody produced in response to different antigens. This is due to sharing of determinants by the two antigens or because the antigenic determinants of the two, although not identical, are closely enough related stereochemically to combine with antibody against any one of them. Heterophile antigen is one such cross reactive antigen. These are antigens which exist on the surface of tissue cells of unrelated plants, animals and bacteria but are identical so that antibodies to one will cross react with the other. Very often these heterophile antigen are polysaccharides and these polysaccharides are structurally similar because of their limited chemical complexity even though they are derived from members of widely separated taxonomic groups. Forssman antigen is one of the heterophile antigen. These are glycolipid antigens, originally described to be present in most tissues of guinea pigs and RBCs of many species such as horse, sheep, dog, cat, chicken and many other organisms. In human, Forssman antigen is found on the gastrointestinal mucosa of some people.

Thymus dependent Antigen

Thymus dependent antigen is one that does not induce an antibody response in an animal which lacks a thymus. Helper T cell cooperation is needed in order B lymphocytes to response to such antigens in producing antibody forming cell. T-cell epitopes are generated by antigen processing, which fragments protein into small peptides that combine with class I or class II MHC molecules to form peptide-MHC complexes that are displayed on the surface of cells. T-cell activation requires the formation of a ternary complex between a T cell's TCR and peptide-MHC on antigen presenting or altered self cells.

Thymus independent Antigen

Thymus independent antigen is one which is able to stimulate B lymphocytes to produce antibody, without the cooperation of T lymphocytes. This includes polysaccharides with repeating antigenic determinants and lipopolysaccharides from Gram negative bacteria. The sizes of B-cell epitopes range widely. Some are quite small (e.g., small peptides or small organic molecules), and are often bound in narrow grooves or deep pockets of the antibody. Protein B-cell epitopes are much larger and interact with a larger, flatter complementary surface on the antibody molecule.

Question Bank

1. Very short answer type questions
   (a) Give 2 examples of heterophile antigens.
   (b) Who discovered blood group antigens?
   (c) Write full form of PAMP.
   (d) Name the biomolecule that can be an antigen.
   (e) Write full form of BSA.
2. Short answer type questions
   (a) Define epitope.
   (b) Define functional valency.
   (c) Define total valency.
   (d) Write short notes on chemical nature of antigen.
   (e) How does solubility affect antigenicity?
   (f) How does molecular weight affect antigenicity?
   (g) Define cross reactive antigens.
   (h) What are Forssman antigen?
   (i) Define haptens.
   (j) Define thymus dependent antigens.
   (k) Define thymus independent antigens.
   (l) Define carrier.
   *(m)*Define heterophile antigens.
3. Long answer type questions
   (a) Describe in detail the essential factors for antigenicity.
   (b) Describe in detail the chemical nature of antigens and antigenic determinants.

Multiple Choice Questions

1. Which is an antigen for human body?
   (a) Bacteria *(b)* Fungi
   (c) Virus *(d)* All of the above

2. Antigen can
   (a) Induce immune response
   (b) React specifically with antibodies
   (c) Both a & b
   (d) None of the above
3. Antigen can be
   (a) Protein *(b)* Carbohydrate
   (c) Lipid *(d)* All of above
4. Hapten is
   (a) Immunogenic
   (b) Non-immunogenic
   (c) Both a & b
   (d) Depends on environment
5. Which sentence is true?
   (a) Hapten is antigen.
   (b) Hapten-protein complex is immunogen.
   (c) Both *(a)* & *(b)* are true.
   (d) None of the above.
6. The part of the antigen with which the antibody reacts is known as-
   (a) Epitope *(b)* Antigenic determinant
   (c) Both a & b *(d)* Paratope
7. The number of epitope per molecule of antigen is referred to as
   (a) Totipotency *(b)* Pluripotency
   (c) Valency *(d)* Transparency
8. How many determinant site/s, is/are present in monovalent antigen?
   (a) One *(b)* Two
   (c) Three *(d)* May vary
9. Which of the following antigen can elicit a stronger immune response?
   (a) Monovalent *(b)* Bivalent
   (c) Trivalent *(d)* Multivalent
10. By which technique you can separate antigens?
    (a) ELISA *(b)* Precipitation
    (c) Electrophoresis *(d)* RIA
11. Higher concentration of antigens are frequently estimated by-
    (a) Spectrophotometry *(b)* Colorimetry
    (c) Nephelometry *(d)* Haemocytometry
12. What are the essential factors for antigenicity?
    (a) Size *(b)* Solubility
    (c) Chemical nature *(d)* All of the above

13. Which statement is true?
    (a) Protein is better antigenic when compared to polysaccharides of the same size.
    (b) Synthetic homopolymers tend to lack immunogenicity.
    (c) Protein organization affects its immunogenicity.
    (d) All above are true.
14. Which of the following is excellent antigen?
    (a) Hemocyanin *(b)* Thyroglobulin
    (c) Tetnus toxin *(d)* All of the above
15. Which statement is true?
    (a) Antigens from related species are less antigenic than that of unrelated species.
    (b) Antigens from members of the same species are less antigenic than that of other species.
    (c) The more distant or foreign the antigen source, the better the antigenicity will be.
    (d) All of the above.
16. Presence of............. amino acid in polypeptide contributes to enhancement of its antigenicity
    (a) Aliphatic *(b)* Cyclic
    (c) Aromatic *(d)* Sulfur
17. Which of the following is poor immunogen?
    (a) Insulin *(b)* Histone
    (c) Both a & b *(d)* Thyroglobulin
18. Which technique can be used to screen for the presence of multiple antigens in a single sample
    (a) Nephelometry *(b)* Antibody microarray
    (c) Colorimetry *(d)* Electrophoresis
19. Which is a self antigen for humans?
    (a) Lens antigen *(b)* Sperm antigen
    (c) Both a & b *(d)* BSA
20. If total valency of an antigen is 20 and the hidden epitopes are 12, then what is the functional valency of that antigen?
    (a) 20 *(b)* 12
    (c) 8 *(d)* 32

Answer Key

Question Number	Answer	Question Number	Answer
1	D	11	C
2	C	12	D

Question Number	Answer	Question Number	Answer
3	D	13	D
4	B	14	D
5	C	15	D
6	B	16	C
7	C	17	C
8	A	18	B
9	D	19	C
10	C	20	C

References

Amigorena S. & Savina (2010) Intracellular mechanisms of antigen cross presentation in dendritic cells. Current Opinion in Immunology 22. 109-177.

Berzofsky, J. A., and J. J. Berkower. 1999. Immunogenicity and antigen structure. In Fundamental Immunology, 4th ed., W. E. Paul, ed., Lippincott-Raven, Philadelphia

Boes M., Stoppelenburg A.J. & Sille F.C.M. (2009) Endosomal processing for antigen presentation by CD1 and class I major histocompatibility complex: roads to display or destruction. Immunology 127, 163-170.

Chapman H.A. (2006) Endosomal proteases in antigen presentation. Current Opinion in Immunology 18, 78-84.

Dale, D., and D. Federman, eds. 1997. Drug allergy. In Scientific American Medicine. Chapter VIII, Hypersensitivity and allergy, p. 27.

Davis S.J. et al. (2003) The nature of molecular recognition bt T-cells. Nature Immunology 4, 217-224.

Demotz, S., H. M. Grey, E. Appella, and A. Sette. 1989. Characterization of a naturally processed MHC class II-restricted Tcell determinant of hen egg lysozyme. Nature 342:682.

Finley D. (2009) Recognition and processing of ubiquitin-protein conjugates by the proteasome. Annual Review of Biochemistry 78, 477-513.

Fraser J.D. & Proft T. (2008) The bacterial superantigen and superantigen like proteins. Immunological Review 255, 226-243.

Godfrey D.I., Rossjohn J. & McCluskey J. (2008) The fidelity, occasional promiscuity, and versatility of T cell receptor recognition. Immunity 28, 304-314.

Grey, H. M., A. Sette, and S. Buus. 1989. How T cells see antigen. Sci. Am. 261(5):56.

Heath W.R. et al. (2004) Cross-presentation, dendritic cell subsets, and the generation of immunity to cellular antigens. Immunological Review 199, 9-26.

Landsteiner, K. 1945. The Specificity of Serological Reactions. Harvard University Press, Cambridge, Massachusetts.

Laver, W. G., G. M. Air, R. G. Webster, and S. J. Smith-Gill. 1990. Epitopes on protein antigens: misconceptions and realities. Cell 61:553.

Moody D.B., Zajonc D.M. & Wilson I.A. (2005) Anatomy of CD1-lipid antigen complexes. Nature Review of Immunology 5, 387-399.

Peiser, L., S. Mukhopadhyay, and S. Gordon. 2002. Scavenger receptors in innate immunity. Curr. Opin. Immunol. 14:123.

Procko E. et al. (2009) The mechanism of ABC transporters: general lesson from structural and functional studies of an antigenic peptide transporter. The FASEB Journal 23, 1287-1302.

Stanfield, R. L., and I. A. Wilson. 1995. Protein-peptide interactions. Curr. Opin. Struc. Biol. 5:103.

Tainer, J. A., et al. 1985. The atomic mobility component of protein antigenicity. Annu. Rev. Immunol. 3:501.

Underhill, D. M., and A. Ozinsky. 2002. Toll-like receptors: key mediators of microbe detection. Curr. Opin. Immunol. 14:103.

CHAPTER 5

Immunoglobulins

Introduction

Immunoglobulins are immunologically active serum proteins formed in response to an antigen and react specifically with that antigen. Immunoglobulins are present on the B-cell membrane and secreted by plasma cells. They are briefly represented as Ig. They are commonly called antibodies (Ab). An antibody or immunoglobulin (Ig) is a glycoprotein that is made in response to an antigen, and can recognize and bind to the antigen that caused its production. Antibodies are present in the blood serum, tissue fluids, and mucosal surfaces of vertebrate animals. Membrane-bound antibody confers antigenic specificity on B cells; antigen-specific proliferation of B-cell clones is elicited by the interaction of membrane antibody with antigen. Secreted antibodies circulate in the blood, where they serve as the effectors of humoral immunity by searching out and neutralizing antigens or marking them for elimination. All antibodies share structural features, bind to antigen, and participate in a limited number of effector functions.

Serum glycoproteins can be separated according to their charge by movement through a gel in an electric field and classified as albumin, alpha-1 globulin, alpha-2 globulin, beta globulin, and gamma globulin. The gamma globulin band is relatively wide because it contains a heterogeneous class of immunoglobulins—namely, IgG, IgA, IgM, and IgD. These differ from each other in molecular size, structure, charge, amino acid composition, and carbohydrate content. Most antibodies in serum are in the IgG class. A fifth immunoglobulin class, the IgE class, has a similar mobility to IgD but cannot be represented quantitatively because of its low concentration in serum. We now know that although immunoglobulin G (IgG), the main class of antibody molecules, is indeed mostly found in the γ globulin fraction, significant amounts of it and other important classes of antibody molecules are found in the α and the β fractions of serum.

Immunoglobulin Structure

Immunoglobulins are immunological missiles produced by the body. They are found in the serum, body fluids and tissues. They are produced by vertebrates only. They are synthesized by lymphocytes and plasma cells. If the blood or plasma is allowed to clot, the fluid phase that remains is called serum. It has been known since the turn of the century that antibodies reside in the serum. The first evidence that antibodies were contained in particular serum protein fractions came from a classic experiment by A. Tiselius and E. A. Kabat, in 1939.

Rodney Porter (1962) proposed the basic structure of immunoglobulin.

Immunoglobulin is a glycoprotein. The antibody molecule is made up of two identical heavy (H) and two identical light (L) chains held together by interchain disulphide (S-S) bond. Each light chain is made up of 214 amino acids and has a mass of approximately 25 kDa. Each heavy chain is made up of450 to 700 amino acids and has a mass of about 50 to 70 kDa. Both the heavy and light chains contain several homologous units of about 100 to 110 amino acids. Within each unit, called a domain, disulfide bonds form a loop of approximately 60 amino acids (figure 5.1).

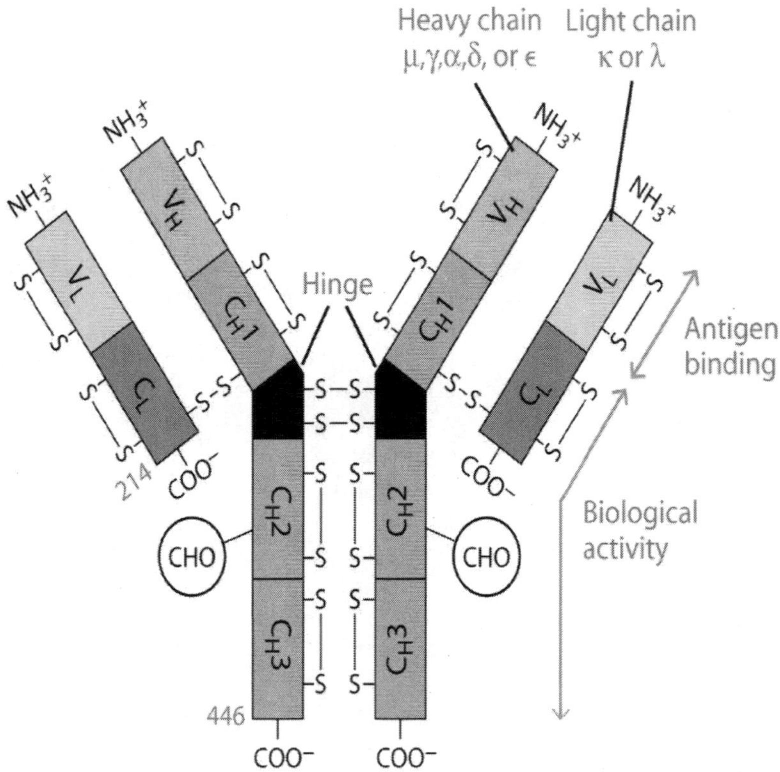

Fig. 5.1 : Structure of an antibody

The immunoglobulin consists of two regions, namely a variable region (V-region) and a constant region (C-region). In the constant region, the amino acid sequence remains constant in most of the immunoglobulins. In the variable region the amino acid sequence shows variability and hence the name. The variable region is located at the extremity of the limbs of Y in the N-terminal end of the immunoglobulin and the constant region is located at the base of the stalk of Y in the C- terminal end. The variable region is formed of both light and heavy chains. Half of the constant region is formed of both light and heavy chains. While the terminal half of the constant region is formed of heavy chains only. Based on the functional aspect, two regions can be recognized in the immunoglobulin. They are Fab fragment or antigen binding fragment and Fc fragment or crystallizable fragment. The Fab is located at the extremity of the two limbs of 'Y'. The Fab fragment reacts with the antigenic determinants and its N-terminal binds with the antigen. The Fc is located at the stalk of the 'Y'. The Fc fragment is involved in complement fixation, attachment to phagocytic cells, degranulation of mast cells, etc. Antibodies are glycoproteins; with few exceptions, the sites of attachment for carbohydrates are restricted to the constant region.

The four chains are interconnected by inter chain disulfide bonds. The two heavy chains are linked by 1 to 13 interchain disulfide bonds. Each light chain is linked to a heavy chain by a single interchain disulfide bond. The light chain has a 2 intrachain disulfide bonds and the heavy chain has 4 intrachain disulfide bonds. These chains can be separated by reduction of the S-S bonds (SH, SH) and acidification. The enzyme papain cleaves just above the interchain disulfide bonds linking the heavy chains, whereas the enzyme pepsin cleaves just below these bonds, so that the two proteolytic enzymes generate different digestion products. Mercaptoethanol reduction and alkylation allow separation of the individual heavy and light chains. The molecule is split by papain to yield two identical fab fragments (fragment antigen binding), each with a single combining site for antigen and a third fragment, fc (fragment crystallizable) which lack the ability to bind antigen. Pepsin acts at a different point and cleaves the IgG into larger fragment f(ab')2 which is still divalent with respect to antigen-binding and a small pFc'. The Fc region contain the carboxyl-terminal of the heavy chain. The ability to cross the placenta and various other biological activities are determined by this region.

The γ, α and δ heavy chains contain an extended peptide sequence between the CH1 and CH2 domains that has no homology with the other domains. This region, called the hinge region. The four chains are arranged in the form of a flexible Y with a hinge region. This hinge region allows the antibody molecule to assume a T shape. The hinge region of the heavy chain is rich in proline residues. The presence or proline confer flexibility any many enable and may enable the two f(ab) region to bind to epitopes which are separated at variable distance. The heavy chain of an antibody molecule determines its types. In humans there are five classes of heavy chains designated by lowercase Greek letters: gamma (γ), alpha (α), mu (μ), delta (δ), and epsilon (ξ). The properties of these heavy chains determine, respectively, the five immunoglobulin classes—IgG, IgA, IgM, IgD, and IgE. Each immunoglobulin class differs in its general properties, half-life, distribution in the body, and interaction with other components of the host's defensive systems.

Only two types of light chains are found in immunoglobulins these are kappa and lambda chains. When the immunoglobulin contains the kappa chains, the immunoglobulin is called K-Type. When it contains the lambda chains, the immunoglobulin is called L- type. Approximately 60% of the serum immunoglobulin molecules are K type, while only 40% are L type.

Detailed comparisons of the amino acid sequences of a large number of VL and VH domains revealed that the sequence variation is concentrated in a few discrete regions of these domains. The pattern of this variation is best summarized by a quantitative plot of the variability at each position of the polypeptide chain.

Each light chain has two domains (regions), namely a variable light chain or VL region and a constant light chain region or CL region. The VL region is located in the N-terminal end and the CL region is located in the C –terminal end. Each heavy chain has 4 domains. The 1st domain is called variable heavy chain region or VH region. It is located at the N-terminal end. The other 3 domains are called constant heavy chain domains or CH regions. They are named CH1, CH2, and CH3. CH3 is located at the C- terminal end (figure 5.1). Immunoglobulins IgM and IgE have an additional constant heavy chain domain called CH4. The specific chemistry, amino acid sequence and the shape of the combining site together constitute the paratope. It is complimentary to the specific shape of the epitope in the antigen.

Antibodies are secreted by plasma cells. All antibody molecule produced by a single plasma cell have identical epitope-specificity. This specificity is conferred by the sequence of the amino acid residue in the f(ab) region which is unique to antibodies produced by single plasma cell. The constant region occupies approximately 75% of the molecule toward the carboxy-terminus. Within the antigen-combining site are restricted regions which are hyper variable i.e. regions where the amino acid residues are even more variable. These regions sometimes known as the hotspots are involved in constructing the antigen combining sites. Three such regions exist in each VL domain and four in each VH domain. These regions are actually involved in the antigen binding site and they are called idiotypic regions. By the folding of the variable domain, the hypervariable regions are brought together to form antigen binding site consisting of 3 hypervariable regions from the light chain and 4 from the adjacent heavy chain.

Within two of the major human immunoglobulin classes, there are three variants viz. allotypes, idiotypes and isotypes.

1. **Allotypes**

   An immunoglobulin (Ig) can be defined by the presence of genetic markers termed allotypes. These markers are different in different individuals and are thus immunogenic when injected into individuals whose Ig lacks the allotypes. Like the ABO blood group antigens, they are determinants which segregate within a species. Allotypes are normally the result of small amino acid differences in IgL- or H-chain constant regions. For example, the Km (Inv) marker is an allotype of human kL chain and is the result of a leucine vs valine difference at position 191. The Gm markers are allotype associated with the IgG H chains. Allotypes are inherited in a strictly Mendelian fashion, and usually have no significance to the function of the antibody molecule, nor are they so immunogenic as to compromise their use in immunotherapy.

2. **Idiotypes**

   Antigenic determinant associated with the binding site of an antibody molecule are called idiotypes and are unique to all antibodies produced by the same clone of B cells. That is, although all antibodies have idiotypic determinants, these determinants are different for all antibodies not derived from the same clone of B cells. Thus, the number of different idiotypes in an individual is at least as numerous as the number of specificities. In fact, one's own idiotypes may be recognized by one's own immune system. Thus idiotypes are immunogenic and can induce immune responses. To that end monoclonal antibodies to idiotypes are being explored as a therapeutic approach to B-cell tumors all of which would express idiotypes on their cell surface.

3. **Isotypes**

   Isotypes refers to the variations in the heavy chain constant regions associated with the different classes that are normally present in all individuals.

Terms associated with antibody

a) **Affinity**

   Different antibody molecules produced in response to a particular antigenic determinant may vary considerably in their tightness of binding to that determinant. The higher the binding constant the less likely the antibody is to dissociate from the antigen. Clearly the affinity of an antibody population is critical when the antigen is a toxin or virus and must be neutralized by rapid and firm combination with antibody. Antibodies formed soon after the injection of an antigen are generally of lower affinity for that antigen, whereas antibodies produced later have dramatically greater affinities.

b) **Antibody Valence**

   The valence of an antibody is the maximum number of antigenic determinants with which it can react. For ex IgG antibodies contain two Fab regions and can bind two molecules of the same antigen or two identical sites on the same particle, and thus have a valence of two. Valence is important for binding affinity, as having two or more binding sites for an antigen can dramatically increase the tightness of binding of the antibody to antigens on a bacteria or virus. This combined effect, avidity results from synergy of the binding strengths of each binding site.

c) **Avidity**

   Avidity is the firmness of association between a multi determinant antigen and the antibodies produced against it. The larger the no. of binding sites per antibody molecule, the larger the no. of bonds formed with an organism, and less likely it will be to dissociate. Thus, an antibody with a poor intrinsic affinity for an antigenic determinant can, as a result of a large no. of combining sites per molecule, be extremely effective in neutralizing a virus or complexing with a microorganism.

Functions of immunoglobulins

Each end of the immunoglobulin molecule has a different role. The Fab region is concerned with binding to antigen, whereas the Fc region mediates binding to host tissue, various cells of the immune system, some phagocytic cells, or the first component of the complement system. The binding of an antibody with an antigen usually does not cause destruction of the antigen or of the microorganism, cell, or agent to which it is attached. Rather the antibody serves to mark and identify the target for immunologic attack and to activate nonspecific immune responses that can destroy the target.

The main function of the immunoglobulins is protection of the body against invading microorganisms. The first and most important function of an antibody molecule is to combine specifically with the epitope it recognizes and then to signal to the other components of the immune system. The class of antibody, the nature of immunogen determines the way in which the immunogen is eliminated from the body. In a primary immune response, when there has been no prior exposure to immunogen, most antibody is of the IgM class. In a secondary response, following a second or subsequent exposure to the same immunogen, IgG makes up the bulk of the antibody.

The protective role is carried out in the following ways-

1. **Agglutination of antigens** - IgG, IgM and IgA are able to agglutinate cells and to precipitate soluble immunogens from solutions. These secondary effects take place because each antibody has atleast two combining sites which can crosslink cells or macromolecules. Agglutination of bacteria or precipitation of harmful proteins serves to localize an infection and allows these immunogens to be more easily removed by phagocytes. As IgM is having 5-10 antigen binding sites it is a very efficient agglutinating antibody molecule. IgG and IgM are the most prevalent antibodies in the blood and provide the main humoral defense against bacteria.
2. **Precipitation of antigens** - Immunoglobulin combines with soluble antigens such as tetanus toxin and the complex thus formed becomes insoluble and precipitates. Thus the toxin is made inactive.
3. **Neutralisation of antigens** - The antibodies cover the toxic sites of the antigenic agents and thus neutralize them (make them inactive).
4. **Lysis of the antigens**- Some potent antibodies are occasionally capable of directly attacking membranes of cellular agents and thereby causing rupture of the cells. It is observed that a single IgM molecule attached to a red blood cell, can bring about lysis by its multiple combining sites, whereas 1000 IgG molecules are required for the same effect.
5. **Opsonisation** - Immunoglobulins specific for particulate antigens such as bacteria play an important role by coating the surface of bacteria and making the antigen more susceptible for phagocytosis. This process is termed as opsonisation. These antibodies are known as opsonising antibodies. IgM performs this role very efficiently than the other immunoglobulins. The actual mechanism of opsonisation is not known but it may be due to the following:
   a) Antibody may alter the surface properties of antigens such as the surface charge and thus may reduce the electrostatic repulsion between the phagocytes and antigens.

b) The Fc fragments of the antibody may have an affinity for the surface of the charge and thus may reduce the electrostatic repulsion between the phagocytes and antigens.

c) One of the product of classical pathway is C3b which strongly activates phagocytosis both neutrophils and macrophages causing them to engulf bacteria attached to the antibody. The process is known as opsonisation.

6. **Tissue fixation** - The ability of the immunoglobulins to attach to tissue cells is a well marked feature which is responsible for various hypersensitivity reactions in human beings. This tissue fixation is mainly carried out by the Fc portion of IgE. IgE, which is usually found in very low concentration in the serum, increases in conditions of hay fever and asthma and these antibodies bind firmly to mast cells independent of any reaction with antigen.

   When an appropriate antigen enters the person, it reacts with the tissue fixed antibody and a chain of events are triggered namely mast cells degranulate, vasoactive amines are released and subsequent clinical symptoms of immediate hypersensitivity such as sneezing and urticaria are produced.

7. **Phagocytosis** - The binding of IgG or IgM to immunogens may activate the complement system which results in lysis of cellular immunogens. Intermediate products of the complement sequence including the glycoproteins C3b, C3a, C5a, stimulate the uptake of antibody antigen complexes by neutrophils and macrophages. Neutrophils and macrophages have cell surface receptors for the Fc region of antigen- bound IgG so that this antibody can form a bridge binding the immunogen to the phagocytic cell resulting in a more efficient phagocytosis.

8. **Chemotaxis** - Large granular lymphocytes possibly the same population as the NK cells also have Fc receptor for IgG. Although these cells are not phagocytic binding to an IgG coated cell triggers the release of toxic granules which destroy the cell. This process is known as antibody – dependent cellular cytotoxicity. Fragments C5a and C3a cause chemotaxis of neutrophils and macrophages which results in the migration of a number of these cells to the regions of antigen-antibody complex accumulation.

9. **Activation of mast cells and basophils** - Fragments C5a and C3a also activate mast cells and basophils resulting in the degranulation. As a result, they release histamines and several other substances, which through different ways immobilize the antigenic agents and also produce inflammation. IgE, which is normally found in low concentration in the plasma is important in the immune responses toward multicellular parasites. IgE can trigger the local release of mediator from the mast cells in the gut, resulting in an inflammation contraction of smooth muscles in the gut, helping to dislodge the intestinal parasites. In addition, an eosinophil chemotactic factor attracts the eosinophils which attract

parasites particularly if the parasites are coated with antibody.

10. **Selective Transport**- The delivery of antibody to the mucosal surfaces of the respiratory, gastrointestinal, and urogenital tracts, as well as its export to breast milk, requires the movement of immunoglobulin across epithelial layers, a process called transcytosis. In human beings, of the five classes of immunoglobulins, only IgG is transported from the mother to the foetus through the placenta which gives passive immunity to the new born baby in the new environment to which it is exposed. The new born is thus passively protected for about 6-9 months, by then the active immunity sets in. All the five class are found in plasma, although IgA is more important as the 'secretory' antibody (which protect the external surface of the body). IgA is also selectively secreted into the saliva, mucous secretions of the respiratory and digestive tracts and also into the colostrums.

Immunoglobulin Classes

IgG is the major immunoglobulin in human serum, accounting for 80% of the immunoglobulin pool. Normal serum concentration of IgG is about 8-16 mg/ml. IgG is present in blood plasma and tissue fluids and is produced particularly during the secondary immune response. The IgG class acts against bacteria and viruses by opsonizing the invaders and neutralizing toxins. It is also one of the two immunoglobulin classes that activate complement by the classical pathway. IgG is the only immunoglobulin molecule able to cross the placenta and provide natural immunity in utero and to the neonate at birth. Germ free animals have low IgG levels but on leaving the germ free environment, the IgG levels rise rapidly. The molecular weight IgG is 150,000 and its sedimentation coefficient is 7S. IgG has a half life of 25 days. The carbohydrate content of IgG is about 3%. The large no. of disulfide bond in IgG3 is associated with a long hinge region consisting of 62 amino acids and this results in the higher molecular weight of IgG 3. Figure 5.2 depicts the structure of IgG.

There are four human IgG subclasses (IgG1, IgG2, IgG3, and IgG4) that vary chemically in their chain composition and the number and arrangement of interchain disulfide (figure 5.3). About 65% of the total serum IgG is IgG1, and 23% is IgG2. IgG is the only immunoglobulin that crosses the human placenta. IgG1, IgG3, and IgG4 readily cross the placenta and play an important role in protecting the developing fetus and thus offers a passive protection to the new born for about 6-9 months. IgG neutralizes toxins and viruses. IgG2 antibodies are opsonic and develop in response to antitoxins. The IgG4 antibodies function as skin sensitizing immunoglobulins. IgG activates the classical complements pathway during antigen antibody reaction IgG3 is the most effective complement activator, followed by IgG1; IgG2 is less efficient, and IgG4 is not able to activate complement at all. By binding to bacteria, IgG opsonises them, thereby enhance their phagocytosis and elimination. This process is known as opsonisation. IgG1 and IgG3 bind with high affinity to Fc receptors on phagocytic cells and thus mediate opsonization. IgG4 has an intermediate affinity for Fc receptors, and IgG2 has an extremely low affinity.

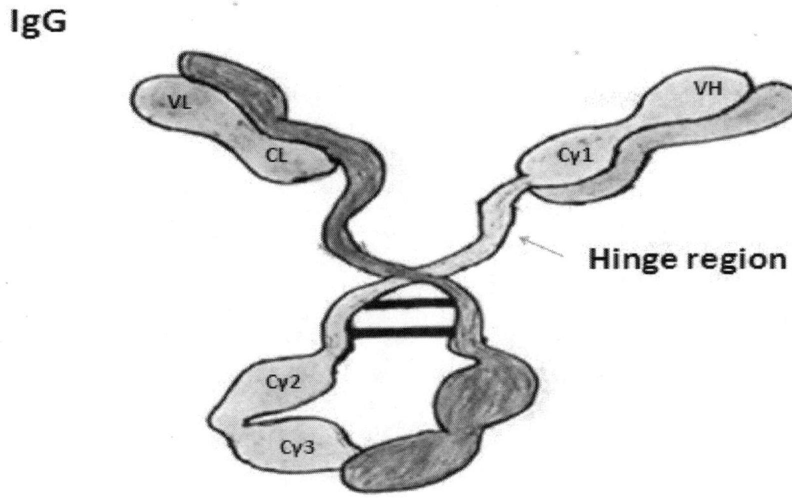

Fig. 5.2 : Structure of IgG

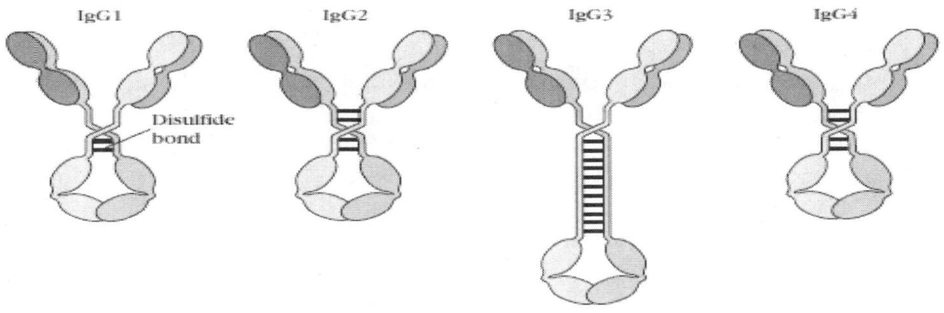

Fig. 5.3 : Types of IgG

IgM accounts for about 10% of the immunoglobulin pool, with an average serum concentration of 1.5 mg/ml. It is usually a polymer of five monomeric units (pentamer), each composed of two heavy chains and two light chains. Monomeric IgM, with a molecular weight of 180,000, is expressed as membrane-bound antibody on B cells. It is often referred as the 'macroglobulin' because of its high molecular weight. The serum level of IgM is very low, about 5 to 2 mg/ml. This low serum level is due to its short half life (5 days) and low synthetic rate (5-8 mg/kg body weight/day). The carbohydrate content is about 10-12%. The sedimentation coefficient of this pentamer is 19S. There are no subclasses for IgM. The monomers are arranged in a pinwheel array with the Fc ends in the center, held together by disulfide bonds and a special J (joining) chain and the ten antigen-binding sites on the periphery of the molecule (figure 5.4). The J chain appears to be required for polymerization of the monomers to form pentameric IgM; it is added just before secretion of the pentamer. Although most IgM appears to be pentameric, around 5% or less of human serum IgM exists in a hexameric form. This molecule contains six monomeric units but seems to lack a J chain. Hexameric IgM activates complement up to twentyfold more effectively than does the normal pentameric form.

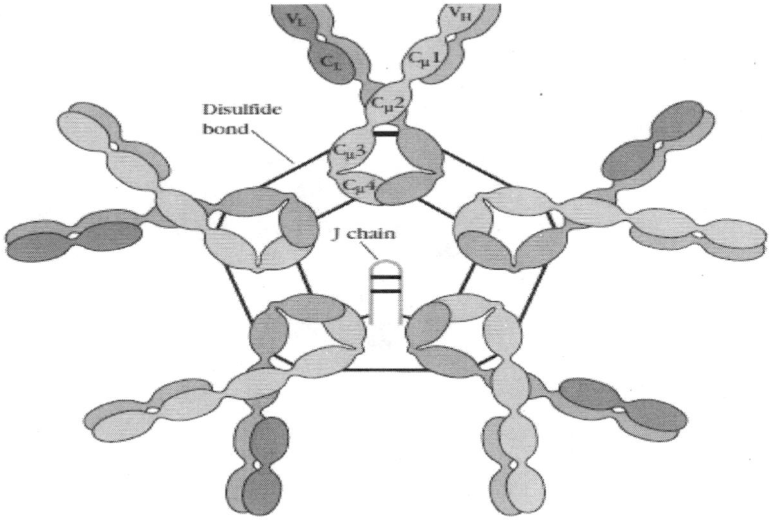

Fig. 5.4 : Structure of IgM

IgM is the first immunoglobulin made during B-cell maturation and is expressed as membrane-bound antibody on B cells. IgM is the first immunoglobulin class produced in a primary response to an antigen, and it is also the first immunoglobulin to be synthesized by the neonate. Since IgM is so large, it does not leave the bloodstream or cross the placenta. Maternal IgM does not cross the placenta but the human foetus can synthesize IgM, if its B cells are antigenically stimulated as in congenital infections. Thus IgM detection in newborn is a useful indicator of intrauterine infections such as congenital syphilis, rubella, taxoplasmosis, etc. An IgM molecule can bind 10 small hapten molecules; however, because of steric hindrance, only 5 or fewer molecules of larger antigens can be bound simultaneously. Because of its high valency, pentameric IgM is more efficient than other isotypes in binding antigens with many repeating epitopes such as viral particles and red blood cells (RBCs). IgM agglutinates bacteria, activates complement by the classical pathway, and enhances the ingestion of pathogens by phagocytic cells. IgM is also more efficient than IgG at activating complement. Complement activation requires two Fc regions in close proximity, and the pentameric structure of a single molecule of IgM fulfills this requirement. Most natural antibodies such as the natural classical ABO blood group isoagglutinins (anti-A and anti-B) many of the natural antibodies to microorganism and also heterophile antibodies are of IgM class.

IgA accounts for about 15% of the immunoglobulin pool. IgA is the second in abundance among the immunoglobulins next to IgG. Some IgA is present in the serum as a monomer of two heavy and two light chains. IgA exists primarily as a monomer, but polymeric forms (dimers, trimers, and some tetramers) are sometimes seen, all containing a J-chain polypeptide (figure 5.5). Two subclasses of

IgA exist namely IgA1 and IgA2. IgA1 has both interchain and intrachain disulfide linkages whereas IgG2 is completely devoid of interchain disulfide bonding between the heavy and light chains. Instead the two chains are held together by non-covalent linkages. The heavy chain of IgA is of alpha type. It has a molecular weight of 160,000. The sedimentation coefficient is 7S. The normal serum level of IgA is 0.6-4.2mg/ml. It has a half life of 6-8 days. Serum IgA has more amount of IgA1 than IgA2. Most IgA, however, occurs in mucous secretions as a polymerized dimer held together by a J chain. IgA has special features that are associated with secretory mucosal surfaces. IgA, when transported from the mucosal-associated lymphoid tissue to mucosal surfaces, acquires a protein termed the secretory component. The secretory piece has a single polypeptide chain of molecular weight 70,000.The J chain is also a polypeptide chain of molecular weight 15,000. The secretory component is produced by epithelial cells of mucous membranes (figure 5.6). It consists of five immunoglobulin-like domains that bind to the Fc region domains of the IgA dimer. This interaction is stabilized by a disulfide bond between the fifth domain of the secretory component and one of the chains of the dimeric IgA.

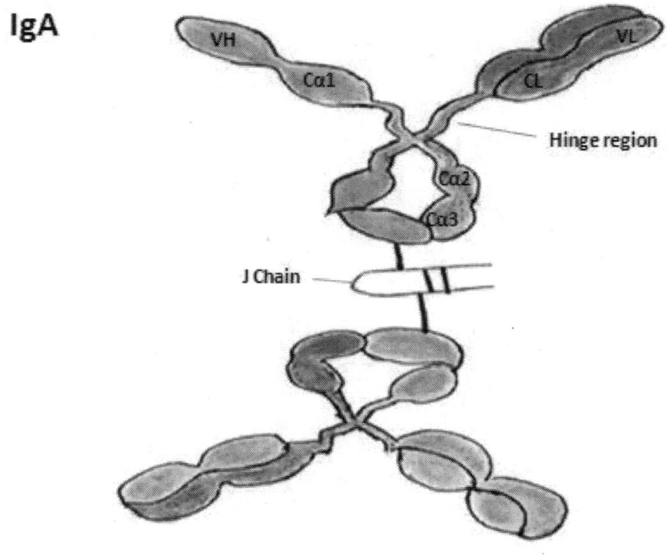

Fig. 5.5 : Structure of IgA

Secretory IgA (sIgA), as the modified molecule is now called, is the primary immunoglobulin of mucosal associated lymphoid tissue. Secretory IgA is also found in saliva, tears, and breast milk. In these fluids and related body areas, sIgA plays a major role in protecting surface tissues against infectious microorganisms by the formation of an immune barrier. For example, in breast milk sIgA helps protect nursing newborns. In the intestine, sIgA attaches to viruses, bacteria, and protozoan parasites such as *Entamoeba histolytica.* This prevents pathogen adherence to mucosal surfaces and invasion of host tissues, a phenomenon known as immune exclusion. In addition, sIgA binds to antigens within the mucosal layer of the small intestine; subsequently the antigen-sIgA complexes are excreted through the adjacent epithelium into the gut lumen (figure 5.6). Along the jejunum of the small intestine, for example, there are more than 2.5 x 10^{10} IgA-secreting plasma cells—a number that surpasses the total plasma cell population of the bone marrow, lymph, and spleen combined! Every day, a human secretes from 5 g to 15 g of secretory IgA into mucous secretions. Complexes of secretory IgA and antigen are easily entrapped in mucus and then eliminated by the ciliated epithelial cells of the respiratory tract or by peristalsis of the gut. This rids the body of locally formed immune complexes and decreases their access to the circulatory system. Secretory IgA has been shown to provide an important line of defense against bacteria such as *Salmonella, Vibrio cholerae,* and *Neisseria gonorrhoeae* and viruses such as polio, influenza, and reovirus. Therefore secretory IgA is termed as the mucosal paint or' antiseptic paint' of the mucous membrane. Secretory IgA also plays a role in the alternative complement pathway, thereby neutralises local toxins, promote phagocytosis and activate bacteriolytic activity. But this occur only in the presence of lysozyme (figure 5.6).

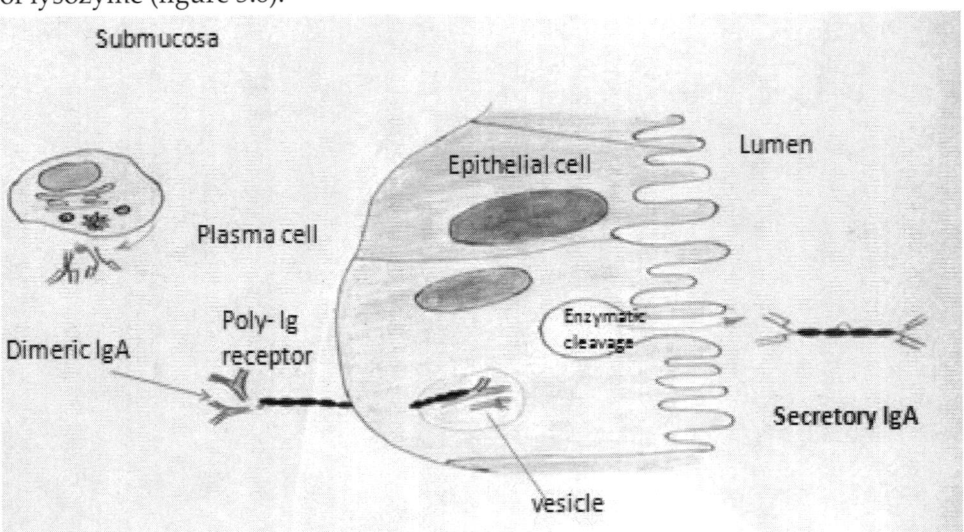

Fig. 5.6 : Formation of secretory IgA

IgD was first discovered when a patient developed a multiple myeloma whose myeloma protein failed to react with antiisotype antisera against the then-known isotypes: IgA, IgM, and IgG. When rabbits were immunized with this myeloma protein, the resulting antisera were used to identify the same class of antibody at low levels in normal human serum. The two heavy chains are of delta type. It has a monomer structure similar to IgG but IgD is slightly larger than IgG, having a molecular weight of 180,000. The large size of the IgD may be associated with an extended hinge region. IgD is limited to the blood serum with serum concentration of 0.03 mg/ml and constitutes about 0.2% of the total immunoglobulin in serum. The average sedimentation coefficient is 7S. IgD is rich in carbohydrates. About 12% of its weight is formed of polysaccharides. The rate of synthesis is 0.4 mg/kg body weight/day. The half life of IgD is 2-3 days. Two subclasses of IgD namely IgD1 and IgD2 have been found. It is found associated with the surface of B lymphocytes. IgD antibodies do not fix complement and cannot cross the placenta, but they are abundant in combination with IgM on the surface of B cells and bind antigens, thus signaling the B cell to start antibody production. Figure 5.7 depicts the structure of immunoglobulin D.

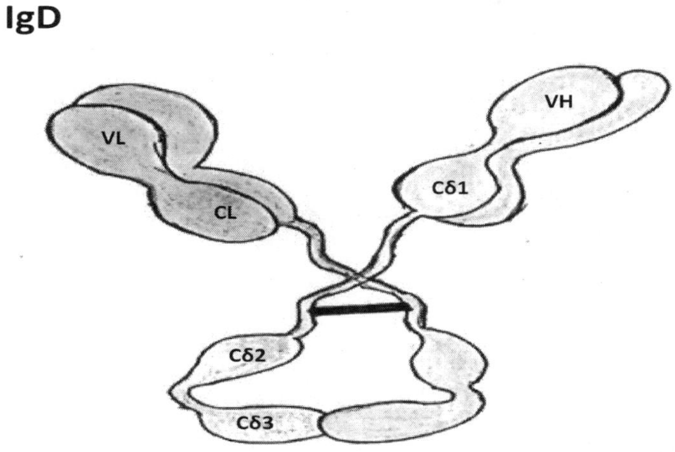

Fig. 5.7 : Structure of IgD

Originally named as Reagin, **IgE** was named in reference to the E antigen of ragweed pollen, which is a potent inducer of this class of antibody. This is the only immunoglobulin without hinge. It has a molecular weight of 190,000 which is slightly higher than that of IgG. It is heat labile immunoglobulin whereas IgG, IgA, IgM, IgD are heat stable. It is found only in traces in the serum and the average serum level is 0.00004mg/ml. IgE has a half life of 2-3 days. Its carbohydrate content is about 12%. The sedimentation coefficient of IgE is 8S. The classic skin-sensitizing and anaphylactic antibodies belong to this class that are responsible for the symptoms of hay fever, asthma, hives, and anaphylactic shock. The P-K reaction (named for its originators, Prausnitz and Kustner), was the basis for the first biological assay for IgE activity. IgE molecules have four constant region domains (Cξ1, Cξ2, Cξ3, and Cξ4) on their heavy chains (figure 5.8). The Fc portion of the Cξ4 chain can bind to special Fcξ receptors on mast cells and basophils. When two IgE molecules on the surface of these cells are cross-linked by binding to the same antigen, the cells degranulate. This degranulation releases histamine and other pharmacological mediators of anaphylaxis. It also stimulates eosinophilia and gut hypermotility (increased rate of movement of the intestinal contents) that aid in the elimination of helminthic parasites. Thus, though IgE is present in small amounts, this class of antibodies has very potent biological capabilities. High level of IgE in children with worm infestation seems to have a protective role. This protective function is either by IgE acting directly on the parasites or by producing vasoactive amines.

IgE

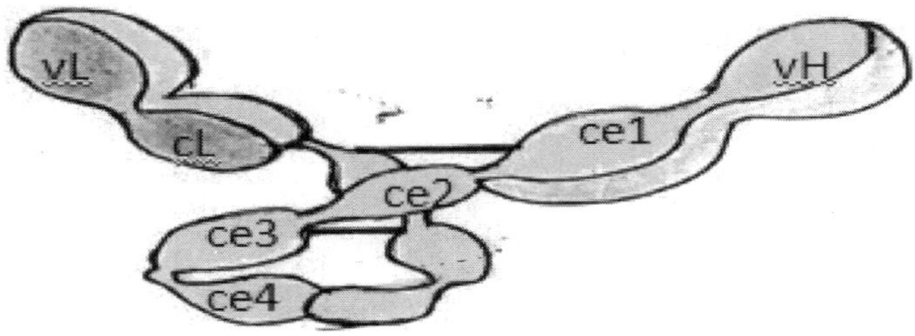

Fig. 5.8 : Structure of IgE

Question Bank

1. Very short answer type questions
   (a) Name the antibody that can cross placenta.
   (b) Name the antibody that is a pentamer.
   (c) Name the antibody that is found on the B cell surface.
   (d) Name the antibody found in milk.
   (e) Name the antibody whose concentration increases during allergy.
   (f) Which antibody is found in highest concentration normally?
   (g) Which antibody is found in highest concentration during infection?
   (h) Name the bonds found in antibody.
   (i) How many types of heavy chains are there?
   (j) How many types of light chains are there?
   (k) Name the amino acids found in hinge region.
2. Short answer type questions
   (a) Define antibody.
   (b) Define paratope.
   (c) Draw a neat labeled diagram of antibody.
   (d) Describe few properties of antibody.
   (e) Define valency.
   (f) Define allotype.
   (g) Define Idiotype.
   (h) Define affinity.
   (i) Define avidity.
   (j) What are hypervariable region?
3. Long answer type questions
   (a) Describe in detail types of antibodies along with their important characteristics.
   (b) Describe in detail the functions of immunoglobulins.
   (c) Describe in detail the ways of creating diversity in antibody.

Multiple Choice Questions

1. Antibodies are secreted by
   (a) T-cells (b) B-cells
   (c) Plasma cells (d) WBC
2. Paratope are found in
   (a) Antigen (b) Antibody
   (c) Plasma cells (d) T-cells
3. Antigenic determinant sites is the term given to
   (a) Epitope (b) Paratope
   (c) Fc part (d) None of the above
4. The shape of antibody resembles letter
   (a) A (b) V
   (c) Y (d) J
5. Variable regions are found in
   (a) Fab part (b) Fc part
   (c) Can be found any where (d) Not specific
6. Antigen binding site is
   (a) Fab (b) Fc
   (c) Both Fab & Fc (d) None of the above
7. How many amino acids are found in light chain?
   (a) 220 (b) 440
   (c) 880 (d) Variable
8. Which chain is responsible for the polymerization of the basic Ig units?
   (a) M chain (b) T chain
   (c) J chain (d) P chain
9. Which antibody is pentamer?
   (a) IgM (b) IgE
   (c) IgA (d) IgD
10. Hinge region is rich in which residues?
    (a) Lysine (b) Tyrosine
    (c) Proline (d) Serine
11. The variable light chain is coded by
    (a) VL (b) JL
    (c) Both a & b (d) VH
12. How many peptide chains are found in one antibody molecule?
    (a) Four (b) Three
    (c) Two (d) One
13. Which bonds are found in between 2 polypeptide chain of antibodies?
    (a) Hydrogen bond (b) Covalent bond

(c) Ionic bond (d) Vander-wal force

14. Which antibody is found most abundant in serum?
(a) IgG (b) IgA
(c) IgD (d) IgE

15. IgG has how many sub- classes?
(a) 2 (b) 3
(c) 4 (d) None

16. Which antibody is found in colostrum?
(a) IgA (b) IgD
(c) IgE (d) Ig M

17. IgM is secreted by plasma cell as a
(a) Monomer (b) Dimer
(c) Trimer (d) Pentamer

18. Which is the major membrane bound immunoglobulin expressed by mature B cells?
(a) IgD (b) IgM
(c) IgA (d) IgE

19. Which antibody participates in immediate hypersensitivity?
(a) IgG (b) IgE
(c) IgM (d) IgD

20. Mast cells and basophils possesses Fc receptors for
(a) IgE (b) IgD
(c)IgM (d) IgA

Answer Key

Question Number	Answer	Question Number	**Answer**
1	C	11	C
2	B	12	A
3	A	13	B
4	C	14	A
5	A	15	C
6	A	16	A
7	A	17	D
8	C	18	A
9	A	19	B
10	C	20	A

References

Bardley L.M., Haynes L. & Swain S.L. (2005) IL-7: maintaining T cell memory and achieving homeostasis. Trends in Immunology 26, 172-176.

Barnes M.J &Powrie F. (2009) Regulatory T cells reinforce intestinal homeostasis. Immunity 31, 401-411.

Batista F.D. & Harwood N.E. (2009) The who, how and where of antigen presentation to B cells Nature Reviews Immunology 9, 15-27.

Beverly P.C.L. (2004) Kinetics and clonality of clonality of immunological memory in humans. Seminars in Immunology 16, 315-321.

Cullen S.P. & Martin S.J. (2008) Mechanism of granule-development killing. Cell Death and Differentiation 15, 251-62.

Fazilleau N, et al. (2009) Follicular helper T cells: lineage and location. Immunity 30, 324-335.

Frazer, J. K., and J. D. Capra. 1999. Immunoglobulins: structure and function. In Fundamental Immunology, 4thed.W. E. Paul, ed. Philadelphia, Lippincott-Raven.

Immunology Today, The Immune Receptor Supplement, 2nd ed. 1997. Elsevier Trends Journals, Cambridge, UK (ISSN 1365-1218).

Kohler, G., and C. Milstein. 1975. Continuous cultures of fused cells secreting antibody of predefined specificity. Nature 256:495.

Korn T., Bettelli E., Oukka M. & Kuchroo V.K. (2009) IL-17 and Th17 Cells. Annual Review of Immunology 27, 485-517.

Littman D.R & Rudensky AY. (2010) Th17 and regulatory T cells in mediating and restraining inflammation . Cell 140, 845-58.

Mitchell D.M & Williams M.A (2010) An activation marker finds a function. Immunity 32, 9-12.

Newman, J. 1995. How breast milk protects newborns. Sci. Am. 273(6):76.

O'Garra A. & Murphy K.M. (2009) From IL-10 to IL-12: how pathogens and their products stimulate APCs to induce TH1 development. Nature Immunology 10, 929-932.

Reth, M. 1995. The B-cell antigen receptor complex and coreceptor. Immunol. Today 16:310.

Stanfield, R. L., and I. A.Wilson. 1995. Protein-peptide interactions. Curr. Opin. Struc. Biol. 5:103.

Wedemayer, G. J., P. A. Patten, L. H. Wang, P. G. Schultz, and R. C. Stevens. 1997. Structural insights into the evolution of an antibody combining site. Science, 276:1665.

Wentworth, P., and Janda, K. 1998. Catalytic Antibodies. Curr. Opin. Chem. Biol. 8:138.

Wilson, I. A., and R. L. Stanfield. 1994.Antibody-antibody interactions: new structures and new conformational changes. Curr. Opin. Struc. Biol. 4:857.

CHAPTER 6

Serological Reaction

Introduction

Immunology like every other branch of science has sophisticated techniques which are very sensitive in solving problems related to the various aspects of immunology. Some of the old techniques have been replaced by more refined modern techniques. Antibodies are useful as reagents for a variety of laboratory procedures, including the detection and quantitation of antigens. Antigens could be used for detecting and quantifying antibodies. Immunoassays have played vital roles in diagnosing diseases, monitoring the level of the humoral immune response, and identifying molecules of biological or medical interest. These assays differ in their speed and sensitivity; some are strictly qualitative, others are quantitative. The branch of medical immunology concerned with antigen-antibody reactions in vitro is serology [serum and -ology]. In vitro reactions, involving antibodies and antigens are widely used in clinical diagnosis, epidemiology and basic research such reactions are termed serological reactions.

The interaction between antigen and antibody is called antigen-antibody reaction. It is abbreviated as ag-ab reaction. Antigen-antibody reaction is the basis of humoral immunity or antibody mediated immune response. Antigen-antibody reaction is characterized by the following salient features:

1. **Immune complex**

   When antigen and antibody are brought together, the antibody binds with the antigen to form a complex molecule called immune complex or antigen-antibody complex (ag-ab complex). An antigen binds to an antibody at the antigen-binding site within the Fab region of the

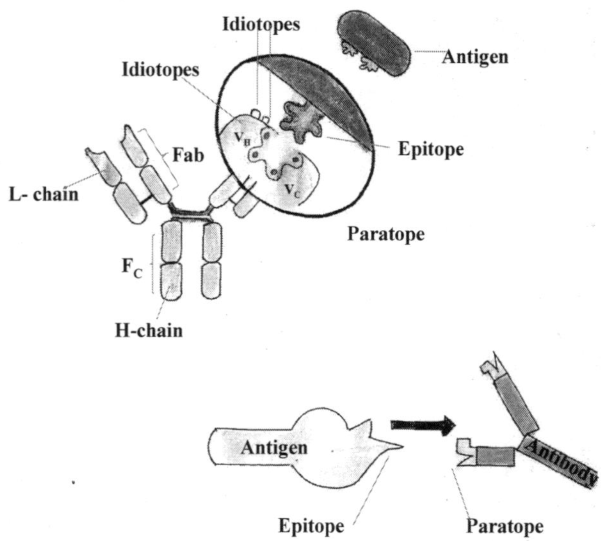

Fig. 6.1 : Immune Complex

antibody. More specifically, a pocket is formed by the folding of the VH and VL regions (figure 6.1)

$$Ag + Ab \longrightarrow Ag\text{-}Ab \text{ complex}$$

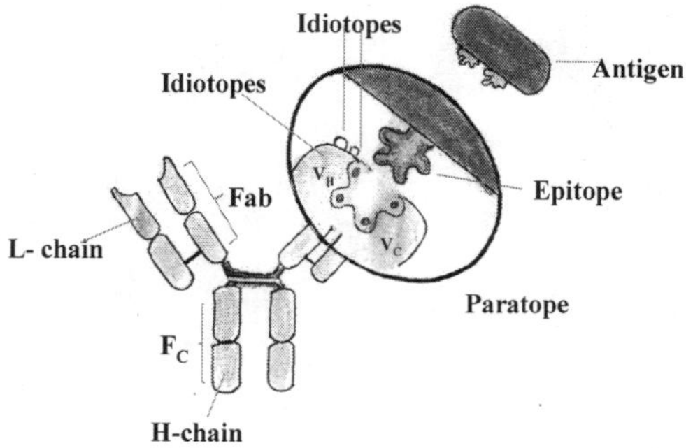

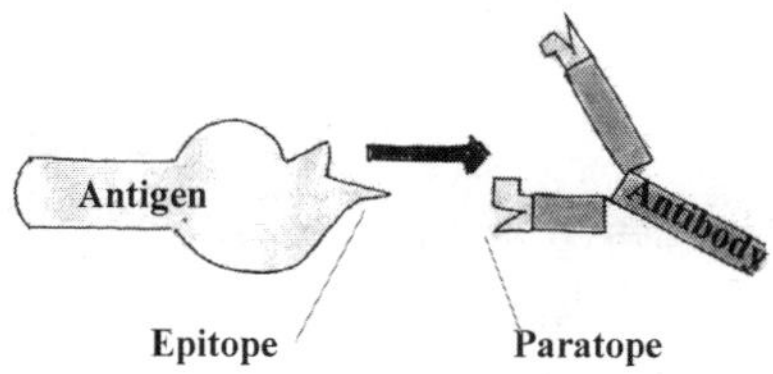

2. **Specificity of Ag-Ab Reaction**

The reaction between antigen and antibody is highly specific. Specificity refers to the discriminate ability of a particular antibody to combine with only one type of antigen. A antibody will combine with the antigen which is the cause for its production. For example, the antibody produced against lens-antigen will bind with lens antigen only and not with any other type of antigen. Similarly, the antibody produced against kidney-antigen will react with only kidney-antigen. Thus, each antigen has a separate antibody for antigen-antibody reaction. The specificity of ag-ab reaction can be compared to lock and key system. A standard lock can be opened by its own key only as one antibody can react with its own antigen.

Although a lock-and-key mechanism normally may operate, in at least one case the antigen-binding site does change shape when it complexes with the antigen (an induced fit mechanism). Regardless of the precise mechanism, antibody specificity results from the nature of antibody-antigen binding.

3. **Binding sites of Antigen and Antibody**

In antigen- antibody reaction, the antibody attaches with the antigen. The part of the antigen which combines with the antibody is called epitope or antigenic determinant. At VH and VL regions site, specific amino acids contact the antigen's epitope or haptenic groups and form multiple noncovalent bonds between the antigen and amino acids of the binding site. The part of the antibody which combines with the antigen is called paratope or antigen binding site. Most of the antibodies are bivalent having two binding sites. But the antibody IgM is monovalent having 5 to 10 binding sites (figure 6.2)

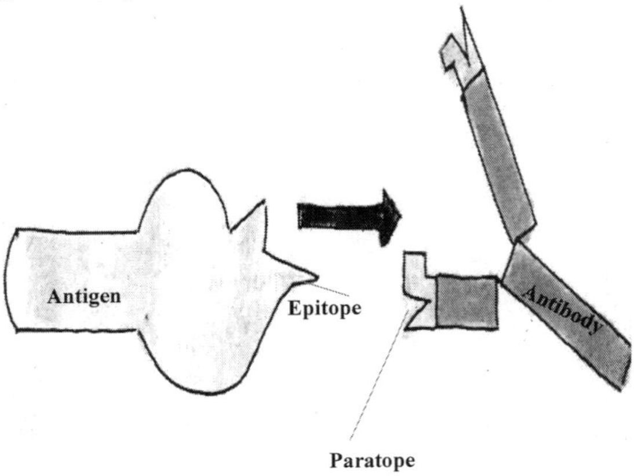

Fig. 6.2 : Epitope and Paratope

4. **Binding forces of antigen and Antibody**

The binding between antigen and antibody in ag-ab reaction is due to three factors. Namely,

a) Closeness between antigen and antibody- when the antigen and antibody are closely fit, the strength of binding is great. When they are apart, the binding strength is low.

b) Intermolecular forces- The forces which operate between two macromolecules, as for example between protein and protein, also exist between antigen and antibody in ag-ab reaction. The intermolecular forces which operate between antigen and antibody are non-covalent forces and are of 4 types.

1. Electrostatic forces
2. Hydrogen bonding
3. Hydrophobic bonding
4. Vander Waals bonding

Because binding is due to weak, noncovalent bonds such as hydrogen bonds and electrostatic attractions, the antigen's shape must exactly match that of the antigen-binding site and a large number of such interactions are required to form a strong Ag-Ab interaction. If the shape of the epitope and binding site are not truly complementary, the antibody will not effectively bind the antigen.

c) Affinity of antibody- The combined strength of the noncovalent interactions between a *single* antigen-binding site on an antibody and a *single* epitope is the affinity of the antibody for that epitope. Antibodies which bind strongly to the antigenic determinant are called high affinity antibodies. Low-affinity antibodies bind antigen weakly and tend to dissociate readily, whereas high-affinity antibodies bind antigen more tightly and remain bound longer. Affinity is used to denote the binding capacity of an antibody with a univalent antigen.

5. Avidity

When complex antigens containing multiple, repeating antigenic determinants are mixed with antibodies containing multiple binding sites, the interaction of an antibody molecule with an antigen molecule at one site will increase the probability of reaction between those two molecules at a second site. The strength of such multiple interactions between a multivalent antibody and antigen is called the avidity. Avidity refers to the capacity of an antiserum containing various antibodies to combine with the whole antigen that stimulated the production of antibodies. Avidity is used to denote the overall capacity of antibodies to combine with multivalent antigen.

$$nAb + mAg \rightleftharpoons AbnAgm$$

where,

nAb=number of antibodies

mAg= number of antigenic determinants

Avidity is the strength of the bond after the formation of antigen-antibody complexes. A noncovalent interaction operates over a very short distance, generally about 1×10^{-7} mm (1 angstrom, Å); consequently, a strong Ag-Ab interaction depends on a very close fit between the antigen and antibody. Such fits require a high degree of complementarity between antigen and antibody, a requirement that underlies the exquisite specificity that characterizes antigen-antibody interactions.

A multivalent antigen has many types of antigenic determinants. When it is injected into the blood, each antigenic determinant stimulates the production of a particular antibody. The various antibodies produced by a single antigen combine with the different antigenic determinants of the antigen.

The avidity of an antibody is a better measure of its binding capacity within biological systems (e.g., the reaction of an antibody with antigenic determinants on a virus or bacterial cell) than the affinity of its individual binding sites. High avidity can compensate for low affinity. For example, secreted pentameric IgM often has a lower affinity than IgG, but the high avidity of IgM, resulting from its higher valence, enables it to bind antigen effectively (figure 6.3).

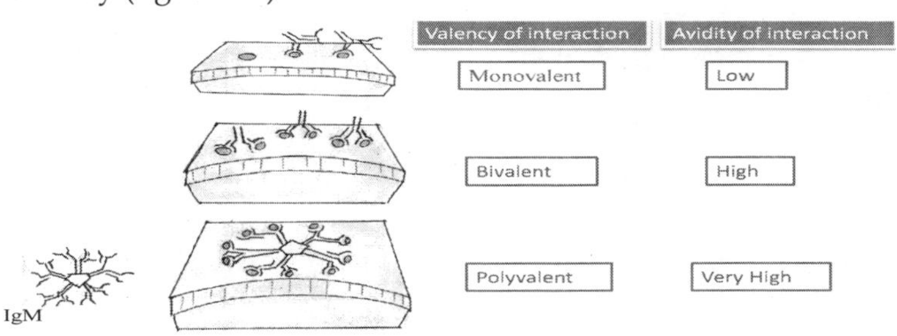

Fig. 6.3 : Valency and avidity of antibody – antigen interaction

6. **Cross Reaction**

An antiserum raised against a given antigen may sometimes react with another closely related antigen. This reaction is called cross reaction and the antigen which produces the cross reaction is called cross reactive antigen. Cross-reactivity occurs if two different antigens share an identical or very similar epitope. In the latter case, the antibody's affinity for the cross-reacting epitope is usually less than that for the original epitope. Cross-reactivity is often observed among polysaccharide antigens that contain similar oligosaccharide residues.

Examples for cross reaction:

1. The antiserum raised against the albumin of hen's egg cross react with the albumin of duck's egg. The antiserum raised against human insulin will react with the insulin of pig, sheep, whale, etc. The antiserum raised against pneumococcal polysaccharide will react with E. coli, blood group A, collagen.
2. Some vaccines also exhibit cross-reactivity. For instance, vaccinia virus, which causes cowpox, expresses cross-reacting epitopes with variola virus, the causative agent of smallpox. This cross-reactivity was the basis of Jenner's method of using vaccinia virus to induce immunity to smallpox.
3. A number of viruses and bacteria have antigenic determinants identical or similar to normal host-cell components. In some cases, these microbial antigens have been shown to elicit antibody that cross-reacts with the host-cell components, resulting in a tissue-damaging autoimmune reaction. The bacterium *Streptococcus pyogenes,* for example, expresses cell-wall proteins called M antigens. Antibodies produced to streptococcal M antigens have been shown to cross-react with several myocardial and skeletal muscle proteins and have been implicated in heart and kidney damage following streptococcal infections. Thus cross-reacting antigens plays an important role in the development of autoimmune diseases.

Agglutination reaction

Agglutination is an antigen-antibody reaction where antibody of serum causes the cellular antigens to adhere to one another to form clumps. It is the clumping of a particular antigen and its antibody. The antibodies that cause agglutination are called agglutinins and the particulate antigens aggregated are called agglutinogens. The particulate antigens include bacteria, viruses, RBC, platelets, lymphocytes, etc. When red blood cells are agglutinated the reaction is called hemagglutination. When bacterial cells are agglutinated the agglutination is called bacterial agglutination.

Agglutination depend on the crosslinking of polyvalent antigens. Excess of antibody can inhibit agglutination reactions; this inhibition is called the prozone effect. Agglutination is brought about by linking of antigens and antibodies. As most of the antibodies are bivalent, an antibody can link two adjacent antigens.

The IgM antibody is multivalent and it contains 5 or 10 combining sites. Hence it can link more number of antigens. Hence IgM antibody has the capacity to make clumps more effectively with a lesser number of molecules than that of IgG antibody molecule. Agglutination test refers to the examination of clump formation when particulate antigen and its antibodies are combined.

Agglutination test has a wide application in the clinical field. It is used to test blood groups and infectious diseases. When microscopic particles aggregate into large clumps as a result of antigen-antibody reaction, the clumps are visible to the unaided eye. When blood cells react with the antigens present on the cells, clumping occurs. Agglutination reactions are routinely performed to type red blood cells (RBCs). In typing for the ABO. Antigens, RBCs are mixed on a slide with antisera to the A or B blood-group antigens. If the antigen is present on the cells, they agglutinate, forming a visible clump on the slide. For ex, blood from a B-group individual is clumped by serum from an A individual but not by serum from B individual. Determination of which antigens are present on donor and recipient RBCs is the basis for matching blood types for transfusions. Direct agglutination reactions are very useful in the diagnosis of certain diseases. For example, the Widal test is a reaction involving the agglutination of typhoid bacilli when they are mixed with serum containing typhoid antibodies from an individual who has typhoid fever. Techniques have also been developed that employ microscopic synthetic latex spheres coated with antigens. These coated microspheres are extremely useful in diagnostic agglutination reactions. For example, the modern pregnancy test detects the elevated level of human chorionic gonadotropin (HCG) hormone that occurs in female urine and blood early in pregnancy. Latex agglutination tests are also used to detect antibodies that develop during certain mycotic, helminthic, and bacterial infections, and in drug testing (figure 6.4).

Immunoprecipitation

Precipitation refers to an antigen-antibody reaction between a soluble antigen and a solution of its homologous antibody, resulting in the formation of insoluble precipitate. The antibody causing precipitation is called precipitin. Mechanism of precipitation: precipitation is due to antigen- antibody complex. Although formation of the soluble Ag-Ab complex occurs within minutes, formation of the visible precipitate occurs more slowly and often takes a day or two to reach completion. The antigen is multivalent and the antibody is bivalent. As each antibody is a bivalent molecule, it can bridge two multivalent antigen molecules. The antibodies link the antigen to form a large antibody-antigen network or lattice that settles out of solution when it becomes sufficiently. When antigen and antibody are in optimal concentration, the precipitation is complete and a large lattice is formed. The reaction becomes visible by the formation of a visible precipitate at the interface of the reactants; but it may be inhibited by an excess of either antigen or antibody (figure 6.5). The most useful precipitin tests provide for the diffusion of the reactants until optimum concentration is reached. If the precipitin reaction takes place in a test tube, a precipitation ring forms in the area in which the optimal ratio or equivalence zone develops (figure 6.6). Formation of an Ag-Ab lattice depends on the valency of both the antibody and antigen. Firstly, the antibody must be bivalent as a precipitate will not form with monovalent Fab fragments. And secondly, the antigen must be either bivalent or polyvalent; that is, it must have at least two copies of the same epitope, or have different epitopes that react with different antibodies present in polyclonal antisera.

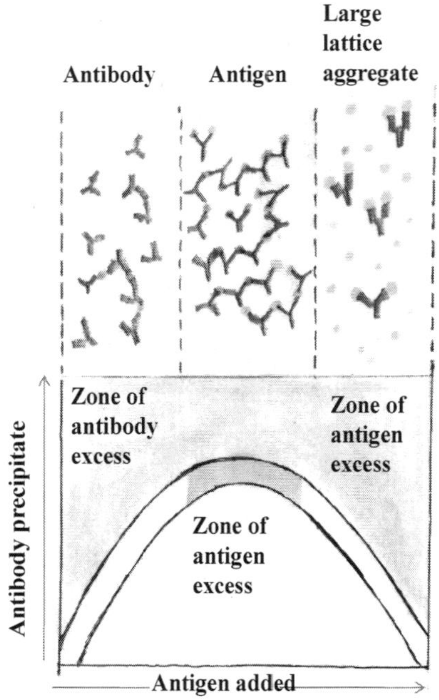

Fig. 6.5 : Lattice formation during Precipitation

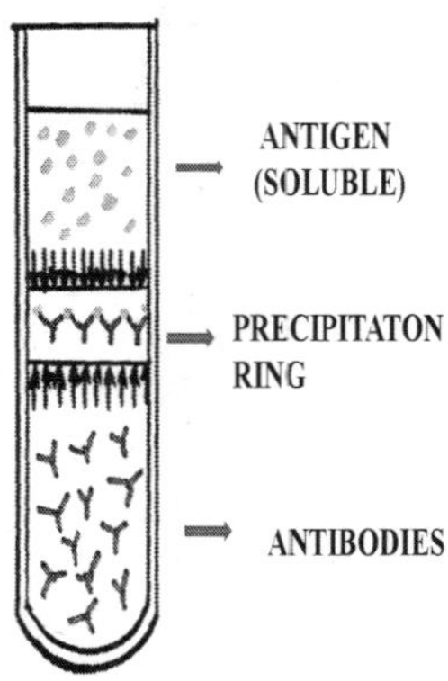

Fig. 6.6 : Immuno-Precipitation

Immunodiffusion test

When a solution of antibodies and a solution of antigens are placed near one another the diffusion of two results in precipitation. One and two dimensional immunodiffusion tests can be conducted. A tube precipitin test can be performed in fluid phase. This is called ring test. The precipitate forms a ring or white disc at the interface between clear solution of antigen and antibody (figure 6). For greater accuracy, ease of handling and preservation of the tests the antibody can be contained in agar gel and the antigen allowed to diffuse it. This is called a single- diffusion method. The method of Oudin directly layers antigen on antibody in agar. Oakley –Fulthrope method separates these two reagents with simple agar this results in the diffusion of both reagents into the agar and formation of precipitin ring with greater accuracy. This method is described as a double-diffusion precipitin test.

When a solution of antibodies and antigens are placed in nearby depressions of a gel, remarkably thin bands of precipitin can be visualized, where antibodies and antigens meet in the zone of equivalence. This simple method for double diffusion in two dimensions was developed by Ouchterlony. In the Ouchterlony method, both antigen and antibody diffuse radially from wells toward each other, thereby establishing a concentration gradient. As equivalence is reached, a visible line of precipitation, a precipitin line, forms. Indeed, immunodiffusion is the term usually applied to this technique which is used to find out whether two antigens share common antigenic determinants. Three wells that form a triangular array are cut in agar gel in a petridish. Serum containing antibody against a certain antigen is placed in a well and the other two wells are filled with a solution of the antigen a continuous precipitin forms in a V-shaped pattern. This V-shaped precipitin is termed the reaction of identity it demonstrates that the antibody molecules bind to the same antigenic determinants in each of the antigen samples. If one of the well is filled with different antigen that shares some determinants with the first antigen a Y-shaped band of precipitin termed reaction of partial identity forms. The stem of the Y is formed by cross-linking those antigenic determinants present in the first antigen but absent in the second (figure 6.7).

Immunoelectrophoresis

Some antigen mixtures are too complex to be resolved by simple diffusion and precipitation. Greater resolution is obtained by the technique of classical immunoelectrophoresis in which antigens are first separated based on their electrical charge, then visualized by the precipitation reaction.

Electrophoresis is a process in which suspended particles or macromolecules with a net electric charge migrate in a solution or agar gel under the influence of an electric current. A characteristic of

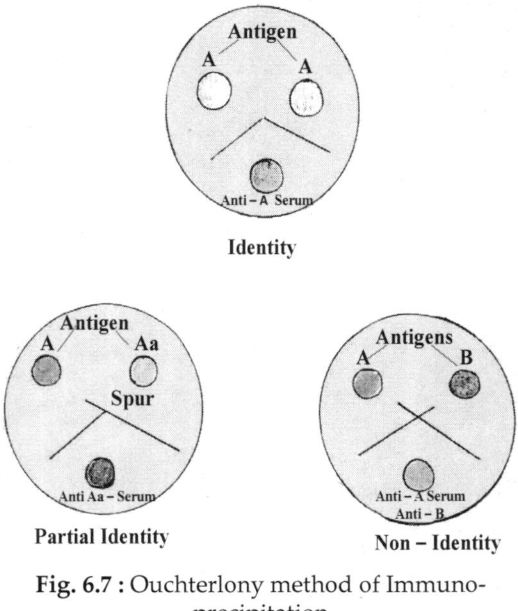

Fig. 6.7 : Ouchterlony method of Immuno-precipitation

living cells in suspension and biological compounds in solutions or a gel is that in an electric field they travel to the positive or negative electrode, depending on the charge of the substances. This movement is called electrophoretic mobility. When electrophoresis is applied to the study of antigen – antibody reactions, it is called immunoelectrophoresis. Here, the techniques of electrophoresis and immunoprecipitation are combined to visualize many individual components in a complex mixture of antigens.

In immunoelectrophoresis, the antigen mixture is first electrophoresed to separate its components by charge. Troughs are then cut into the agar gel parallel to the direction of the electric field, and antiserum is added to the troughs. Antibody and antigen then diffuse toward each other and produce lines of precipitation where they meet in appropriate proportions (figure 6.8).

Immunoelectrophoresis is used in clinical laboratories to detect the presence or absence of proteins in the serum. This technique is useful in determining whether a patient produces abnormally low amounts of one or more isotypes, characteristic of certain immunodeficiency diseases. It can also show whether a patient overproduces some serum protein, such as albumin, immunoglobulin, or transferrin. Because immunoelectrophoresis is a strictly *qualitative* technique that only detects relatively high antibody concentrations (greater than several hundred g/ml), it utility is limited to the detection of quantitative abnormalities only when the departure from normal is striking, as in immunodeficiency states and immunoproliferative disorders.

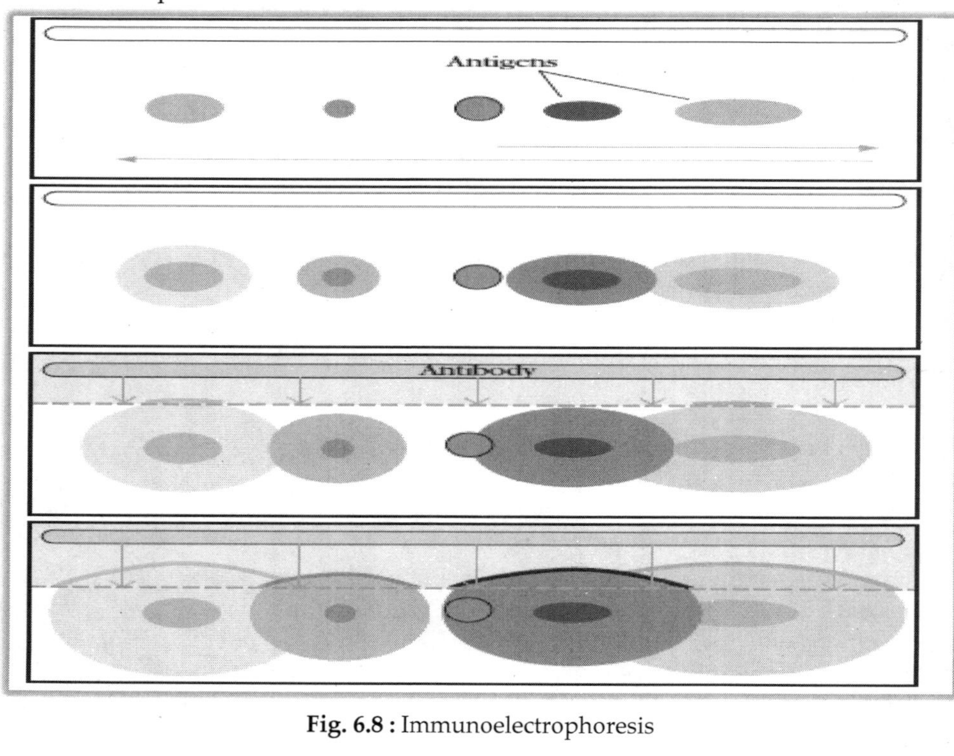

Fig. 6.8 : Immunoelectrophoresis

Rocket immunoelectrophoresis

A combination of immunoelectrophoresis assay and Mancini assay results in rocket immunoelectrophoresis. In rocket immunoelectrophoresis, antigen from wells migrates elctrophoretically into an agar gel which contain specific antiserum. This results in rocket-shaped precipitated. The height of each rocket is proportional to the concentration of the antigen in the well. In electrophoresis the antigen migrates in the electric field into the antibody-containing gel. The antigen combines with antibody to form immune complexes. The complexes continue migration but migration stops completely when the aggregates become large enough to be retained by the pores. One limitation of rocket electrophoresis is the need for the antigen to be negatively charged for electrophoretic movement within the agar matrix. Some proteins, immunoglobulins for example, are not sufficiently charged to be quantitatively analyzed by rocket electrophoresis; nor is it possible to measure the amounts of several antigens in a mixture at the same time.

Radio-immuno assay

Radio-immuno assay is a procedure in which serological methods are used for the detection and quantification of a specific substance. It is one of the most sensitive techniques for detecting antigen or antibody. The technique was first developed in 1960 by two endocrinologists, S. A. Berson and Rosalyn Yalow, to determine levels of insulin–anti-insulin complexes in diabetics. Indeed, Rosalyn Yalow won the 1977 Nobel Prize in Physiology or Medicine for its development. This is sensitive technique which revolutionized hormone research. The *r*adio *i*mmuno *a*ssay (RIA) technique has become an extremely important tool in biomedical research and clinical practice (e.g., in cardiology, blood banking, diagnosis of allergies, and endocrinology). The technique is especially useful for assay hormone. Although their technique encountered some skepticism, it soon proved its value for measuring hormones, serum proteins, drugs, and vitamins at concentrations of 0.001 *micrograms* per milliliter or less and that's why RIA technique is a tracer procedure used to measure trace amounts of any substance having antigenic properties. Depending on the specific activity of the labeled compounds, quantities of antigens that are as low as 10 picograms.

RIA uses a purified antigen that is radioisotope-labeled and competes for antibody with unlabeled standard or antigen in experimental samples. The radioactivity associated with the antibody is then detected by means of radioisotope analyzers and autoradiography (photographic emulsions that show areas of radioactivity). If there is much antigen in an experimental sample, it will compete with the radioisotope-labeled antigen for antigen-binding sites on the antibody, and little radioactivity will be bound. A large amount of bound radioactivity indicates that there is little antigen present in the experimental sample.

The principle of RIA involves competitive binding of radiolabeled antigen and unlabeled antigen to a high-affinity antibody. The labeled antigen is mixed with antibody at a concentration that saturates the antigen-binding sites of the antibody. Then test samples of unlabeled antigen of unknown concentration are added in progressively larger amounts. The antibody does not distinguish labeled from unlabeled antigen, so the two kinds of antigen compete for available binding sites on the antibody. As the concentration of unlabeled antigen increases, more labeled antigen will be displaced from the binding sites. The decrease in the amount of radiolabeled antigen bound to specific antibody in the presence of the test sample is measured in order to determine the amount of antigen present in the test sample. The antigen is generally labeled with a gamma-emitting isotope such as ^{125}I, but beta-emitting isotopes such as tritium (^{3}H) are also routinely used as labels. The radiolabeled antigen is part of the assay mixture; the test sample may be a complex mixture, such as serum or other body fluids, that contains the unlabeled antigen.

ELISA

The *e*nzyme-*l*inked *i*mmuno*s*orbent *a*ssay (ELISA) has become one of the most widely used serological tests for antibody or antigen detection. It is the most common alternative to RIA. ELISA is more sensitive then RIA. ELISA is a rapid and convenient. It does not cause health hazards or deterioration of reagents through radiation damage as no radio-active isotopes are used. This test involves the linking of various "label" enzymes to either antigens or antibodies. An enzyme conjugated with an antibody reacts with a colorless substrate to generate a colored reaction product. Such a substrate is called a chromogenic substrate. A number of enzymes have been employed for ELISA, including alkaline phosphatase, horseradish peroxidase, and galactosidase. These assays approach the sensitivity of RIAs and have the advantage of being safer and less costly. Two basic methods are used: the double antibody sandwich assay and the indirect immunosorbent assay (figure 6.9).

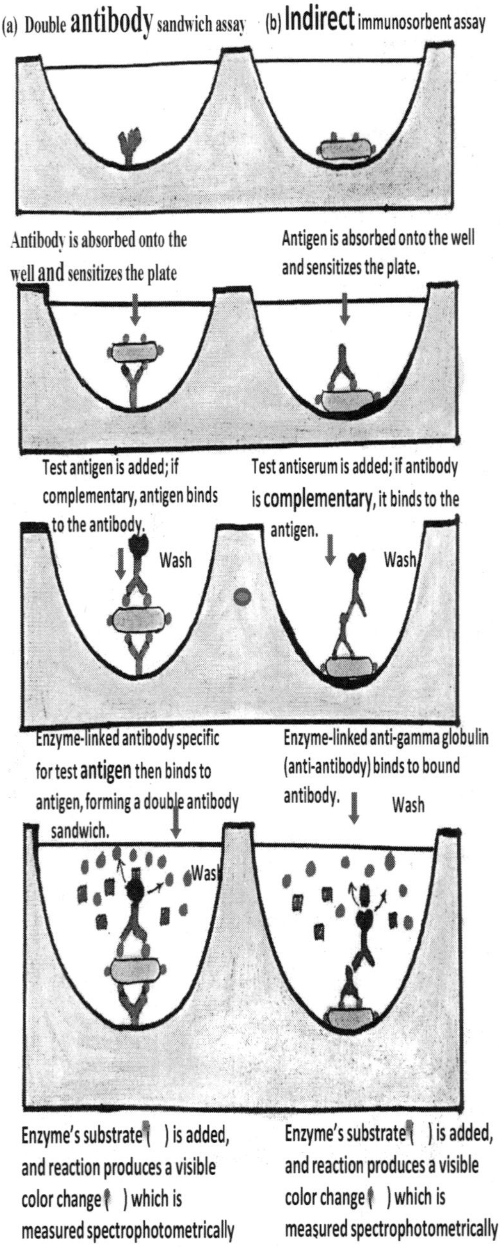

Fig. 6.9 : Enzyme Linked immune- Sorbent Assay (ELISA)

ELISA is used for testing human pregnancy. HCG is a hormone produced by the placenta it is detectable in maternal urine a few days after conception. In the ELISA an antibody specific for HCG is attached to the bottom of a well in a plastic tray to this a few drops of urine are added. If any HCG is present, it will blind to the antibody molecules. The tray is then washed, and a second antibody (which is also specific for another epitope of the HCG) is added. The amount of second antibody bound to the tray is proportional to the quantity of the antigen present in the sample and bound to the first antibody. This second antibody is linked to an enzyme that catalyzes the conversion of the colourless compound to a coloured compound. The amount of coloured compound produced provides a sensitive measure of the amount of hormone present. Thus, not only the presence of any hormone can be detected, but also the amount of hormone can be determined. The ELISA has been adapted for use in determining the amount of specific protein in tissue sample, in blood, or in urine.

Immunofluorescence

In 1944, Albert Coons showed that antibodies could be labeled with molecules that have the property of fluorescence. Immunofluorescence is a process in which dyes called fluorochromes are exposed to UV, violet, or blue light to make them fluoresce or emit visible light. When antibodies are mixed with fluorescent dyes such as fluorescein or rhodamine, they emit radiation. This phenomenon of emitting radiation by antibodies labeled with fluorescent dyes is called immunofluorescence. The immunofluorescence can be observed by a fluorescent microscope. Dyes such as rhodamine B, phycoerythrin or fluorescein isothiocyanate (FITC) can be coupled to antibody molecules without changing the antibody's capacity to bind to a specific antigen. Fluorochromes also can be attached to antigens. Each of the fluorochromes below absorbs light at one wavelength and emits light at a longer wavelength:

1. **Fluorescein,** an organic dye that is the most widely used label for immunofluorescence procedures, absorbs blue light (490 nm) and emits an intense yellow-green fluorescence (517 nm).
2. **Rhodamine,** another organic dye, absorbs in the yellow-green range (515 nm) and emits a deep red fluorescence (546 nm). Because it emits fluorescence at a longer wavelength than fluorescein, it can be used in two-color immunofluorescence assays. An antibody specific to one determinant is labeled with fluorescein, and an antibody recognizing a different antigen is labeled with rhodamine. The location of the fluorescein-tagged antibody will be visible by its yellow green color, easy to distinguish from the red color emitted where the rhodamine-tagged antibody has bound. By conjugating fluorescein to one antibody and rhodamine to another antibody, one can, for example, visualize simultaneously two different cell-membrane antigens on the same cell.
3. **Phycoerythrin** is an efficient absorber of light (~30-fold greater than fluorescein) and a brilliant emitter of red fluorescence, stimulating its wide use as a label for immunofluorescence.

The immunofluorescence test can be applied in three methods, namely direct method, indirect method and sandwich method.

1. Direct method - In this method the antibody labeled with fluorescent dye is applied directly on the tissue sections. The labeled antibody binds with specific antigen. This can be observed under the fluorescent microscope. Direct immunofluorescence is used to identify antigens such as those found on the surface of group A streptococci and to diagnose enteropathogenic *Escherichia coli, Neisseria meningitidis, Salmonella typhi, Shigella sonnei, Listeria monocytogenes, Haemophilus influenzae* type b, and the rabies virus.
2. Indirect method - In indirect method unlabelled antibody is directly applied on the tissue sections. The unlabelled antibody binds with its specific antigen. Then, anti-immunoglobulin antibody labeled with fluorescent dyes, is applied on the tissues. The labeled anti-immunoglobulin antibody is highly specific for unlabelled antibody and hence it binds with the already linked unlabelled antibody. In this method cell or tissue antigens as well as specific antibodies can be detected. Indirect immunofluorescence is used to identify the presence of *Treponema pallidum* antibodies in the diagnosis of syphilis (treponemal antibody absorption, FTA-ABS) as well as antibodies produced in response to other microorganisms.
3. Sandwich method - This is an immunofluorescence method used to test the number of cells producing antibodies for a specific antigen. The cells producing antibodies for example lymphocytes are fixed in ethanol. The fixed cells are treated with the polysaccharide antigen of pneumococcus. This antigen will specifically combine with those lymphocytes which have the capacity to produce antibody against pneumococcus polysaccharide antigen. Now fluorescent labeled antibody is added. The labeled antibody will bind to the antigen which has already linked to the antibody producing lymphocyte. In this test the antigen is sandwiched between the antibody present in the lymphocytes and the fluorescent labeled antibody. Hence this test is called sandwich test.

Immunofluorescence has the following applications:

a) It is used to locate and identify antigens in tissues.

b) Certain pathogenic bacteria can be identified.

c) This technique helps to identify a number of subpopulations of lymphocytes, notably the $CD4^+$ and $CD8^+$ T-cell subpopulations.

d) Antibodies directed to cell or tissue antigen can be detected.

e) Detecting Ag-Ab complexes in autoimmune disease, detecting complement components in tissues, and localizing hormones and other cellular products stained in situ

f) Localization of antigens in tissue sections or in subcellular compartments.

Complement fixation test

Complement fixation test is a technique used for the detection of unknown antigen or antibody with the help of complement. Complement fixation tests are very sensitive and can be used to detect extremely small amounts of an antibody for a suspect microorganism in an individual's serum.

The binding of complement to antigen- antibody complex is called complement fixation. When complement is added to a serum containing an antigen and its antibody, the complement is activated and immediately it binds to the antigen-antibody complex and the complement is said to be fixed. In this system, the complement does not remain free. The complement fixation test involves two immune systems. One system is a known reaction containing sensitized RBC and it acts as an indicator and determines the complement activity. It is called the indicator system. The other system is the unknown reaction under investigation. It is called the test system.

In a typical complement fixation test, the serum to be tested for antibody is allowed to react with a known antigen and an optimal amount of complement. On the other hand, if the specific antibodies are present in the test serum and complement is consumed by the immune complexes, insufficient amounts of complement will be available to lyse the indicator cells. Absence of lysis shows that specific antibodies are present in the test serum (figure 6.10).

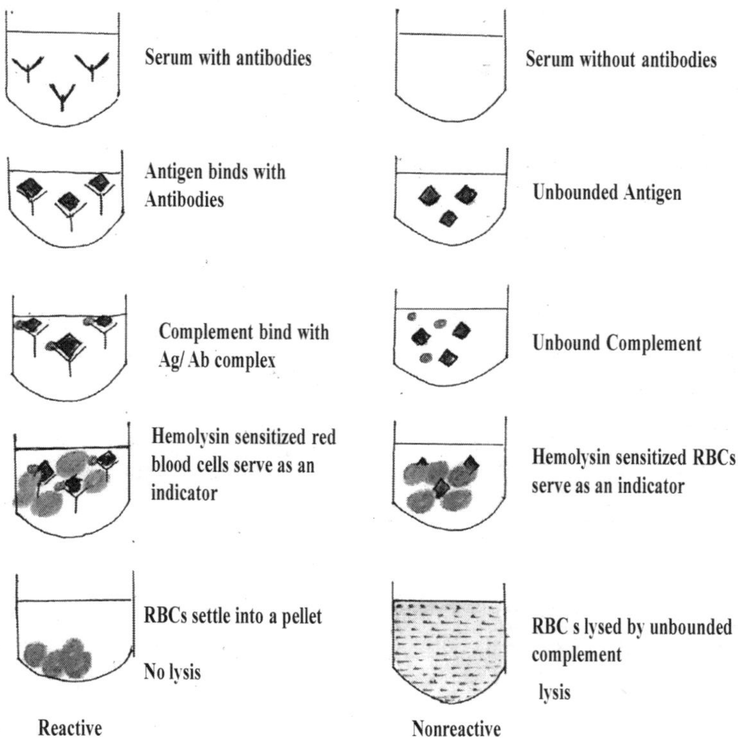

Fig. 6.10 : Compliment Fixation Test

Haemolysis is a visible manifestation of the second reaction. The absence of free complement is due to its binding with the ag-ab complex of the test system. Hence the test serum contains the specific antibody. So the absence of haemolysis is a positive test showing the presences of specific antibody. If the test serum does not contain specific antibody, the antigen-antibody complex will not form and hence the complement is not fixed and its remains free in the test system. When the RBC and its antibody are added to this test system, the freely available complement of the test system combines with the antigen (RBC) antibody complex and the RBC is lysed. Thus the occurrence of haemolysis indicates the absence of specific antibody in the test serum and hence it is a negative test (figure 10). In the complement test, the second reaction indicates the presences or absence of specific antibody through its haemolysis. Hence the second reaction is called indicator system. Complement fixation was once used in the diagnosis of syphilis (the Wassermann test) and is currently used in the diagnosis of certain viral, fungal, rickettsial, chlamydial, and protozoan diseases.

Question Bank

1. Very short answer type questions
   (a) Write the full form of ELISA.
   (b) Write the full form of RIA.
   (c) Write the full form of IFA.
   (d) Name one isotope used in radio immunoassay.
   (e) Name one enzyme used in ELISA.
   (f) Name the indicator used in complement fixation.
   (g) Name one hormone that can be detected by ELISA.
   (h) Name few chemicals measured by RIA.
   (i) What is the shape of band formed in test for detecting unrelated antigens?
2. Short answer type questions
   (a) What is Ouchterlony test?
   (b) What is Oudin test?
   (c) What is Oakelyfulthrope test?
   (d) Define zone of equivalence.
   (e) Define Agglutination.
   (f) Define immunoelectrophoresis.
   (g) Define serology.
3. Long answer type questions
   (a) Describe in detail the mechanism of agglutination with suitable example.
   (b) What is immunoflourescence? Describe its applications and methods.
   (c) Distinguish between precipitation and agglutination.
   (d) Describe in detail immunoelectrophoresis with an example.
   (e) Describe in detail ELISA and its applications.

Multiple Choice Questions

1. The reaction between antigen and antibody is
(a) Non- specific (b) Specific
(c) Highly specific (d) Depends on environment
2. The part of antigen which combines with antibody is called
(a) Epitope (b) Antigenic determinant
(c) Both a & b (d) Paratope
3. The part of antibody which combines with the antigen is called
(a) Paratope (b) Antigen binding site
(c) Both a & b (d) Epitope
4. The overall capacity of antibody to combine with mulivalent antigen is known as
(a) Affinity (b) Avidity
(c) Specificity (d) Stereo specificity
5. An antiserum raised against a given antigen may sometimes react with another closely related antigen. This process is known as
(a) Affinity (b) Avidity
(c) Cross- reaction (d) Specificity
6. In serology, the antigen – antibody reaction are carried out in
(a) In - situ (b) In- vivo
(c) De - novo (d) In- vitro
7. Clumping of particulate antigen and its antibody is known as
(a) Precipitation (b) Electrophoresis
(c) Agglutination (d) Radial diffusion
8. Agglutinins are
(a) Antibodies (b) Antigen
(c) Bacteria (d) Virus
9. Examples of agglutinogens are
(a) Bacterial (b) Viruses
(c) RBC (d) All of the above
10. In hemagglutination, agglutinogens are
(a) RBC (b) WBC
(c) Platelets (d) All of the above
11. How many combining sites are found in IgM?
(a) 4 (b) 6
(c) 8 (d) 10
12. How many combining sites are found in dimer IgG?
(a) 4 (b) 6
(c) 8 (d) 10

13. Widal is the for detection of
    (a) Syphilis (b) Typhoid
    (c) Pneumonia (d) AIDS
14. RPR is the test for detection of
    (a) Typhoid (b) Malaria
    (c) Syphilis (d) Typhus
15. The reaction between soluble antigen and its antibody is known as
    (a) Ouchterlony reaction (b) Precipitation
    (c) Agglutination (d) Electrophoresis
16. Lattice formation is the characteristic of
    (a) Precipitation (b) ELISA
    (c) RIA (d) None of them
17. Ouchterlony test is
    (a) Single diffusion in 1Dimension (b) Single diffusion in 2Dimension
    (c) Double diffusion in 1Dimension (d) Double diffusion in 2Dimension
18. Shape of band in partial identity is
    (a) V (b) X
    (c) Y (d) T
19. Name the indicator used in complement fixation test
    (a) RBC (b) WBC
    (c) Platelets (d) Monocyte
20. Radio immunoassay was developed by
    (a) Alec Jeffrey (b) Burnet
    (c) Yalow and Berson (d) Ouchterlony

Answer Key

Question Number	Answer	Question Number	Answer
1	C	11	D
2	C	12	A
3	C	13	B
4	B	14	C
5	C	15	B
6	D	16	A
7	C	17	D
8	A	18	C
9	D	19	A
10	A	20	C

References

Alkan S.S. (2004) Monoclonal antibodies: the story of a discovery that revolutionized science and medicine. Nature Reviews Immunology 4,153-156.

Altman J.D. &Davis M.M. (2003) MHC-peptide tetramers to visualize antigen-specific T cells. Current Protocols in Immunology Chapter 17, Unit 17.3, John Wiley &Sons.

Ansubel F.M., Brent R., Kingston R.E., Moore D.D., Seidman J.G., Smith J.A. & Struhl K. (eds.) (2010) Current Protocols in Molecular Biology. John Wiley, New york.

Berzofsky, J. A., I. J. Berkower, and S. L. Epstein. 1991. Antigen antibody interactions and monoclonal antibodies. In Fundamental Immunology, 3rd ed W. E. Paul, ed. Raven Press, New York.

Bonifacino P. (1998) The increasing power of immunohistochemistry and immunocytochemistry. Journal of Immunological Method 216, 49-67.

Brannigan J.A. & Wilkinson A.J. (2002) Protein engineering 20 years on. Nature Reviews Molecular and Cell Biology 3,964-970.

Coligan J.E., Bierer B.E., Margulies D.H., Shevach E.M. &Strober W.(eds.) (2010) Current Protocols in immunology. John Wiley, New York.

Coligan, J. E., A. M. Kruisbeek, D. H. Margulies, E. M. Shevach, and W. Strober. 1997. Current Protocols in Immunology. Wiley, New York.

George A.J. Lee L. & Pirzalis C. (2003) Isolating ligands specific for human vasculature using in vivo Phage Selection. Trends in Biotechnology 5, 199-203.

Harlow, E., and D. Lane. 1999. Using Antibodies: A laboratory manual. Cold Spring Harbor Laboratory Press.

Herzenberg, L. A., ed. 1996. Weir's Handbook of Experimental Immunology, 5th ed. Oxford, Blackwell Scientific Publications. Rose, N. R., E. C. de Macario, J. D. Folds, C. H. Lane, and R. M. Nakamura. 1997. Manual of Clinical Laboratory Immunology.

Huppi K. Martin S.E. & Caplen N.J. (2005) Defining and assaying RNAi in mammalian cells. Molecular Cell 17,1-10.

Letsch A. & Scheibenbogen C. (2003) Quantification and characterization of specific T cells by antigen-specific cytikine production using ELISPOT assay or intracellular cytokine staining .Methods 31,143-149.

Liu M. et al. (2004) Gene- based vaccines and immunotherapeutics. Proceedings of the National Academy of Science USA 101, Suppl.2, 14567-14571.

Rose, N. R., E. C. de Macario, J. D. Folds, C. H. Lane, and R. M. Nakamura. 1997. Manual of Clinical Laboratory Immunology. American Society of Microbiology, Washington, D.C.

Stites, D. P., C. Rodgers, J.D. Folds, and J. Schmitz. 1997. Clinical laboratory detection of antigens and antibodies. In Medical Immunology, 9th ed., D. P. Stites, A. I. Terr, and T. G. Parslow, eds., Appelton and Lange, Stamford, CT.

Wild, D., ed. 2001. The Immunoassay Handbook. Nature Publishing Group, NY.

CHAPTER 7

Major Histocompatibility Complex

Introduction

An individual's immune system tolerates "self-makers" the native molecules. Among the important "self-makers", are a collection of molecules called the major Histocompatibility complex (MHC). The major histocompatibility complex is a collection of genes arrayed within a long continuous stretch of DNA on chromosome 6 in humans and on chromosome 17 in mice. This term is derived from the Greek word for tissue [*histo*] and the ability to get along [compatibility]. The MHC is referred to as the human leukocyte antigen (HLA) complex in humans and as the H-2 complex in mice. MHC molecules in man are called HLA molecules (human leukocytes antigen) since they were first discovered on the surface of leukocytes. Molecules within this complex were originally defined by their ability to provoke vigorous rejection of graft exchanged between different members of a species.

General Organization and Inheritance of the MHC

Major Histocompatibility Complex refers to a cluster of genes responsible for immune response, transplantation antigens and proteins if the complement system. It is abbreviated as MHC. It was discovered by Gorer in 1930. Histocompatibility gene was the name given by Snell. The major histocompatibility complex produces a set of proteins called histocompatible molecules. These molecules are located on the cell membranes of nucleated cells of the body as well as in the blood serum. These molecules are responsible for allograft rejection, immune recognition, complement levels, etc. The gene segment is named as major histocompatibility complex because its original discovery was based on transplantation experiments. These are the major barrier to transplantation of nucleated cells. MHC molecules are expressed on all nucleated cells the body and their physiological function is to direct T cells to carry out their function. However, like the locus coding for the major blood group antigens and unlike the majority of the other gene products, genes coding for MHC molecules are polymorphic. In contrast to the ABO system, each MHC locus can encode for a very large number of different allelic forms and, to further increase the complexity, there are six different loci. In humans, these loci are found on chromosomes 6 this is called the human leukocyte antigen (HLA) system since in humans the antigens were first discovered on leukocytes. These molecules are glycoproteins (proteins with carbohydrates attached to them) embedded in plasma membranes of cells (figure 7.1). MHC molecules are important in determining the ability of an animal to mount an immune response. A family of genes code for the MHC proteins because there are at least 50 alleles for each gene, it is virtually impossible for any two people, except identical twins, to have matching sets of MHC makers on their cells. Thus the major contains histocompatibility complex is a biochemical fingerprint unique to each individual. The combinations of the many different allelic variants which are co- dominantly expressed means that the chance of two unrelated individuals having completely identical set of alleles is extremely remote. Thus the different allelic variants of the donor organ/tissue will be foreign to the recipient who does not have them and will therefore generate an immune response to them.

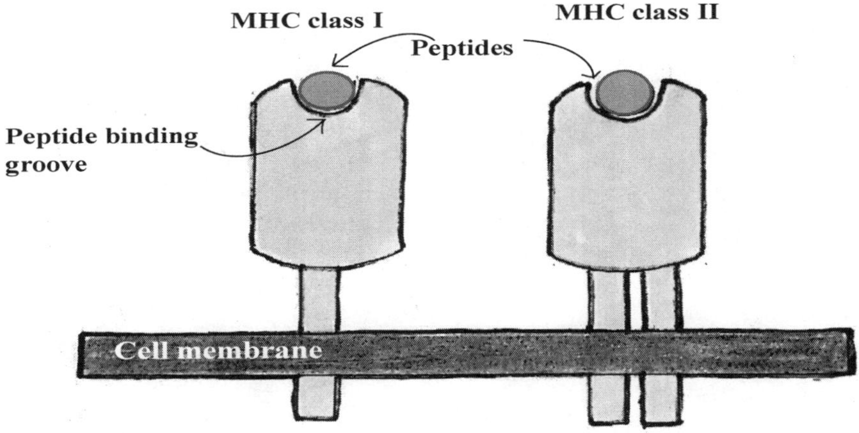

Figure 7.1 – MHC I and MHC II

Gene encoding MHC molecules

Both MHC class I and class II molecules are encoded by genes that are polymorphic and are closely linked together in chromosome 6 in man. These and other genes are critical to antigen processing and presentation, as suggested from their distribution within the MHC gene locus. Note that in man there are three different loci for MHC class I genes (HLA-A, B and C) and four loci for MHC class II genes (HLA-DP, DQ, and DR, and another no polymorphic locus for HLA-DM (involved in antigen processing). MHC class III genes include those coding for some complement components and tumor necrosis factors and are not directly involved in antigen processing and presentation. The many alternative (allelic) forms of genes for each sub-region of the MHC locus gives rise to many different forms of class I and II molecules each with a binding groove that can bind a different antigenic peptide. The combination of the encoded alleles within the MHC locus is referred to as the haplotype (for haploid, as opposed to diploid). Because genes within the MHC are closely linked, haplotypes are usually inherited intact.

The MHC Encodes Three Major Classes of Molecules

Although the arrangement of genes is somewhat different, in both cases the MHC genes are organized into regions encoding three classes of molecules. The MHC contains three groups of genes known as classes I, II and III. Class I and II genes code for integral membrane proteins, whereas class III genes code for some serum proteins.

Class I MHC genes encode glycoproteins expressed on the surface of nearly all nucleated cells; the major function of the class I gene products is presentation of peptide antigens to T- cytotoxic (Tc) cells. Class I MHC molecules consist of a complex of two protein chains, one with a mass of 45 kDa (the heavy chain) and the other with a mass of 12 kDa (β2-microglobulin). The two chains contain four regions. The outer segment of the heavy chain can be divided into three functional domains, designated $\alpha1$, α 2, and α 3. β_2-microglobulin is similar to $\alpha3$. The β2 microglobulin (β2m) protein and α 3 segment of the heavy chain are noncovalently associated with one another and are close to the plasma membrane (figure 7.2). A small segment of the heavy chain is attached to the membrane by a short amino acid sequence that extends into the cell interior, but the rest of the protein protrudes to the outside. $\alpha1$ and $\alpha2$ form peptide binding cleft and fits peptide of about 8-10 amino acid long. $\alpha3$ is highly conserved among MHC I molecules. The Class I region is encoded by another three another three loci named DP, DQ and DR. These alleles are codominant, which means that the products of both the alleles are expressed in cells. The enzyme papain cleaves the α chain just 13 residues proximal to its transmembrane domain, releasing the extracellular portion of the molecule, consisting of α 1, α 2, α 3, and β2-microglobulin.

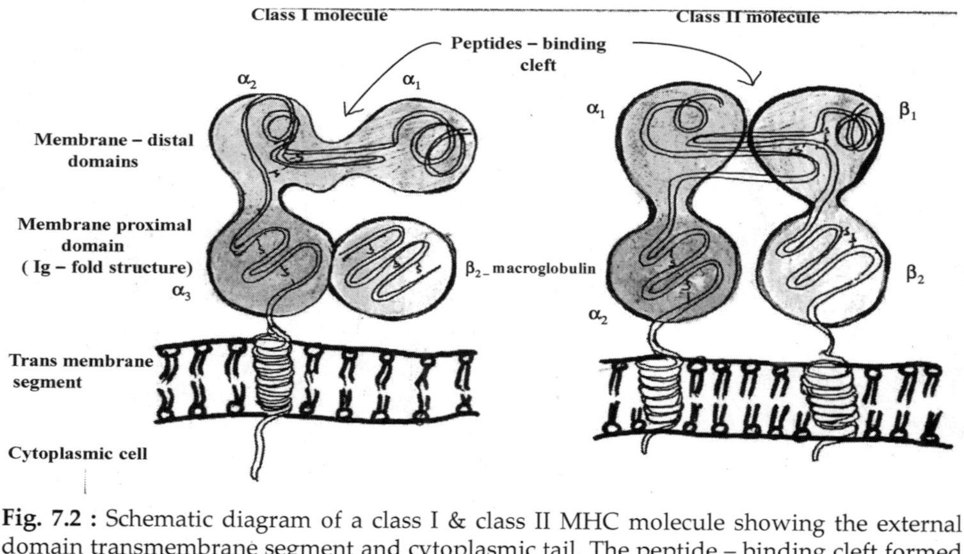

Fig. 7.2 : Schematic diagram of a class I & class II MHC molecule showing the external domain transmembrane segment and cytoplasmic tail. The peptide – binding cleft formed by the membrane – distal domain in both class I & class II molecule. The membrane proximal domain posses the basic immunoglobulin fold structure , thus class I & class II MHC molecule are classified as membrane of the immunoglobulin superfamily.

In the absence of β2-microglobulin, the class I MHC α chain is not expressed on the cell membrane. This is illustrated by Daudi tumor cells, which are unable to synthesize β2-microglobulin. These tumor cells produce class I MHC α chains, but do not express them on the membrane. However, if Daudi cells are transfected with a functional gene encoding β2-microglobulin, class I molecules appear on the membrane.

Class II MHC genes encode glycoproteins expressed primarily on antigen-presenting cells (macrophages, dendritic cells, and B cells), where they present processed antigenic peptides to T- helper (Th) cells. Class II MHC molecules are restricted to macrophages and B- lymphocytes; they play an important role in interactions between cells of the immune system. Class II MHC molecules are also transmembrane proteins consisting of α and β chains of mass 34 kDa and 28 kDa, respectively. Both chains are folded to give two domains. $\alpha1$ and $\alpha2$ (α chain) and $\beta1$ and $\beta2$ (β chain). $\alpha1$and $\beta1$ form antigen binding cleft. CD4 molecule binds $\alpha2/\beta2$ domains.

When T-lymphocytes respond to an antigen, they recognize cell surface proteins also; these proteins are encoded by genes within the MHC. Antigen recognition by T-cells is important when antigen presenting cells are stimulating Th cells and also for the cytotoxic lymphocytes (Tc) to destroy virus-infected cells. If the MHC proteins are not also recognized, then the immune response does not occur.

Two main classes of MHC molecules mark cells as self" Class I or Class II MHC molecules are located on all nucleated cells- almost every cell of the body. MHC proteins lie embedded in the plasma membrane they tenaciously grip bound peptides so that they can be touched and scrutinized by T- cell receptors on the surface of a killer cell. CD8 on killer T- cells and CD4 on helper T- cells act in concert with T- cell receptors. The molecules that direct T-cell to different targets are the integral membrane proteins CD8 and CD4, which serves as co-receptors. Each chain in the CD8 dimer contains a domain that resembles an immunoglobulin variable domain CD4, which is monomeric, contains four such immunoglobulin-like domains (figure 7.3).

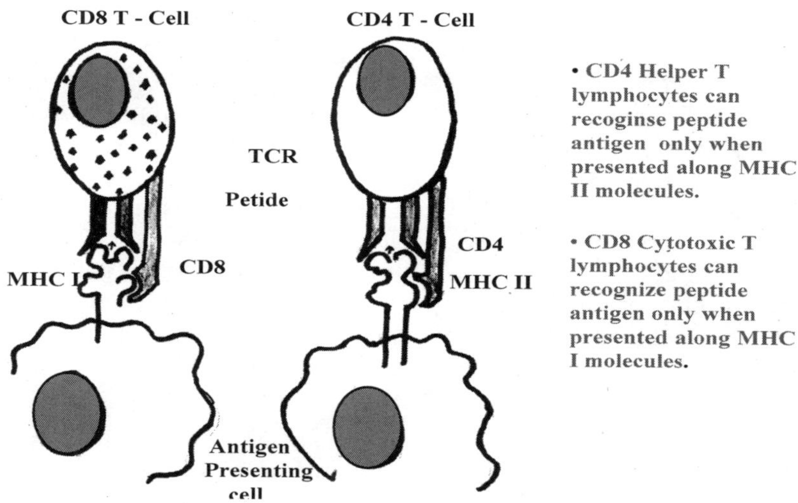

Fig. 7.3 : Association of MHCs with their respective CDs and T- lymphocytes

Class III MHC genes encode, in addition to other products, various secreted proteins that have immune functions, including components of the complement system and molecules involved in inflammation. Class III products are heterogeneous but include complement components linked to the formation of C3 convertase, heat shock proteins and tumor necrosis factors.

Difference between MHC Class I & II

MHC class I MHC class II

Present on the surface of all nucleated cells	Present on the surface of antigen presenting cells
Consist of 2 non-identical chains (1- long alpha & 1-short beta)	Consist of two identical chains (1-alpha & 1- beta)
Mainly interacts with cytotoxic T cell	Mainly interacts with T-helper cell
Alpha chain is coded on chromosome 6 and beta chain is coded on chromosome 15	Both the chains are coded on chromosome 6
Encoded by HLA-A, B & C gene	Encoded by HLA-D gene
Responsible for graft rejection and clearance of endogenous antigens	Responsible for graft rejection and clearance of exogenous antigens

Cellular distribution of MHC molecules

MHC Class I and MHC Class II molecules have a distinct distribution on cells that directly reflects the different effector functions that the cells play. Furthermore, under some conditions e.g. (cytokine activation), the expression of MHC Class I and or II molecules may be induced or enhanced. Essentially, all nucleated cells carry classical class I molecules. These are abundantly expressed on both lymphoid and myeloid cells, less so on liver, lung and kidney and only sparsely on brain and skeletal muscle. In the human, the surface of the placental extravillous cytotrophoblast lacks HLA-A and –B, although there is now some evidence that it may express HLA-C. What is well established is that the extravillous cytotrophoblast and other placental tissues bear HLA-G, a molecule that generally lacks allodeterminants and that does not appear on most other body cells, except for medullary and subcapsular epithelium in the thymus, and on blood monocytes following activation with γ-interferon. The role of HLA-G in the placenta is not fully resolved, but it appears to function as a replacement for classical class I molecules serving to inhabit immune responses against paternal MHC alleles carried by the foetus. MHC class I molecules are expressed on virtually all cells in humans except for red blood cells. The expression of MHC class I molecules on all nucleated cells permits the immune system to survey these cells for infection by intracellular pathogens and allows their destruction via class I- restricted cytotoxic T lymphocytes (CTLs). It is interesting to note that the absences of class I MHC molecules on RBC may allow the unchecked growth of Plasmodium, the agent responsible for malaria.

Class II molecules, on the other hand, are highly restricted in their expression, being present only on B cells, dendritic cells, macrophages and thymic epithelium. However, when activated by agents such as γ-interferon, capillary endothelia and many epithelial cells in tissues other than the thymus express surface class II and increased levels of class I. When B cells take up antigen through their B cell receptors (BCR), they upregulate their MHC class II molecules to prepare for presentation of peptides to Th cells. Other cells that express MHC class II molecules (dendritic cells, macrophages) are efficient antigen presenting cells for the activation of Th cells. Table 7.1 depicts the expression of MHC class I and II molecules on various cells and tissues.

Table 7.1 - Expression of MHC class I and II molecules

Tissue / cells	MHC Class I	MHC Class II
T cells	+++	_
B cells	+++	+++
Monocytes	+++	+
Macrophages	+++	++
Dendritic cells	+++	+++
Neutrophils	++	_
Liver cells	+	_
Kidney cells	++	_
Brain cells	+	_
Red Blood cells	_	_

Nature of MHC binding peptide

Polymorphic residues within the peptide-binding groove/site of each of MHC molecules make contact with the antigenic peptide. The peptides that are bound by MHC class I and Class II molecules are short, ranging from 8 to 10 amino acid residues (for MHC Class I) and 10 to 20 amino acids residues (for MHC Class II). The sites on the peptides that fasten the peptide to the MHC molecules are the anchor residues. The peptide residues in the MHC- binding groove are the same for each allelic form of the MHC molecules. Therefore, each allelic form MHC molecules is only able to bind peptides bearing specific anchor residues. Thus, depending on the MHC molecules that are inherited, a person might not be able to bind with specific peptides form, for example, a virus. If a person's MHC molecules cannot bind the peptide generated from a specific virus, then they will be unable to mount a CD8 response to the cells infected with virus. This forms at least one basics for the genetic control of immune response. That is, the MHC molecules inherited by an individual ultimately determine to which peptides that individual can elicit T-Cell- mediated immune responses, and at the population level, the polymorphism increases the chance of survival of at least some individuals.

Functions of MHC

The MHC performs the following functions:

1. Production of HLA: The MHC genes control the production of antigens located on the nucleated cells such as lymphocytes. These antigens are called human leucocytes antigens or graft rejection antigens or transplantation antigens.
2. Production of immune associated antigens: The MHC genes control the production of immune associated antigens (Ia) located on the surface of

B- cells, macrophages, monocytes, antigen presenting cells and activated T- cells.

3. Control of the levels of components: The MHC genes are responsible for the control of the levels of complements of the classical pathway and factor B of alternative pathway.
4. HLA complex help in T-cell recognition: T- Cells recognize foreign antigen only in the presences of MHC Class I molecules as well as MHC class II molecules.

   Cytotoxic T- cells need class I molecules; Helper and suppressor T- cells need class II molecules.

   MHC restriction is the recognition of foreign antigen located in the surface of a cell, e.g. a virus infected cell by T Lymphocytes. It occurs, only in association with self-antigens of major histocompatibility complex.

   Cytotoxic T lymphocytes usually respond to foreign antigen in association with Class I MHC antigen, whereas T helper cells respond to foreign antigen in association with Class II (Ia) antigens.

   The presentation of antigens by macrophages to T cells appears to be very specific. The macrophages that present antigens to T helper cells (TH) should have Class II MHC antigens on the surface, whereas macrophages that present antigens to T cytotoxic cells (Tc) should have the Class I MHC antigens. When the macrophage bears a different MHC antigen, it cannot cooperate and thus antigen presentation cannot occur and this is known as MHC restriction.
5. Graft Rejection: Graft rejection is an immunological reaction. It is mediated by lymphocytes. The MHC is responsible for intense graft reactions. This reaction occurs when genetically dissimilar lymphocytes interact.
6. Non-immunological function of MHC: The MHC has several non-immunological functions such as the control of body weight in mice, egg production in chickens, etc.

Question Bank

1. Very short answer type questions
   (a) In humans, MHC genes are located in which chromosomes?
   (b) Give full form of MHC.
   (c) Give examples of antigen presenting cells.
   (d) Give examples of cytokines.
   (e) Give full form of CD.
   (f) Give full form of IL.
   (g) Give full form of INF.
   (h) Which domains of α and β chains forms antigen binding cleft in MHCII?
   (i) Which domains of α chains forms antigen binding cleft in MHC I?
   (j) Define agretope.

2. Short answer type questions
   (a) Why are MHC products highly polymorphic?
   (b) Describe the classes of MHC.
   (c) Draw well labelled diagram of MHC I and MHC II.
   (d) How does MHC I interact with Tc cells?
   (e) How does MHC II interact with Th cells?
   (f) Differentiate between MHC class I & II.
   (g) What are the functions of MHC?

   Q3. Long answer type questions
   (a) Describe in detail the expression of MHC Class I.
   (b) Describe in detail the expression of MHC Class II.
   (c) Describe in detail the classes of MHC their expression, function along with well labelled diagram.
   (d) Describe in detail how does MHC interacts with T lymphocytes.

Multiple Choice Questions

1. MHC participates in the development of
   (a) Humoral immunity (b) Cell mediated immunity
   (c) Both a & b (d) None of the above
2. MHC was discovered by
   (a) Hershey (b) Metchnikoff
   (c) Gorer (d) Berson
3. In humans MHC is found on chromosome
   (a) 10 (b) 12
   (c) 6 (d) 3
4. MHC products are
   (a) Monomorphic (b) Dimorphic
   (c) Polymorphic (d) Highly Polymorphic
5. Endogenous peptides are associated with
   (a) Class I MHC (b) Class II MHC
   (c) Class III MHC (d) None of the above
6. Exogenous peptides are associated with
   (a) Class I MHC (b) Class II MHC
   (c) Class III MHC (d) None of the above
7. Class I MHC, gene present processed antigen to
   (a) Th (b) Tc
   (c) Ts (d) B cells
8. Class II MHC gene present processed antigen to
   (a) Th (b) Tc
   (c) Ts (d) B Cells

9. Antigen presenting cells have
   (a) Class I MHC
   (b) Class II MHC
   (c) Class III MHC
   (d) All of the above
10. All nucleated cells have
   (a) Class I MHC
   (b) Class II MHC
   (c) Class III MHC
   (d) All of the above
11. Class I MHC genes are found in region
   (a) A (b) B
   (c) C (d) All of the above
12. Class II MHC genes are found in region
   (a) DP (b) DD
   (c) DZ (d) DS
13. β2 – macroglobulin is found in
   (a) Class I MHC (b) Class II MHC
   (c) Class III MHC (d) None of the above
14. α1, α2 and α3 are found in which molecule?
   (a) Class I MHC (b) Class II MHC
   (c) Class III MHC (d) None of the above
15. α1, α2 and β1, β2 are found in which molecule?
   (a) Class I MHC (b) Class II MHC
   (c) Class III MHC (d) None of the above
16. MHC class I is expressed via .... pathway
   (a) Exogenous (b) Endogenous
   (c) membrane (d) nucleus
17. MHC class II is expressed via ....pathway
   (a) Exogenous (b) Endogenous
   (c) membrane (d) nucleus
18. MHC II molecule and antigen molecules is recognized by
   (a) CD4 (b) CD8
   (c) Helper T cell (d) Both a & c
19. MHC I molecules and antigen molecules is recognized by
   (a) CD4 (b) CD8
   (c) Cytotoxic T cell (d) Both b & c
20. α and β chains of MHC Class II are coded on chromosome no.
   (a) 2 (b) 3
   (c) 5 (d) 6

Answer Key

Question Number	Answer	Question Number	Answer
1	C	11	D
2	C	12	A
3	C	13	A
4	D	14	A
5	A	15	B
6	B	16	B
7	B	17	A
8	A	18	D
9	B	19	D
10	A	20	D

References

Biassoni R. (2009) Human natural killer receptors, co- operators, and their ligands. Current Protocols in Immunolog. Chapter 14 Unit 14.10.John Willey and Sons.

Braud V.M., D.S.J. and Mc Michael A.J. (1999) Function of non classical MHC and non- MHC- encoded class I molecules. Current Opinion in Immunology 11,100- 108.

Call M.E. and Wuchpfenning K.W. (2005) The T cell receptor: crictical role of the membrane environment in receptor assembly and function. Annual Review of Immunology 23,101-125'

Clark D.A. (1999) Human leukocyte antigen –G: Newrols for old. American Journal of Reproductive Immunology 41,117-120.

Drakesmith, H., and A. Townsend. 2000. The structure andfunction of HFE. BioEssays. 22:595.

Fahrer, A. M., et al. 2001. A genomic view of immunology. Nature409:836.

Horton R. et al (2004) Gene map of the extended human MHC Nature Review Genetics 5, 889-899.

International Human Genome Sequencing Consortium. 2001.Initial sequencing and analysis of the human genome. Nature409:860. International Human Genome Sequencing Consortium. 2001.

Kumar V. and McNerney M.E. (2005) A New self :MHC class I – independent naturalkiller cell self- tolerance.Nature review of Immunology 5,363-374.

Margulies, D. 1999. The major histocompatibility complex. InFundamental Immunology, 4th ed. W. E. Paul, ed. LippincottRaven, Philadelphia.

Meyer, D., and G. Thompson. 2001. How selection shapes variationof the human major histocompatibility complex: a review.Ann. Hum. Genet. 65:1.

MHC Sequencing Consortium (1999) complete sequence and gene map of a human major histocompatibility complex. Nature 401, 921-923.

Natarajan, K., et al. 1999. MHC class I molecules, structure and function. Revs. in Immunogenetics 1:32.

Parham, P. 1999. Virtual reality in the MHC. Immunol. Revs.167:5.

Rothenberg, B. E., and J. R. Voland. 1996. Beta 2 knockout mice develop parenchymal iron overload: A putative role for class I genes of the major histocompatibility complex in iron metabolism. Proc. Natl. Acad. Sci. U.S.A. 93:1529.

Rouas-Freiss, N., et al. 1997.Direct evidence to support the role of HLA-G in protecting the fetus from maternal uterine natural killer cytolysis. Proc. Natl. Acad. Sci. U.S.A. 94:11520.

Yung,Y. C., et al. 2000. The human and mouse class III region: a parade of 21 genes at the centromeric segment. Immunol. Today21:320.

CHAPTER 8

Immunoprophylaxis

Introduction

Immunoprophylaxis refers to the prevention of disease by immunization. Bacterial and viral diseases are prevented and controlled by immunization. Immunization is a process of rendering an individual resistant to infections. The resistance to infection can be brought about by two methods, namely active immunization and passive immunization.

Passive immunization

One way of protecting an individual against an infectious disease is to provide that individual with performed antibodies (or immune cells, but this is much less practical and rarely done) directed against the infecting agent. This is referred to as passive immunization. This refers to the short-lived protection afforded by injection of preformed antibodies against a variety of bacterial or viral antigens. Passive immunization refers to the development of resistance to an infection in a non-immune individual by the administration of sensitized lymphocytes or serum antibodies. However, this form of immunization should be used only when absolutely necessary because of the risks involved such as developing anaphylaxis, serum sickness, or a type III hypersensitivity reaction. Passive immunization is routinely administered to individuals exposed to certain microbial pathogens that cause diseases such as botulism, diphtheria, hepatitis, measles, rabies, and tetanus as well as to protect them against snake and spider bites. Passive immunization could give immediate relief or rapid protection in an emergency. Passive immunization is of two types-

a) **Natural Passive Immunization** - The immunity transferred from the mother to the child passively is known as natural passive immunization. Before birth the antibodies of mother pass into the blood of newborn through the placenta. Only IgG antibodies are transferred through the placenta, since the other types of antibodies cannot pass through the placenta. After birth antibodies are passively transferred to the babies through colostrums*. The breast fed babies can absorb the antibodies directly from the intestine. Till 3 months of age the baby does not develop any proper immune mechanism. However, the baby is well protected upto 5 months against various infections by the maternal antibodies, it had received.

b) **Artificial Passive Immunization** - The artificial transfer of antibodies and sensitized lymphocytes from an immunized donor to a nonimmune recipient is called artificial passive immunization. The antibodies transferred in artificial passive immunity may be homologous antibodies or heterologous antibodies. When the antibodies are transferred between two individuals of the same species, that is man to man, the antibodies are called homologous antibodies. When antibodies of one species of animal are transferred to another species, that is from horse to man or vice versa, the antibodies are called heterologous antibodies.

The importance of immunoglobulins in preventive medicine are anti-toxins and human gamma globulins. The anti toxins are prepared by the immunization of horses against diphtheria, tetanus, etc. Certain people are hypersensitive to horse serum. Hence antitoxins are not generally used. Human gamma globulin gives only passive immunity. To be effective, it must be given in the incubation period. Human gamma globulin is used for the prophylaxis of viral hepatitis A, measles, small pox, mumps tetanus and chicken pox.

Passive immunization is the administration of preformed antibodies, usually IgG, either intravenously or intramuscularly. These may be derived from individuals who have high antibody titers to particular microbes and can thus provide rapid protection against infections such as Diphtheria, rabies, or those caused by Clostridium species. They are also very useful in the event of accidental exposure to certain pathogens such as hepatitis B. Transplacental transfer of maternal antibodies is an example of passive immunization – this plays an important role in protecting babies from infection in the first 6 months of life, as their own immune system matures. Passive immunization is also used to provide protection in immunocompromised individuals who are unable to make appropriate antibody responses or in some instances incapable of making any antibody at all, that is, in severe combined immunodeficiency. Antibodies given to immune-deficient patients are usually of the IgG class and are derived from pooled normal plasma. These antibodies must be given on a continuous basis, ideally every three weeks, because they are continuously catabolized and are only effective for a short period.

The protection transferred in this way is immediate, but it only lasts as long transferred antibodies last. The antibodies may be human in origin, i.e. derived from blood donors – or may have been purposefully raised in an animal. The former has the potential risk of all material derived from blood donors- possible contamination with blood– borne viruses or even prions, whereas the latter carries the risk of inducing an immune response to the foreign proteins injected. Antibodies preformed in animals, notably horses, are also administered for some disease, but with repeated injection there is the danger of immune –complex formation and serum sickness. Antisera are usually injected intramuscularly, but can be given intravenously in extremely acute conditions. Indications for the use of passive immunization by the injection of preformed antibody are shown in table 8.1.

Table 8.1- Passive immunization

Disease / Infection	Source of antiserum	Indications
Tetanus	Immune human; horse	Post-exposure (plus
Diphtheria	Horse	vaccine)
Gas gangrene	Horse	Post-exposure
Botulism	Horse	Post-exposure
Varicella- zoster	Immune human	Post-exposure
Rabies	Immune human	Post-exposure in
Hepatitis B	Immune human	immunodeficiency
Prophylactic treatment	Pooled human lg	Post-exposure (plus
Hepatitis A	Immune human	vaccine)
Measles	Horse	Post-exposure
Snakebite	Pooled human lg	Prophylaxis
Some autoimmune diseases		Post-exposure in infants
		Post-bite
		Acute thrombocytopenia
		Autoimmune neutropenia

Active immunization

This refers to the process whereby an individual is deliberately exposed to key microbial antigens, in order to induce cellular and/ or humoral immune responses to protect the individual against future exposure to the agent from which the antigens were derived. Active immunization is the protection of susceptible humans and domestic animals from communicable diseases by the administration of vaccines (vaccination). The preparation of antigens is referred to as the vaccine. Vaccine-induced protection is not immediate- it takes a finite time for the host system to mount a response to an antigenic challenge. However, active immunization yields much longer- lasting protection than passive immunization, as some immune cells become memory cells, able to be stimulated years later if challenged with the antigen. Vaccination works because such a challenge generates a secondary immune response, rather than a primary one and secondary responses are faster, of higher affinity, and greater titer than primary ones.

In active immunization, the individual is injected with an antigen to induced an immune response against an infection. This immunization has brought direct benefit to human beings and domestic animals. For example, active immunization with cowpox vaccine is responsible for the complete eradication of small pox from human beings, Similarly, active immunization with vaccines against tetanus, diphtheria and poliomyelitis has made these diseases rare in many countries. The active immunization may be of two types namely natural immunization and artificial immunization.

a) **Natural Active Immunization** - Natural active immunization refers to the development of resistance to infection due to naturally occurring infections. For example a person attacked by measles or small pox develops natural immunity as he recovers from the disease. The immunity acquired by way of such infections is long lasting and the person will not contract the same disease for the second time during his life.

b) b. **Artificial Active Immunization** - Artificial active immunization refers to the development of resistance to infections owing to vaccines. Administration of vaccines containing microbial products with or without adjuvants in order to obtain long –term immunological protection against the offending microbe is termed active immunization. Immunization can be given via two different routes. They are systemic immunization and mucosal immunization

1. Systemic immunization

This is the method of choice at present for most vaccinations and is usually carried out by injecting the vaccine subcutaneously or intramuscularly into the deltoid muscle. Ideally all vaccines would be given soon after birth, but some are deliberately delayed, for various reasons. The common systemic vaccines for measles, mumps, and rubella are usually given at 1 year of age because, if given earlier, maternal antibody could decrease their effectiveness. The carbohydrate, vaccines for Pneumococcus, Meningococcus, and Hemophilus infections are usually given at about 2 year of age, as before this age they respond poorly to polysaccharides unless they are associated with protein components that can act to recruit T- cell help for the development of anti-polysaccharide antibody, for example hen egg albumin.

2. Mucosal immunization

Most infectious agents gain entry to the body through mucosal surfaces, sites that are also associated with the largest source of lymphoid tissue. Thus current vaccination approaches have focused on immunization either orally or through nasal-associated immune tissue. This approach has become more efficient and available for public use, obviating the need for painful injection, and permitting self- administration of certain vaccine (e.g., for immunization against influenza). Adjuvant vaccines and live vectors have also been successfully used to target the mucosal immune system. Moreover, in animal models attenuated strains of Salmonella act as a powerful immune stimulus and, as carriers of foreign antigen, can be used to immunizes mucosal surfaces against herpes simplex virus and human papillomavirus. Furthermore, bacterial toxins, for example those derived from Vibrio cholera, Escherichia coli, and Bordetella pertussis, have immunomodulatory properties that are being exploited in the development of mucosally active adjuvants. Pertussis toxin augments the co-stimulatory molecules CD86 on B cells and CD28 on T cells and increase IFNγ production.

Principles of vaccination

Edward Jenner, a country physician in England, noticed that dairymaids who frequently contracted cowpox were often immune to the ravages of smallpox, leading him to develop an approach whereby cowpox was used to vaccinate people against smallpox. The term vaccination eventually is derived from the Latin word vaccinus meaning "from cows." Vaccination eventually resulted in the complete eradication of smallpox (in 1980) and has been generalized as a reliable method of protection against many pathogens. The aims of vaccination are to induce memory in T and/or B lymphocytes through the injection of a nonvirulent antigen preparation. Thus, in the event of an actual infection, the infectious agent and/or its toxin are met by a secondary rather than a primary response. Figure 8.1 depicts a schematic view of the relative contributions of humoral & cellular immunity during primary or secondary viral infection. The ideal vaccine would protect the individual and ultimately eliminate the disease, but most vaccines simply protect the individual. A standard set of vaccines is now in use worldwide, some of which are (or should be) given to everyone, others to those particularly at risk (Table 8.2). The timing of vaccination depends on the likelihood of infection, vaccines against common infections being given as early as possible, allowing for the fact that some vaccines do not work properly in very young infants.

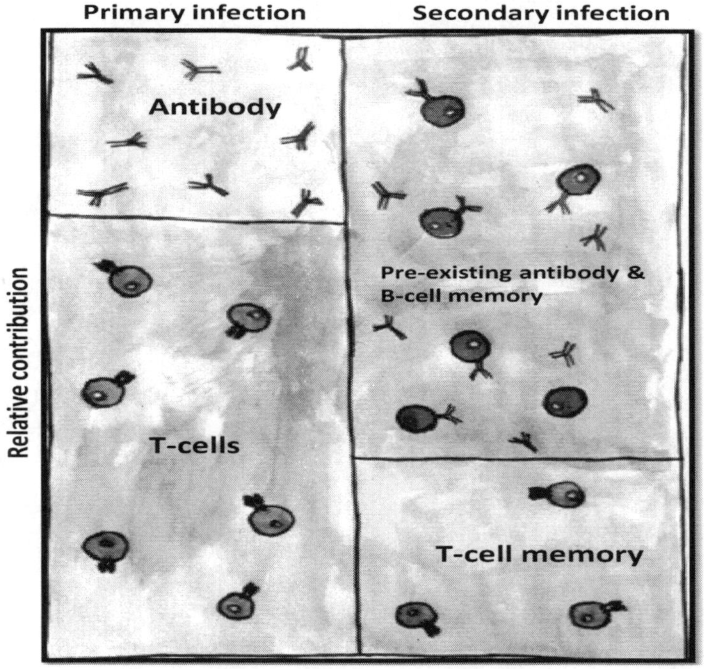

Fig. 8.1 : A schematic view of the relative contributions of humoral & cellular immunity during primary or secondary viral infection.

Herd Immunity

Herd immunity results from the vaccination of a significant proportion of the population, which probably causes disruption to the chain of infection. Protecting individuals reduces the number of infectious organisms and decreases the chances of non-vaccinated individuals being infected. Where a disease depends on human transmission, immunity in just a proportion of the population can help the whole community if it leads to a fall in the reproduction rate (i.e. the number of further cases produced by each infected individual) to less than one; under these circumstances the disease will die out: witness, for example, the disappearance of diphtheria from communities in which around 75% of the children have been immunized. But this figure must be maintained; there is no room for complacency.

Table 8.2 - Vaccine recommendations

Recommended for	Vaccine	**When given/to whom**
All	Measles	From 1 year(6 months in tropics), boost at 10-14 years
	Mumps	
	Rubella	
	Diphtheria	From 2 to 3 months old
	Tetanus	Dip/tet boost at 5 years
	Pertusis	
	Polio(Sabin)	2-6 months (oral)
	(or Salk *)	Parenterally
	BCG**	Varies, see footnote
Those at risk	Hepatitis B	Travelers, children (some countries) at risk.
	Hepatitis A	Travelers, people with chronic liver disease, institution etc.
	Influenza	Aged, doctors, nurses etc., annual boost needed.
	Rabies	Travelers, post-exposure: vaccine + antibody
	Meningococcal	Children: 2-10 years
	Pneumococcal	Elderly
	Haemophilus influenza type b	Infants 2-15 months
	Varicella-zoster	Children with leukemia
At risk (travel)	Typhoid	Travelers
	Cholera	Travelers
	Yellow fever	Travelers: boost at 10-year intervals

Vaccines and their types

A **vaccine** [Latin *vacca,* cow] is a preparation from an infectious agent that is administered to humans and other animals to induce protective immunity. Vaccination is still one of the most cost-effective weapons for microbial disease prevention, and vaccines arguably constitute one of the greatest achievements of modern medicine.

Vaccination is the safest and most cost- effective method of disease preventions; however, developing and introducing protective vaccines against infectious disease is not an easy task. Several factors determine the development and licensing and vaccines, including the prevalence of disease, seriousness to health or economy, and the availability of safe and protective antigen preparations There are numerous serious infectious conditions where preventive vaccines would be highly desirable, but protective preparations are not yet available for most of these.

There are many form of vaccine available (figure 8.2), each with advantages and disadvantages. Vaccines may consist of viable but attenuated organism, nonviable whole cell mixtures or fragments (subunit) of organism. Only highly protective vaccines against relatively common and serious disease with proven safety records are introduced into the routine childhood immunization programmes. Partially protective vaccines are made available to certain high- risk groups. Vaccinomics, the application of genomics and bioinformatics to vaccine development, is bringing a fresh approach to the Herculean problem of making vaccines against various microorganisms and parasites.

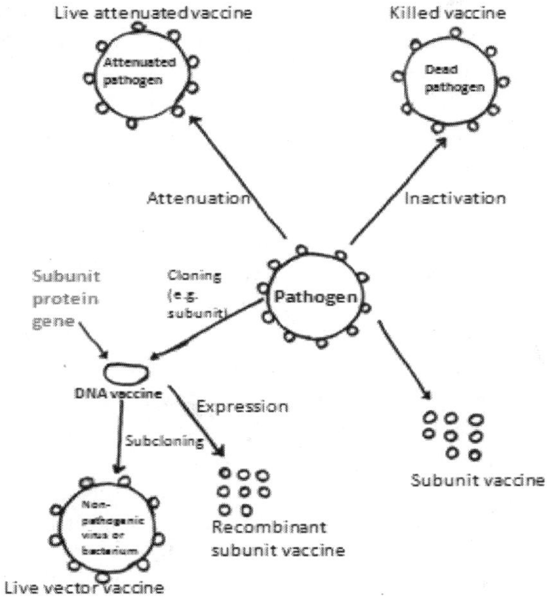

Fig. 8.2 : Classical vaccine approaches

1. **Live attenuated** organisms generate both humoral and cellular immune responses to a wide range of antigens within the organism under consideration, but they require a secure cold chain, i.e. they must be kept at low temperatures until administration, as otherwise they become nonviable. Exposure to live and fully virulent organisms often acts as an effective vaccination (provided the host survives the initial attack). For example, patients who recover from hepatitis A virus infection remain solidly immune to further attacks throughout life. Live attenuated vaccines stimulate a broad immune response (i.e. both humoral and cellular) to a wide range of microbial antigens, both structural and nonstructural. They should be attenuated to a sufficient degree that they do not of themselves give rise to serious disease. Ideally, they should be administered through the natural route of infection, and thereby stimulate protective immune response in relevant parts of the body (e.g. live attenuated poliovirus vaccine is given by mouth, and stimulates protective immunity in the gut). Effectiveness of live attenuated vaccines must be partly because the replication of the living microbe confronts the host with the larger and more sustained dose of antigen and that, with budding viruses,

infected cells are required for the establishment of good cytotoxic T-cell memory. BCG, Bacille Calmette-Guerin, an attenuated mycobacterium used to vaccinate against tuberculosis. This was first prepared by two French workers *Calmette* and *Guerin,* hence the name. Here, the bacilli are attenuated by cultivating in glycerol-bile- potato medium. Another significant advantage of using live organisms is that the immune response takes place largely at the site of natural infection. This is well illustrated by the nasopharyngeal IgA response to immunization with polio vaccine. In contrast with the ineffectiveness of parenteral injection of killed vaccine, intranasal administration evoked a good local antibody response; however, whereas this declined over a period of 2 months or so, per oral immunization with live attenuated virus established a persistently high IgA antibody level.

2. **Killed organism as vaccine-** The simplest way to destroy the ability of microbe to cause disease, yet maintain their antigenic constitution, is to prevent their replication by killing in an appropriate manner. Inactivated whole organism vaccines are more stable, but less immunogenic, therefore requiring multiple doses, administered by injection. Inactivated vaccines, both whole viruses and whole-cell- killed bacteria, are administered by injection. Inactivated vaccines are effective, but they often require several boosters and normally do not adequately stimulate cell-mediated immunity or secretory IgA production. In contrast, attenuated vaccines usually are given in a single dose and stimulate both humoral and cell-mediated immunity. However, they are more stable than live vaccines, which require maintenance of the cold chain prior to administration, i.e. they must be kept at low temperature in order to prevent loss of viability. The immune response to inactivated vaccines is skewed to the humoral, rather than the cellular arm of the immune system. Parasitic worms and, to a lesser extent, protozoa are extremely difficult to grow up in bulk to manufacture killed vaccines. This problem does not arise for many bacteria and viruses and, in these cases, the inactivated microorganisms have provided a number of safe antigens for immunization. Examples are influenza, cholera and inactivated poliomyelitis (Salk) vaccines. Care has to be taken to ensure that important protective antigens are not destroyed in the inactivation process.

3. **Subunit vaccines** consist of only a key part of the organism. Whole organisms have a multiplicity of antigens, some of which are not protective, may induce hypersensitivity or might even be immunosuppressive. These also require multiple doses, and, as with inactivated whole organism vaccines, induce much better humoral than cellular responses. A few of the common risks associated with whole-organism vaccines can be avoided by using only specific, purified macromolecules derived from pathogenic microorganisms. Currently, there are three general forms of macromolecule vaccines: (1) capsular polysaccharides, (2) recombinant surface antigens, and (3) inactivated exotoxins called toxoids. Toxins to be used as subunit vaccines must first be inactivated, e.g. by treatment

with formaldehyde, thereby yielding toxoid (figure 8.3). Formaldehyde detoxicated tetanus toxin of tetanus bacteria is used in prophylactic immunization against tetanus. It is given by repeated subcutaneous dose. This forms a part of triple vaccine. Diphtheria toxoid is toxoid vaccine prepared by formalin treatment of the bacterial toxin producing diphtheria. This is also used most commonly in the form of *triple vaccine.* Subunit vaccines (also nonviable) consist of one or more highly protective components of the organism, selected and purified in the laboratory. These are also administered by injection, and multiple doses are required. The antigens represent key virulence or survival factors of the organism which can generate neutralizing or bactericidal antibodies. The hepatitis B surface antigen particle is a classical example of effective subunit viral vaccine. Many successful bacterial vaccines target glycans on the surface of the organism using glycoconjugate preparations. DNA encoding the proteins from a pathogen can be injected directly into muscle to generate the proteins in situ and produce immune response (figure 8.4). The advantages are stability, ease of production and cheapness.

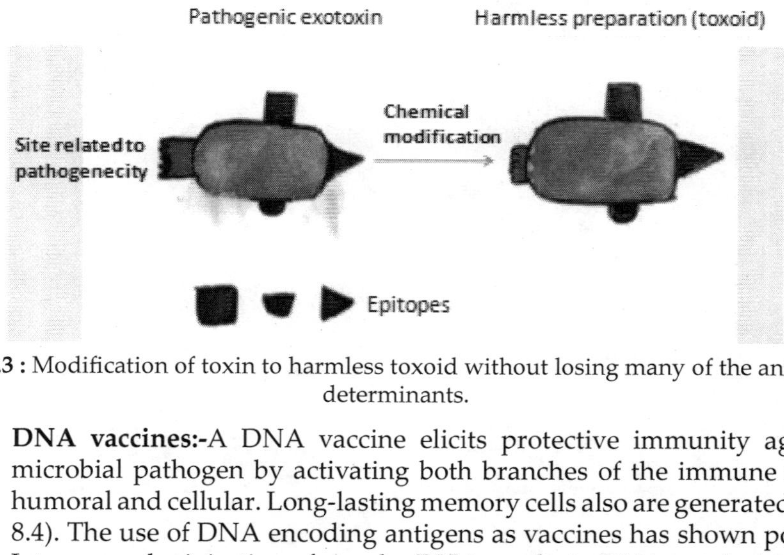

Fig. 8.3 : Modification of toxin to harmless toxoid without losing many of the antigenic determinants.

4. **DNA vaccines:-**A DNA vaccine elicits protective immunity against a microbial pathogen by activating both branches of the immune system: humoral and cellular. Long-lasting memory cells also are generated (figure 8.4). The use of DNA encoding antigens as vaccines has shown potential. Intramuscular injection of circular DNA results in DNA uptake by muscle cells, expression of the encoded protein and induction of both humoral and cell-mediated immunity. The immunization procedure begins with the injection into muscle of a plasmid preparation that contains genes for pathogen antigens. The plasmids are taken up by muscle cells, enter the cell nuclei, and express their antigen genes. The muscle cells commence protein synthesis and produce the pathogen's antigenic proteins. At present, there are human trials under way with several different DNA vaccines against malaria, AIDS, influenza, hepatitis B, and herpesvirus. Vaccines against a number of cancers (lymphomas, prostate, colon) are also being tested.

5. **Recombinant vaccines:-**Genetic vaccines are quite different in structure from whole organism vaccines. It is now possible to isolate genes that encode major antigens from a pathogen and insert them into nonvirulent viruses or bacteria. Using molecular genetics, selective recombinant proteins with defined epitopes can be prepared that can induce protective immunity to pathogens (figure 4). This approach overcomes the problem of disease complication that may occur with modified live vaccines. The vaccines are usually delivered by needle injection or by a device called a gene gun. The attenuated microorganism serves as a vector, replicating within the host and expressing the gene product of the pathogen–encoded antigenic proteins. The antigens can elicit humoral immunity when they escape from the vector, and they can also elicit cellular immunity when they are broken down and properly displayed on the cell surface (just as occurs when cells harbor an active pathogen). Recently several microorganisms have been used in the production of these **recombinant-vector vaccines.** Examples include adenovirus, vaccinia virus, canarypox virus, attenuated poliovirus, and attenuated strains of *Salmonella* and *Mycobacterium.*

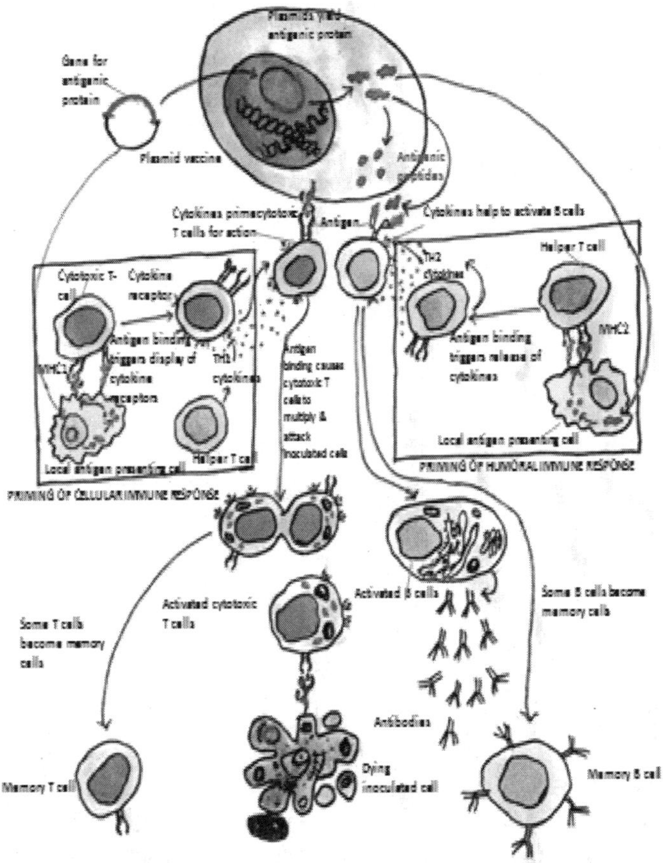

Fig. 8.4 : Pathway for stimulation of B and T cell immunity and cell memory

6. **Nanoparticle vaccines** - Nanoparticles consisting of synthetic resins, polystyrenes, carbon particles, silica, iron, or polyethylenes are currently being investigated for suitability as adjuvants in vaccine delivery. They offer potential advantages over current vaccines in that they are easily manipulated and may be give through the mucosal route or systemically.
7. **Cytokines** - Cytokines can be added at the time of immunization to skew the immune response to a Th1- or Th2-type response depending on the kind of response needed for protection against a particular pathogen. Cytokines that might be useful are IL-12 or IFNγ, which favor a Th 1 response, or IL-4 and IL-10 which favor a Th2 response. Table 8.3 illustrates the composition of currently available vaccines.

Table 8.3 Composition of currently available vaccines.

Type of microbe	Vaccine content	**Infection**
Viruses	Live attenuated	Polio (Sabin vaccine), measles, mumps, rubella, varicella-zoster, smallpox (vaccinia), yellow fever
	Inactivated	Polio (Salk vaccine), influenza, hepatitis A, Japanese encephalitis, tick-borne encephalitis, rabies
	Subunit	Hepatitis B, influenza
Bacteria	Live attenuated	BCG, typhoid
	Whole-cell killed	Pertussis, typhoid, plague, Q-fever, cholera
	Single protein (toxoid)	Diphtheria, tetanus
	Multiple proteins	Pertussis, anthrax
	Capsule (carbohydrate)	Haemophilus influenza type b, Neisseria meningitidis Group C, typhoid, Pneumococcus

Many vaccines are administered together with an adjuvant, something which enhances the local immune response to the vaccine antigens, e.g. aluminum hydroxide. Nonliving vaccines, especially those consisting of small molecules, require the inclusion of adjuvants to enhance their effectiveness. These include microbial, synthetic, and endogenous preparations having adjuvant activity; at present only aluminum and calcium salts are used in humans. Adjuvants should preserve antigen integrity, enable antigens to be slowly released, and permit effective targeting of antigen-presenting cells. Biologically active toxins, such as diphtheria or tetanus toxins, are rendered into toxoids by inactivation with formaldehyde before being introduced to humans, otherwise they may cause serious damage. Adjuvants generate enhanced longer- lived immune responses. They are generally not required for live attenuated vaccines but are crucial for protein subunit vaccines. Adjuvants function by immunostimulation and antigen delivery or both. Immunostimulation arises by the action of molecules such as cytokines and bacterial exotoxins to directly enhance immune responses, particularly involving the dendritic cell. Antigen delivery vehicles prevent antigen dispersal and promote slow release. They include mineral salt and emulsion. Certain adjuvants such as cholera toxin are potent at stimulating mucosal responses, which may be most appropriate for certain pathogens infecting via mucosal surfaces. The most widely used adjuvant in humans are based on gels formed by aluminum salts and are referred to collectively as "alum" adjuvants. Antigens are adsorbed on aluminum particles and the appropriate adjuvant formulation selected based on immunogenicity. The activity of alum is ascribed to depot effects and immunostimulatory effects based on particle formation and induction of inflammation. Alum is used in several licensed vaccines, including hepatitis A, human pappilomavirus (HPV), diphtheria- pertusis-tetanus (DPT), Haemophilus influenza b and inactivated polio.

Time of Immunization

Immunization is carried out in two ways, namely routine immunization and immunization under special circumstances.

1. Routine Immunization

Routine immunization is the fixed and regular way of doing immunization. The children are protected from disease like polio, tetanus, whooping cough, small pox etc, by subjected to routine immunization. The WHO (World Health Organization) in the year 1970 has given a schedule of immunization for children. This schedule is carried out in almost all the countries. Children in both the USA and UK are routinely immunized with diphtheria and tetanus toxoid and acellular pertussis (DPT triple vaccine), attenuated strains of measles, mumps and rubella (MMR), inactivated polio, and the capsular polysaccharides of H. influenza type b linked to a carrier (table 8.4). Although in the UK and many other countries, BCG is given at 10-14 years of age, or for high- risk infants immediately after birth, it is not used routinely in the USA.

Table 8.4 - Routine childhood immunization program in the UK.

Age group	Number of doses	Vaccines
First 6 months of life	3	Diphtheria, pertusis, tetanus, polio,
By 15 months	1	Haemophilus influenza type b (Hib),
By school entry	1 (booster dose)	meningococcus Group C
By 10-14 years	1	Measles, mumps, rubella (MMR)
Before leaving	1	Diphtheria, polio, MMR, tetanus
School		BCG
		Polio, tetanus, diphtheria

2. Immunization on Special Circumstances

When there occur sudden outbreaks of certain diseases, they are prevented by mass immunization in the affected areas. For example during flood, there is possibility for the outbreak of cholera. In such areas cholera vaccines are given. Similarly, vaccination for plague, typhoid fever, influenza, yellow fever, etc. are given on certain occasion. When mass camps are conducted, the participants are given vaccinations against infectious diseases. People are travelling by air, sea and land to all parts of the world for commercial, cultural and recreational purposes. These international travelers are usually immunized against diseases, like small pox, yellow fever, cholera, and plague.

Depending on the country of travel, international travelers are routinely immunized against cholera, hepatitis, plague, polio, typhoid, typhus, and yellow fever. Health care personnel and people exposed through life-style patterns are immunized against hepatitis B. Immunization against anthrax is reserved for individuals (veterinarians or agricultural workers) who might come into contact with infected animals or products from the animals. Veterinarians, forest rangers, and others whose jobs involve contact with animals are vaccinated against rabies, plague, and Lyme disease. Table 8.5 highlights the vaccines available to those at risk of infection

Table 8.5 - Other vaccines available to those at risk of infection.

Risk group	Vaccine
Previously unimmunized individuals	Polio, tetanus, diphtheria
Seronegative women before pregnancy	Rubella
Minority groups at high risk of acquiring infection	Hepatitis A, Hepatitis B, BCG, varicella, anthrax
Elderly, Immunocompromised, patients with organ failure	Influenza, Pneumococcus
Travellers to certain parts of Africa	Yellow fever Meningococcus Group A, C, W135,
Travellers to developing countries	Thyphoid, hepatitis A and B, cholera, polio, rabies, Japanese encephalitis, tick-borne encephalitis, and many other depending on the country

Before any vaccine is introduced to routine immunization programmes, rigorous checks are made in the laboratory, in animals, and in a large number of human volunteers. Licensing only occurs once the vaccine is considered safe and free of serious side-effects.

Contraindications – There are very few genuine reasons why certain individuals should not be given certain vaccines. These are referred to as contraindications:

1. Acute illness. If an individual is acutely ill at the time when they present for vaccination, the procedure should be postponed until he/ she has recovered.
2. Allergy to a component of the vaccine. Vaccines may contain a variety of substances other than the relevant antigens. Influenza vaccine is grown in hen's eggs and may contain a trace of egg proteins. Antibiotics are added to some vaccines to prevent bacterial contamination.
3. Pregnancy. If at all possible, it is sensible to postpone vaccination until the end of pregnancy, although there will be circumstances where the risk of possible damage to the fetus is outweighed by the risk of not vaccinating, e.g. yellow fever vaccination for someone visiting a yellow fever endemic area.

4. Immunosuppression, from whatever cause. Live vaccines in particular should be avoided in immunocompromised patients, as the absence of a fully functioning immune system may allow the attenuated organism to become an opportunistic pathogen.
5. No immune procedure is entirely free from the risk of adverse reactions. The following adverse reactions may occur during immunization: As a result of inoculation local reaction such as pain, redness, tenderness and development of a small nodule at the site of injection may occur. After inoculation general reactions like fever, malaise, headache, etc may occur. When improperly sterilized syringes and needles are used infection like Staphylococcus, Streptococcus, etc. may occur. Administration of antisera may sometimes cause serum sickness and anaphylactic shock. Small pox vaccine may cause encephalitis and encephalopathy.

In addition to the above genuine contraindications, there are, unfortunately, a wide range of false beliefs and myths about vaccination, which collectively mean that large numbers of individuals are being denied the benefits of vaccination.

Question Bank

1. Very short answer type questions
   (a) Give the full form of BCG.
   (b) Give examples of live vaccines.
   (c) Give examples of killed vaccines.
   (d) Give examples of recombinant vaccines.
   (e) Give examples of toxoid.
   (f) Give full form of DPT.
   (g) Give examples of an adjuvant.
   (h) Give are example of triple vaccine.
   (i) Give full form of MMR.
   (j) Give are example of cellular vaccine.
   (k) Give are example of freeze dried vaccine.
2. Short Answer type Questions
   (a) Define active immunization.
   (b) Define passive immunization.
   (c) What is sabin? Give example.
   (d) What is salk vaccine?
   (e) Define vaccines.
   (f) Define homologous vaccines.
   (g) Define heterologous vaccines.
   (h) What are subunit vaccines?
   (i) Define immunoprophylaxis.
   (j) Define serum sickness.

3. Long Answer type Questions
   (a) Describe in detail the time schedule of immunization as specified by WHO.
   (b) Describe in details the complications related with Immunization.
   (c) Describe in details the type of vaccines.
   (d) Classify vaccination.
   (e) Describe in detail the role of memory cell in immunization.
   (f) What are the complications associated with passive immunization?

Multiple Choice Questions

1. Which diseases are controlled by immunoprophylaxis?
   (a) Bacterial (b) Viral
   (c) Fungal (d) All of the above
2. Antigens are administrated in
   (a) Active immunization (b) Passive immunization
   (c) Both a & b (d) None of the above
3. Development of resistance to infection owing to vaccine comes under
   (a) Natural active immunization (b) Artificial active immunization
   (c) Natural passive immunization (d) Artificial passive immunization
4. Vaccines prepared from one microbe and used against the same is known as
   (a) Homologous (b) Cellular
   (c) Heterologous (d) Subunit
5. What is administrated in passive immunization?
   (a) Sensitized lymphocytes (b) Serum antibodies
   (c) Antigens (d) Both a and b
6. Immunization either orally or through nasal associated immune tissue is carried out in
   (a) Systematic immunization (b) Mucosal immunization
   (c) Passive immunization (d) None of the above
7. Which immune responses are induced in active immunization?
   (a) Cell mediated (b) Humoral
   (c) Both a & b (d) None of the above
8. Development of resistance to infection due to naturally occurring infection comes under
   (a) Natural active immunization (b) Artificial active immunization
   (c) Natural passive immunization (d) Artificial passive immunization
9. Immediate protection is provided by
   (a) Active immunization (b) Passive immunization
   (c) Both a & b (d) None of the above

10. Which sentence is true about vaccine?
(a) Protection is not immediate
(b) Long lasting immunity
(c) Finite time is taken to develop immunity
(d) All above are true
11. The term vaccination is derived from word *Vacca*, which means
(a) Sheep (b) Buffalo
(c) Cow (d) Goat
12. When toxins and chemicals are used for vaccine preparation, they are known as
(a) Cellular vaccines (b) Sub cellular
(c) Toxoid (d) Recombinant vaccines
13. Sabin vaccine is given
(a) Intramuscularly (b) Peritoneally
(c) orally (d) Intrathecally
14. Pertusis is a _________ vaccine
(a) Live (b) Killed
(c) Toxoid (d) None of the above
15. Which condition may be associated with passive immunization?
(a) Anaphylaxis
(b) Serum sickness
(c) Type III hypersensitivity reaction
(d) All of the above
16. In case of snake & spider bite, which immunization is suitable?
(a) Active immunization (b) Passive immunization
(c) Both a & b (d) None of the above
17. Which diseases are treated by passive immunization?
(a) Hepatitis (b) Measles
(c) Rabies (d) All of the above
18. The immunity transferred from mother to the child is
(a) Natural active immunization (b) Artificial active immunization
(c) Natural passive immunization (d) Artificial passive immunization
19. Person will not contact the same disease for the second time when immunized with
(a) Natural active immunization (b) Artificial active immunization
(c) Both a & b (d) None of the above
20. When whole microbe is used for vaccine production, it is known as
(a) Cellular vaccine (b) Sub cellular vaccine
(c) Homologous vaccine (d) Heterologous vaccine

Answer Key

Question Number	Answer	Question Number	Answer
1	D	11	C
2	A	12	B
3	B	13	C
4	A	14	B
5	D	15	D
6	B	16	B
7	C	17	D
8	A	18	C
9	B	19	C
10	D	20	A

References

Allen A. (2008) Vaccine: the controversial story of medicine's greatest life saver. W.W. Norton & Company, New York.

Amanna I.J. & Slifka M.K. (2009) Wanted, dead or alive: new viral vaccines. Antiviral Research 84, 119-130

Amanna I.J., Messaoudi I. & Slifka M.K. (2008) Protective immunity following vaccination: how is it defined? Human Vaccines 4, 316-319

Astronomo R.D. & Burton D.R. (2010) Carbohydrate vaccines: developing sweet solutions to sticky situations? Nature Review Drug Discovery 9, 308-324

Benoist, C., and D. Matis. 2001. Autoimmunity provoked by infection: how good is the case for T cell epitope mimicry? Nat Immunol. 2:797.

Birkett A.J. (2010) PATH Malaria Vaccine Initiative (MVI): perspectives on the status of malaria vaccine development. Human Vaccines 6, 139-145

Erikson, J., et al. 1998. Self-reactive B cells in nonautoimmune and autoimmune mice.Immunol. Res. 17:49.

Hausmann, S., and K. W. Wucherpfennig. 1997. Activation of autoreactive T cells by peptides from human pathogens. Curr. Opin. Immunol. 9:831.

Horwitz, M.S., et al.1998.Diabetes induced by Coxsackie virus: initiation by bystander damage and not molecular mimicry. Nature Med. 4:781.

King, C., and N. Sarvetnick. 1997. Organ specific autoimmunity. Curr. Opin. Immunol. 9:863.

Levin, M. C., et al. 2002.Autoimmunity due to molecular mimicry as a cause of neurological disease. Nat Med. 8:509.

O'Garra, A., L. Steinman, and K.Gijbels.1997.CD4+ T-cell subsets in autoimmunity. Curr. Opin. Immunol. 9:872.

Plotkin S.A. (2010) Correlates of protection of induced by vaccination. Clinical Vaccine & Immunology 17, 1055-1065

Sinden R.E. (2010) A biologists perspective on malaria vaccine development. Human Vaccines 6, 3-11.

Taylor K.M Nguyen A. & Steohenne J. (2009) The need for new vaccines. Vaccine 27, G3-G8.

Virgin H.W. & Walker B.D. (2010) Immunology & the elusive AIDS vaccine. Nature 464, 224-231

Vyse, T. J., and B. L. Kotzin. 1998. Genetic susceptibility to systemic lupus erythematosus. Annu. Rev. Immunol. 16:261.

Welsh R.M., Che J.W., Brehm M.A. & Selin L.K. (2010) Heterologous immunity between viruses. Immunological Reviews 235, 244-266

Wucherpfennig, K. W. 2001.Mechanisms for the induction of autoimmunity by infectious agents. J Clin. Invest. 108:1097.

Zhao, Z-S, et al. 1998. Molecular mimicry by herpes simplex virus type-1: autoimmune disease after viral infection. Science 279:1344.

CHAPTER 9

Immunohaematology

Introduction

Immunohaematology refers to the study of blood groups, blood transfusion, blood group antigen, blood group antigen-antibody reactions and the blood group disorder. Ever since the beginning of transfusion of blood from one person to another, the transfusions were sometimes successful and were fatal at times. It was because of the lack of knowledge about blood groups. Karl Landsteiner first of all in 1900 discovered that the red blood cells of humans were not all antigenically alike. He reported four different immunological human blood types, that is A, B, AB and O. These blood groups are called Landsteiner groups or ABO blood groups. Landsteiner was awarded with Nobel prize in1932 for his discovery.

Blood Groups

1. ABO Blood Groups

Based on the presence or absence of antigens and antibodies human beings are classified into four groups namely A, B, AB, and O, A group persons contain antigen A and antibody b. B group persons contain antigen B and antibody a: AB group persons contain both antigens A and B, but no antibody; O group person contain no antigen, but both antibodies a and b are present. O group person is called the universal donor because he / she can donate blood to any group. As there is no antigen in the O group there will not be any reaction. AB group person is called universal recipient because he can receive blood from any group. As there is no antibody in the AB group, there will not be any reaction (figure 9.1).

2. Rh Blood Group System

The second major blood group system is the Rhesus (Rho) system. Landsteiner and Wiener (1940) discovered the existence of a special type of antigen in the RBC of Rhesus monkey. Since this factor was first discovered in Rhesus monkey, it was named Rhesus factor or Rh factor.

The Rh factor is also present in the RBC of some human beings and it is absent from others. Based on the presence or absence of Rh factor, the human beings are classified into two groups. They are Rh positive (Rh^+) and Rh negative (Rh^-). The Rh+ person has Rh antigen on the RBC; the Rh- person has no Rh antigen. D is the main antigen of the Rhesus system.

In the European countries 85% of the human beings are Rh+ and remaining 15% are Rh; in India 93% are Rh+ and 7% are Rh-. In China 99.5 are Rh+ and only 0.5% are Rh-. Approximately 85% of the Caucasian populations are Rho (D) positive.

Human red blood cells are classified as Rho (D) positive or Rho (D) negative depending upon the presence or absence of D (Rho) antigen on them. The D phenotype is variant of D (Rho) antigen and is recognized by performing the antiglobulin test. About 60% of the D's now classified as weak or partial D's, may react with Anti-D(Rho) (IgM) in slide tests and about 90% may be detected by the tube technique. The Rh and antigen has no natural antibody. However, Rh antibody can be produced artificially. An Rh- person develops Rh antibody when he receives blood from an Rh+ person. Even a small amount of Rh+ blood (as small as 0.05 ml) can evoke the production of Rh antibody in the Rh- person. The antibody once formed remains throughout the life.

Genetics of blood groups

1. ABO Blood Groups

The ABO blood group is inherited by a set of multiple alleles. The synthesis of antigen A is controlled by a dominant alleles represented by L^A (the letter L is used to honor the discoverer of blood groups, *Landsteiner*). Antigen B synthesis is controlled by another dominant allele B represented by L^B. The absence of antigen is due to the presence of recessive alleles represented by L^0. The inheritance of blood groups follows simple Mendelian principle. A and B allele are dominant over O and codominant with one another. In general, persons with blood types A, B and AB inherit a gene for the enzymes that adds a certain terminal sugar to the basic RBC receptor. Type O persons do not have such an enzyme and lack the terminal sugar. The specific enzymes produced by RBCs of types A, B and AB add sugars N-acetyl-galactosamine, D-galactose and both N-acetyl-galactosamine and D-galactose respectively to the receptors.

The major blood group ABO antigens are mainly present on the surface of erythrocytes (although they are also expressed on the endothelial cells of the kidney) and the gene encoding them are polymorphic, that is, there is more than one allele coding for the gene product. This is in contrast to most protein, for example albumin, which are coded for by non-polymorphic genes or genes which lack allelic variation. The major blood group alleles A and B code for enzymes which create different sugars on proteins and lipids on the surface of erythrocytes. Blood group O is a null allele and does not add sugars. These alleles are inherited in a simple Mendelian inheritance pattern and are co-dominantly expressed (i.e. both allelic products are expressed on the erythrocyte surface, table 9.1). An individual can be either homozygous (the same) or heterozygous (different) for the inherited alleles.

The major blood groups ABO are mainly present on the surface of erythrocytes (except those having AB blood group) have antibodies (isohemagglutinins) to these blood group antigen (table 9.1). These isohemagglutinins are usually IgM and probably belong to class of "natural antibodies", they would be boosted through contact with antigen of the gut flora that are structurally similar to the blood group carbohydrate, so that the antibodies formed cross-react with the appropriate red cell type.

The reason for development of these antibodies is unclear, but is probably due to cross-reactivity of AB antigens with those of certain ubiquitous microbes. These antibodies had no effect on the RBC of the same individual but when mixed with the RBC antigen(s) of different blood types, i.e. during transfusion, a violent, incompatible reaction may result and may be fatal. In other words we can say that transplantation of blood to a recipient who has serum isohemagglutinins can result in a severe transfusion reaction mediated by a type II hypersensitivity reaction that can lead to death. Thus blood typing is a prerequisite to blood transfusion.

Clinical refractoriness to platelet transfusions is frequently due to HLA alloimmunization, but one can usually circumvent this problem by depleting the platelets of leukocytes.

Table 9.1 - Blood group antigen and isohemagglutinins

Blood group	A	B	AB	O
Genotype Isohemagglutinins	AA or AO Anti-B	BB or BO Anti-A	AB None	O or O Anti-A and B

2. Rh Blood Group System

Genetically, a person's Rh type results from a combination of two possible alleles – a dominant one that produces the factor and a recessive one that does not. There are several varieties of Rh antigen and of antibody. The commonest Rh antigen is called antigen D and controlled by multiple alleles. The antigen D is produced by a dominant gene represented by R .When this gene is recessive it cannot produce the antigen. Hence the Rh+ persons may be homozygous dominant (RR) or heterozygous (Rr). The Rh- person are always homozygous recessive (rr). The Rh factor follows the Mendelian principle of inheritance. The blood type of the children can be easily visualized by knowing the blood type of parents. A person inheriting at least one Rh gene will be Rh+, and only those persons inheriting two recessive genes are Rh-.

Blood Transfusion

Blood transfusion refers to the transfer of blood from one person to another. The person receiving the blood is called recipient and the person giving blood is called donor. Blood transfusion saves life when a person loses blood in accident, delivery and surgery. The blood of the donor and recipient should be typed for ABO and Rh blood groups. The mismatched groups should not be transfused. Before transfusion, cross matching should be performed to ensure that the donor cells are compatible with the recipient plasma.

The transfer of blood from one person to another person is called blood transfusion. The person receiving blood is called recipient. The person donating blood is called donor. In blood transfusion the ABO grouping should be tested. When a recipient receives a wrong blood group, agglutination of blood occurs in the body of the recipient and this leads to his death (table 9.2). In blood transfusion the two most important blood group systems are the ABO system and the Rhesus system. The ABO system divides the blood group into four major groups A, B, AB, and O depending on the presence or absence of the A or B antigens on the red blood cells.

In blood transfusion, one must consider the antibodies of the recipient; the antibodies of the donor have no effect because it is diluted before transfusion. The recipient plasma should not contain any antibody that will damage the donor's red blood cells. Before transfusion, the blood must be screened from infectious disease such as AIDS, hepatitis, syphilis, malaria etc.

A group person can receive blood from another A group person and O group person. He cannot receive blood from AB group person because A group person contains antibody B which reacts with the antigen B of AB group person. Similarly B group person can receive blood from another B group and O group, but not from AB group. AB group person can receive blood from all four groups. O group person can receive blood only from O group and not from any other group. The AB group person is called a universal recipient because he can receive blood from all group. The O group person is called universal donor because he can donate his blood to any group (figure 9.1).

An Rh positive person can safely receive either Rh positive or Rh negative blood. The Rh negative person should be given only Rh- blood. When the recipient is Rh negative, the Rh blood group must be tested. The Rh- individual, receiving Rh+ blood may form antibodies against the Rh antigen. A subsequent transfusion with Rh- blood may cause reaction.

Consequences of mismatched blood transfusion

The donor red cells should not contain antigen that is lacking in the recipient. When the transfused cell contains a foreign antigen, it will stimulate an immune response in the recipient.

It is common practice to give blood transfusion in cases blood loss. Most individuals have IgM antibodies to the major blood group antigen A and B that are expressed on the surface of erythrocytes. Individuals who are blood group A have antibodies to B antigen, those who are blood group B will have anti-A antibodies, and those who are AB will have neither. Those who are blood group O will have both antibodies (figure 9.2). It is therefore important to do blood group typing on transfusion donors and recipients. In most cases, this is done accurately. But occasionally accidents occur whereby blood is given to a recipient who has the reactive isohemagglutinins. This can result in a transfusion reaction which manifests itself as a complement-mediated massive intravascular life – threatening hemolysis.

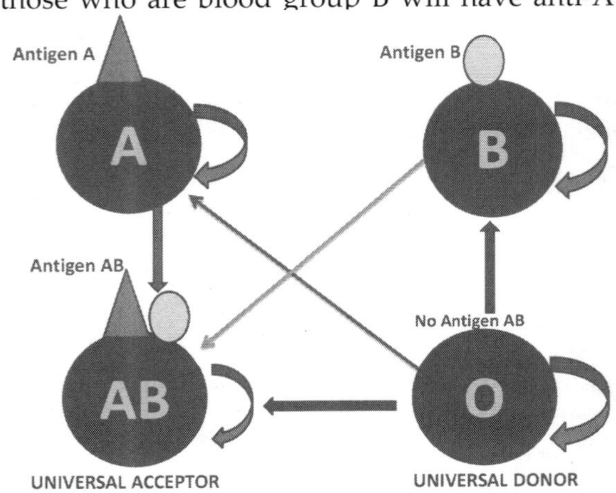

Fig. 9.1 : Blood transfusion. Curved arrows indicate blood transfusion to similar blood group and straight arrows indicates, blood transfusion to other blood groups.

Antibody, alone or together with complement, can cause hypersensitivity reactions that usually result in the direct lysis or removal of cells, hence the alternative name of cytotoxic hypersensitivity. Disease caused by this type of hypersensitivity often involves erythrocytes (autoimmune diseases). Cell death (or lysis) is mediated through normal mechanisms by which antibodies and complement carry out their function including phagocytosis, lysis, and antibody-dependent cellular cytotoxicity. Incompatible transfusion may lead to the clumping and heamolysis of red blood cells.

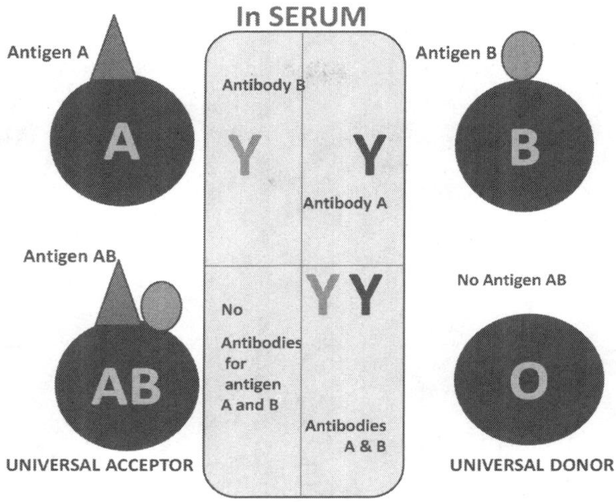

Fig. 9.2 : Antibody/ies found in serum of various blood group antigens

Incompatible transfusion leads to certain clinical symptoms such as shivering, tingling sensation, bursting headache, and severe lumbar pain, cyanosis, feeble pulse, jaundice, oliguria and anuria may also follow.

A negative woman should not be given Rh positive blood because sensitization of negative woman leads to haemolytic disease of the newborn. Rhesus D (RhD) antigen is carried by erythrocytes. Children born to RhD– mother and RhD+ father may express RhD on their erythrocytes. The mother can become sensitized to RhD antigen prior to pregnancy through blood transfusion, or during pregnancy, and especially at birth, by the baby's RhD+ erythrocytes coming into contact with the mother's immune system. Some pass across the placenta but most are released into the maternal circulation during placental shedding. Since RhD is not present in the mother, her immune system responds to it as a foreign antigen and makes antibodies (figure 9.3).

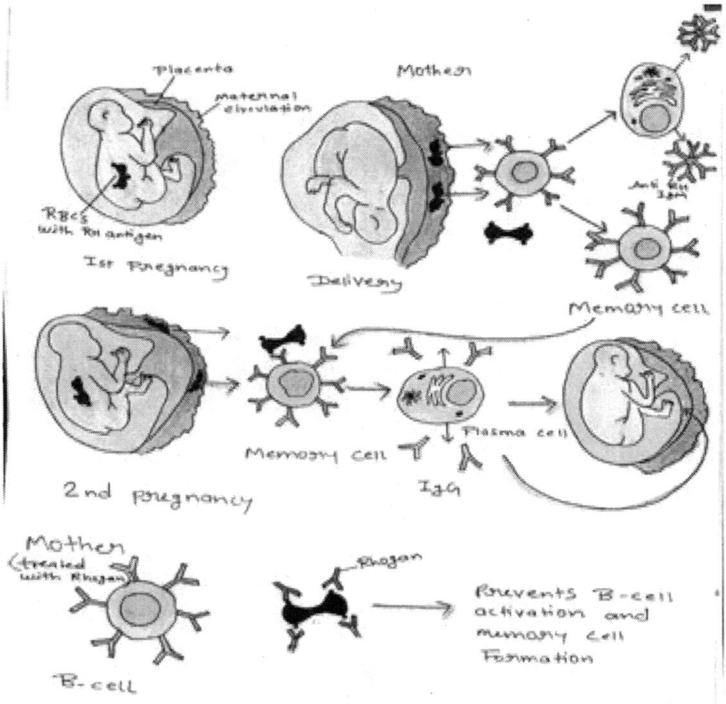

Fig. 9.3 : Rh incompatibility during pregnancy

This is often not a problem during the first pregnancy but in subsequent pregnancies small amounts of erythrocytes passing across the placenta stimulate a memory response leading to specific anti-RhD antibody production. IgG antibodies pass across the placenta and bind to the fetal erythrocytes leading to their opsonization and lysis. If not prevented, this result in hemolytic disease of the newborn (HDN). The destruction of RBC leads to haemolytic jaundice and anemia. The dead RBCs are carried to liver for disintegration. As more work is given to the liver, the liver is heavily damaged. Hydrops foetalis refers to the abnormal accumulation of serous fluid in the tissues or in the body cavity. This causes the death of the baby.

These anti-D antibodies fail to agglutinate RhD+ red cells *in vitro* ("incomplete antibodies") because the low density of antigenic site does not allow sufficient antibody bridges to be formed between the negatively charged erythrocytes to overcome the electrostatic repulsive forces. Erythrocytes coated with anti-D can be made agglutinate by addition of an anti-immunoglobulin serum.

If a mother has natural isohemagglutinins that can react with any fetal erythrocytes reaching her circulation, sensitization to the D- antigens is likely due to "deviation" of the red cells away from the antigen sensitive cells. For example, a group O RhD– mother with a group A RhD+ baby would destroy any fetal erythrocytes with her anti-A before they could immunize to produce anti-D. In an extension of this principle, RhD– mothers are treated prophylactically with IgG anti-D at 28 weeks and 34 weeks gestation and then again at the time of birth if the baby is RhD+. This greatly reduces the risk of sensitization.

Generally, mothers at risk are detected during pregnancy at early routine checks and monitored thereafter. Following each pregnancy with an RhD+ fetus, RhD-mothers are given antibodies to RhD to remove the fetal erythrocytes from the blood stream and suppress the development of a subsequent anti-RhD immune response. Haemolytic disease does not affect all issues of Rh incompatible marriages. Its incidence is much less than the expected figures. This is because of the following factors:

a) Immunological unresponsiveness to the antigen: Certain Rh- individuals will not produce Rh antibodies even after repeated injection of Rh antigens. They are called non – responders. The Rh+ foetus on non –responders will not be affected by haemolytic disease.

b) Foetomaternal ABO incompatibility: when the mother and foetus possess the same ABO group, Rh immunization easily occurs. When Rh and ABO incompatibility coexist, Rh sensitization in the mother is rare. In such instance, the foetus cells entering the maternal circulation are believed to be destroyed rapidly by the ABO antibodies before they can induce Rh antibodies.

c) Number of pregnancies: Usually the first child is not affected by haemolytic disease because the Rh antigen enters the mother only during its delivery. The risk to the foetus increases with the number of pregnancies.

d) Zygosity of the father: When the father is homozygous dominant (DD) for Rh blood group, all his children will meet the risk. But when he is heterozygous (Dd), only 50% of his children will meet the risk because the other 50% will be Rh-.

Hemolytic disease of the newborn caused by Rh incompatibility in a subsequent pregnancy can be almost entirely prevented by administering antibodies against the Rh antigen to the mother within 24–48 h after the first delivery. These antibodies, called Rhogam, bind to any fetal red blood cells that enter the mother's circulation at the time of delivery and facilitate their clearance before B-cell activation and ensuing memory-cell production can take place. In a subsequent pregnancy with an Rh+ fetus, a mother who has been treated with Rhogam is unlikely to produce IgG anti-Rh antibodies; thus, the fetus is protected from the damage that would occur when these antibodies crossed the placenta.

The development of hemolytic disease of the newborn caused by Rh incompatibility can be detected by testing maternal serum at intervals during pregnancy for antibodies to the Rh antigen. A rise in the titer of these antibodies as pregnancy progresses indicates that the mother has been exposed to Rh antigens and is producing increasing amounts of antibody. The presence of maternal IgG on the surface of fetal red blood cells can be detected by a Coombs test. Isolated fetal red blood cells are incubated with the Coombs reagent, goat antibody to human IgG antibody. If maternal IgG is bound to the fetal red blood cells, the cells agglutinate with the Coombs reagent.

If hemolytic disease caused by Rh incompatibility is detected during pregnancy, the treatment depends on the severity of the reaction. For a severe reaction, the fetus can be given an intrauterine blood-exchange transfusion to replace fetal Rh+ red blood cells with Rh– cells. These transfusions are given every 10–21 days until delivery. In less severe cases, a blood-exchange transfusion is not given until after birth, primarily to remove bilirubin; the infant is also exposed to low levels of UV light to break down the bilirubin and prevent cerebral damage. The mother can also be treated during the pregnancy by plasmapheresis. In this procedure, a cell separation machine is used to separate the mother's blood into two fractions, cells and plasma. The plasma containing the anti-Rh antibody is discarded, and the cells are reinfused into the mother in an albumin or fresh-plasma solution.

Another disease resulting from transplacental passage of maternal antibodies is neonatal alloimmune thrombocytopenia. The fall in platelet numbers is greatly ameliorated by intravenous injections of pooled human IgG. The efficacy of Fcγ fragments and of anti- FcγR suggests that this works by blockade of the Fcγ receptors.

Blood Typing

ABO typing of blood is based on the principle of agglutination, type of reaction that occurs between particulate antigen and specific antibodies (agglutinins) that leads to clumping or agglutination of cells. When the cells involved are RBC, the reaction is reaction is termed as hemagglutination. The presence of Rh factor in human blood is determined by agglutination reaction between anti-D typing serum and red blood cells.

Monoclonal antibodies are derived from hybridoma cell lines, created by fusing mouse antibody producing B lymphocytes with mouse myeloma cells of through Epstein-Barr virus (EBV) transformation. Each hybridoma cell line produces homogenous antibodies of only one immunoglobulin class, which are identical in their chemical structure and immunological activity. Since monoclonal antibodies only recognize one epitope, they generally have low cross reactivity with non-specific antigens. Their epitope specificity, limited cross reactivity, and long term yield make monoclonal antibodies attractive for use in many biological assays and application (photograph 1).

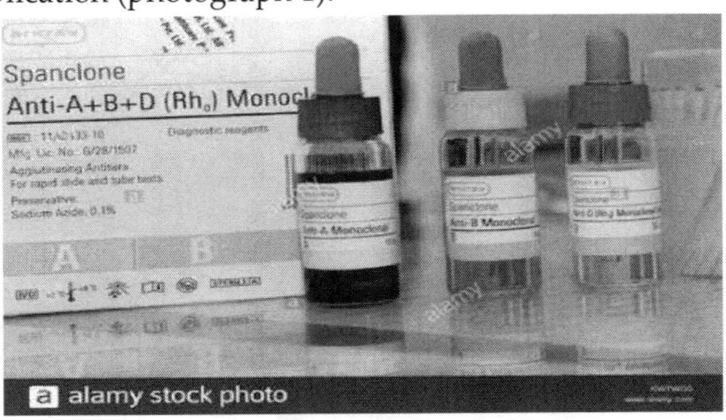

Photograph 1 : Monoclonal antibodies (Anti-A, Anti-B and Anti-D), employed in detection of blood groups.

Human red blood cells possessing A, B and D (Rho) antigen will agglutinate in the presence of antibody directed towards the antigen (table 9.2). Agglutination of red blood cells with Anti-A, Anti-B and Anti-D (Rho) (IgM) reagent is a positive test result and indicates the presence of the corresponding antigen. Absence of agglutination of red blood cells with Anti-A, Anti-B and Anti-B and Anti-D (Rho) (IgM) reagent is a negative test result and indicates the absence of the corresponding antigen (figure 9.4).

Table 9.2- Presence and absence of agglutination reaction upon blood transfusion

		RECIPIENT			
D		A	B	AB	O
O	A	_	+	_	+
N	B	_	_	_	+
O	AB	+	+	_	+
R	O	_	_	_	_

+ Agglutination

- No agglutination

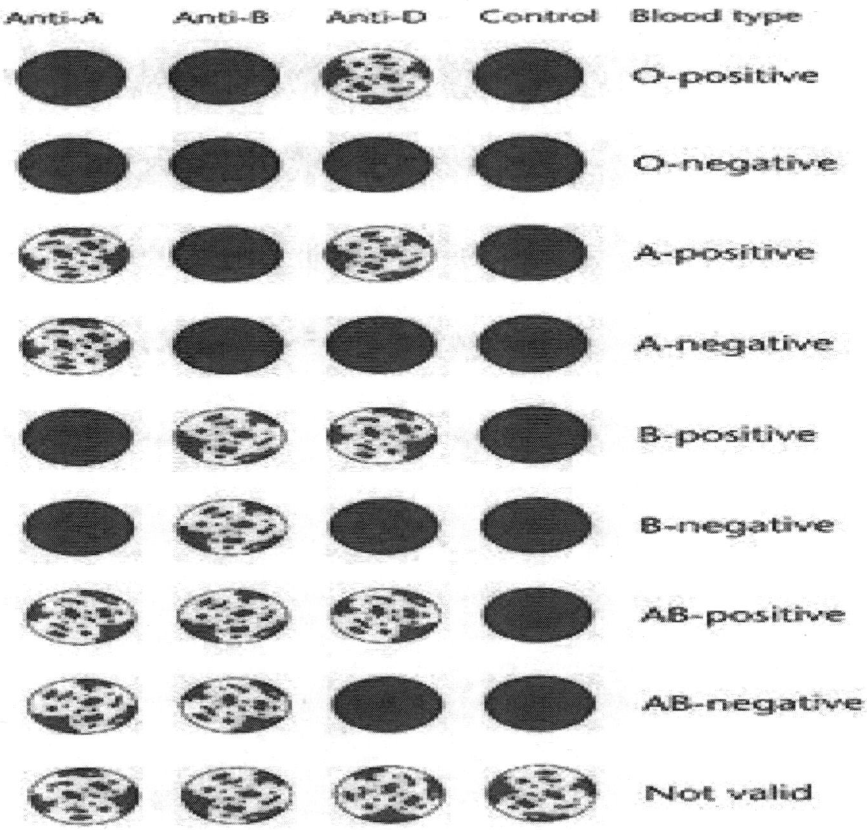

Fig. 9.4 : Visual interpretation of blood groups based on agglutination

How blood grouping is performed?

Reagent and sample are brought to room temperature before testing. Two tests can be performed, slide test and tube test. In slide test one drop each of Anti-A, Anti-B, and Anti-D (Rho) (IgM) reagent is placed on a clean glass slide. To each reagent drop, one small drop (50 μl) of whole blood is added. Mixing is done with a mixing stick uniformly over an area of approximately 2.5cm^2. The slide is gently rocked, back and forth. Agglutination is observed microscopically at two minutes.

In tube test, a 2-3% suspension of the red cells is prepared to be tested in isotonic saline. One drop each of Anti-A, Anti-B, Anti-D (Rho) (IgM) reagent is placed into corresponding labeled test tube. One drop (50 μl) of the test red cell suspension is pipette into each of the test tube, and mixed well. Centrifugation is done for 1 minute at 1000 RPM (125g) or 20 seconds at 3400 RPM (1000g). Agglutination is observed macroscopically.

Agglutination is a positive test result and indicates the presence of the respective red blood cell antigen. Peripheral drying or fibrin are not interpretated as agglutination. No agglutination is a negative test result and indicates the absence of red blood cell antigens (figure 9.3).

Question Bank

1. Very short answer type questions
   (a) Name universal donor.
   (b) Name universal acceptor.
   (c) What is the structure of RBC?
   (d) Name the pigment found in RBC.
   (e) What will be the genotype of blood group A?
   (f) What will be the genotype of blood group B?
   (g) What will be the genotype of blood group AB?
   (h) What will be the genotype of blood group O?
   (i) Who discovered blood group?
2. Short answer type questions
   (a) Define immunohematology.
   (b) Define monoclonal antibodies.
   (c) Why AB blood group is universal recipient?
   (d) Why O blood group is universal donor?
   (e) Why RBC is non-nucleated?
   (f) Define isoantibodies.
   (g) Define isoantigens.
   (h) Define Rhesus factor.
   (i) What is antigen D?
   (j) Define haemagglutination.

3. Long answer type questions
   (a) Describe in detail the blood groups and their significance.
   (b) Describe in detail Erythroblastosis fetalis.
   (c) Describe the importance of Rh factor.
   (d) How is the blood group compatibility checked?
   (e) What are the medical applications of blood groups?
   (f) Describe in detail the genotype and phenotype of all blood groups.

Multiple Choice Questions

1. Rh blood group system was discovered in
   (a) 1941 (b) 1940
   (c) 1939 (d) 1938
2. ABO blood group was discovered by
   (a) Paul Ehlrich (b) Landsteiner
   (c) Gell & Coomb (d) Metnikoff
3. Which antigen is found on surface of RBC of person who has blood group A?
   (a) A (b) B
   (c) AB (d) O
4. Which antibody is found in serum of person with blood group A?
   (a) A (b) B
   (c) AB (d) O
5. Which antigen is found on surface of RBC of person who has blood group B?
   (a) A (b) B
   (c) AB (d) O
6. Which antibody is found in serum of person with blood group B?
   (a) A (b) B
   (c) AB (d) O
7. Which antigen found on surface of RBC of person with blood group AB?
   (a) A (b) B
   (c) AB (d) O
8. Which antibody is found in serum of person with blood group O?
   (a) A (b) B
   (c) AB (d) O
9. Rh positive person has which antigen on his RBC surface?
   (a) A (b) B
   (c) D (d) C
10. Rh negative person does not have this antigen on their RBC surface
    (a) A (b) B
    (c) D (d) O

11. If mother is Rh- and father is Rh+, what will be the blood group of child?
    (a) Rh+ *(b)* Rh-
    (c) May vary *(d)* None of above
12. If the mother's blood group is A and father's blood group is O, what will be the blood group of child?
    (a) A *(b)* B
    (c) AB *(d)* O
13. If the mother's blood group is B and father's blood group is O, what will be the blood group of child?
    (a) A *(b)* B
    (c) AB *(d)* O
14. If the mother's blood group is A and father's blood group is B, what will be the blood group of child?
    (a) A *(b)* B
    (c) AB *(d)* O
15. Which blood group is common?
    (a) Rh+ *(b)* Rh-
    (c) O *(d)* None of above
16. Which blood group is rare?
    (a) A *(b)* B
    (c) AB *(d)* O
17. Which element is required for the formation of blood?
    (a) Co *(b)* Zn
    (c) Fe *(d)* Al
18. Which pigment is found in human blood?
    (a) Haemocyanin *(b)* Haemoglobin
    (c) Erythrocynin *(d)* Phycobillin
19. Which serological test is used to identify blood group?
    (a) Precipitation *(b)* Agglutination
    (c) ELISA *(d)* RIA
20. Blood transfusing needle should be
    (a) Clean *(b)* Washed
    (c) Sterilized *(d)* None of above

Answer Key

Question Number	Answer	Question Number	Answer
1	B	11	A
2	B	12	A
3	A	13	B

Question Number	Answer	Question Number	Answer
4	B	14	C
5	B	15	A
6	A	16	C
7	C	17	C
8	C	18	B
9	C	19	B
10	C	20	C

References

Alcorn J.E., Crowe C.R. &Kolls J.K. (2010) TH 17 cells in asthma and COPD. Annual Review of Physiology 72, 495-516.

Ansari, A. A., et al. 1989. Human immune responsiveness to Loliumperenne pollen allergen Lol p III (rye III) is associated with HLA-DR3 and DR5. Hum. Immunol. 25:59.

Aubry, J. P., et al. 1992. CD21 is a ligand for CD23 and regulates IgE production. Nature 358:505.

Barnes, K.C., and D. G. Marsh. 1998. The genetics and complexity of allergy and asthma. Immunol. Today 19:325.

Bonnefoy, J. Y., et al. 1993. A new pair of surface molecules involved in human IgE regulation. Immunol. Today 14:1.

Borish, L. 1999. Genetics of allergy and asthma. Ann. Allergy Asthma Immunol. 82:413.

Broide D.H. (2009) Immunomodulation of allergic diseases. Annual Review of Medicine 60, 279-291.

Busse, W., and W. Neaville. 2001. Anti-immunoglobulin E for the treatment of allergic disease. Curr. Opin. in Allergy &Immunol.1:105.

Chang, T.W. 2000. The pharmacological basis of anti-IgE therapy. Nat. Biotech. 18:157.

Chapel H., Haeney M., Misbah S. & Snowden N. (2006) Essential of Clinical Immunology,5thedn. Blackwell Publishing Oxford.

Daser, A., et al. 1995. Role and modulation of T-cell cytokines in allergy. Curr. Opin. Immunol. 7:762.

Finkelman, F.D., et al. 1988. IL-4 is required to generate and sustain in vivo IgE response. J. Immunol. 141:2335.

Frew A.J. (2008) Sublingual immunotherapy. New England Journal of Medicine 358

Holt, P. G. 1994. Immunoprophylaxis of atopy: light at the end of the tunnel? Immunol. Today 15:484.

Hoyne, G. F., et al. 1995. Peptide modulation of allergen-specific immune responses. Curr. Opin. Immunol. 7:757.

Kuhn, R., K. Rajewsky, and W. Muller. 1991. Generation and analysis of interleukin-4 deficient mice. Science 254:707.

Lympany, P., et al. 1992. Genetic analysis of the linkage between chromosome 11q and atopy. Clin. Exp. Allergy 22:1085.

Marsh, D. G., et al. The Collaborative Study on the Genetics of Asthma (CSGA). 1997. A genome-wide search for asthma susceptibility loci in ethnically diverse populations. Nat. Genet.15:389.

Marsh, D. G., et al. 1994. Linkage analysis of IL-4 and other chromosome 5q31.1 markers and total serum immunoglobulin E concentrations. Science 264:1152.

Medoff B.D., Thomas S.Y. &Luster A.D. (2008) T cell trafficking in allergic asthma: the ins and outs. Annual Review of Immunology 26, 205-232.

Metzger, H. 1999. It's spring, and thoughts turn to . . . allergies. Cell 97:287.

Meyer E.H., DeKruyff R.H., &Umetsu D.T. (2008) T cells and NKT cells in the pathogenesis of asthma. Annual Review of Medicine 59, 281-292.

Novak, N., S. Kraft, and T. Bieber. 2001. IgE receptors. Curr. Opinion in Immunol. 13:721.

Palomares O. et al. (2010) Role of T regulatory cells in immune regulation of allergic diseases. European Journal of Immunology 40, 1232-1240.

Paul-Eugène, N., et al. 1993. Functional interaction between _2-adrenoceptor agonists and interleukin-4 in the regulation of CD23 expression and release and IgE production in humans. Molec. Immunol. 30:157.

Razin, E., I. Pecht, and J. Rivera. 1995. Signal transduction in the activation of mast cells and basophils. Immunol. Today 16:370.

Romagnani, S. 2001. T-cell responses in allergy and asthma. Curr. Opin. in Allergy &Clin. Immunol. 1:73.

Rosenstreich, D. L., et al. 1997. The role of cockroach allergy and exposure to cockroach allergen in causing morbidity among inner-city children with asthma.N. Engl. J. Med. 336:1356.

Sicherer S.H. & Sampson H.A. (2009) Food allergy: recent advances in pathophysiology and treatment. Annual Review of Medicine 60, 261-277.

Teixeira, M.M., T. J. Williams, and P. G. Hellewell. 1995.Mechanisms and pharmacological manipulation of eosinophil accumulation. Trends Pharmacol. Sci. 16:418.

Thomas, P., et al. 1992. Glycosylation-inhibiting factor from human T cell hybridomas constructed from peripheral blood lymphocytes of a bee venom–sensitive allergic patient. J. Immunol.148:729.

Valenta R. et al. (2010) From allergen genes to allergy vaccines. Annual Review of Immunology 28, 211-241.

CHAPTER 10

Hypersensitivity

Introduction

The immune system normally responds to a variety of microbial invaders with little or no damage to host tissues. However, in some situations, immune responses (especially to some antigens) can lead to more severe tissue-damaging reactions (immunopathology). This "inappropriate response" by the immune system to antigens is referred to as hypersensitivity and is by no means restricted to antigens of microbial origin since it also included both inert and self-antigens (autoimmunity). Immune response is always directed towards the protection of host. But in hypersensitivity the immune response becomes injurious to the host. Hence the immune response becomes a destructive process in hypersensitivity. In protective immune response, the antigens are bacterium or virus is killed or neutralized. But in hypersensitivity, the cells of the host are killed or the host itself is damaged or killed. Hypersensitivity is an exaggerated immune response that results in tissue damage and is manifested in the individual on second or subsequent contact with an antigen. Although the word *hypersensitivity* implies an increased response, the response is not always heightened but may, instead, be an inappropriate immune response to an antigen. Hypersensitive reactions may develop in the course of either humoral or cell-mediated responses. The factors causing hypersensitivity are called allergens. In clinical terms, hypersensitivity is called allergy.

Classification of Hypersensitivity

Paul Portier and Charles Richet coined the term *anaphylaxis,* loosely translated from Greek to mean the opposite of *prophylaxis*. Richet was subsequently awarded the Nobel Prize in Physiology or Medicine in 1913 for his work on anaphylaxis. Hypersensitivity reactions can be classified as either immediate or delayed. In immediate hypersensitivity, the symptoms are manifested within minutes or hours after a sensitized recipient encounters antigen (table 10.1). Delayed-type hypersensitivity (DTH) is so named in recognition of the delay of symptoms until days after exposure. The main difference between immediate and delayed type hypersensitivity is in the nature of the immune response to the antigen. Realizing this fact, Peter Gell and Robert Coombs developed a classification system for reactions responsible for hypersensitivities in 1963. Gell and Coombs proposed a classification scheme in which hypersensitive reactions are divided into four types. Three types of hypersensitivity occur within the humoral branch and are mediated by antibody or antigen-antibody complexes: IgE-mediated (type I), antibody-mediated (type II), and immune complex–mediated (type III). A fourth type of hypersensitivity depends on reactions within the cell-mediated branch, and is termed delayed-type hypersensitivity, or DTH (type IV). Each type involves distinct mechanisms, cells, and mediator molecules. Their system correlates clinical symptoms with information about immunologic events that occur during hypersensitivity reactions.

Table 10.1 - Classification of Hypersensitivity

Time of appearance	Type	Immune mechanism
2-30 min (Immediate)	I	IgE antibodies (acute inflammatory response)
5-8 h (Cytotoxic)	II	Antibody and complement
2-8 h (Immune complex)	III	Antibody- antigen complexes
24-72 h (Delayed)	IV	T-cell mediated
Chronic	V	(can be granulomatous)
		Antibody-mediated stimulation

Factors Causing Hypersensitivity

Factors leading to the development of hypersensitive states include environment, genetics, and age. Moreover, some antigens can induce more than one type of tissue damaging reaction. For example, penicillin can induce type I, II, III, and IV hypersensitivity reactions. Hypersensitivity is caused by numerous factors. These factors causing allergy are called allergens. They may be extrinsic factors (introduced into the body from outside) or intrinsic factors (factors which remain within the body).

They are the following:

1. Drugs such as penicillin, sulphamide, aspirine, etc.
2. Airborne particle such as pollen grains, house dust mite, spores, animal danders (scales and feathers of animals), etc.
3. Food stuffs such as shell fish, strawberries, brinjal, etc.
4. Infectious organisms like bacteria, viruses, fungi, parasite, etc.
5. Blood transfusion of mismatched blood.

Hypersensitivity reactions occur when the normally protective immune system responds abnormally, potentially harming the body. Various autoimmune disorders as well as allergies fall under the umbrella of hypersensitivity reactions, the difference being that allergies are immune reactions to exogenous substances (antigens or allergens), whereas autoimmune diseases arise from an abnormal immune response to endogenous substances (autoantigens). A symptomatic reaction only occurs in sensitized individuals, i.e., they must have had at least one prior asymptomatic contact with the offending antigen. Hypersensitivity reactions are commonly classified into four types. Type I hypersensitivity reactions are immediate allergic reactions (e.g., food and pollen allergies, asthma, anaphylaxis). Type II hypersensitivity reactions are referred to as cytotoxic, as they involve antibodies that are specific to particular tissues within the body and cause destruction of cells in these tissues (e.g., autoimmune haemolytic anaemia, Goodpasture syndrome). Type III hypersensitivity reactions are immune complex-mediated, with tissue damage caused by antigen-antibody complex deposition (e.g., many vasculitides and glomerulonephritides). Type IV hypersensitivity reactions (e.g., TB skin tests, contact dermatitis) are delayed and cell-mediated and are the only hypersensitivity reaction that involves sensitized T lymphocytes rather than antibodies.

Type I Hypersensitivity

Some antigens (allergens), such as insect venom, foods, pollen, and dust mite, can induce the formation of IgE antibodies in individuals with a corresponding predisposition. The IgE antibodies bind via Fc receptors to mast cells (sensitization). If the individual is re-exposed to the allergen, cross-linkage of the membrane-bound IgE occurs (figure 10.1). This results in the immediate release of mediators (e.g., histamine, kininogen), which induce vasodilation, smooth-muscle contraction, mucus secretion, edema, and/or skin blisters. Most allergens are small proteins that can easily diffuse through the skin or mucosa. They are frequently proteases and are active at very low doses. IL-4 favours differentiation of TH2 cells. The exact mechanism that leads B cells to produce IgE is not known.

Type II Hypersensitivity

The immunization of individuals to erythrocyte antigens during pregnancy is a typical example of a type II reaction. Children who inherit the RhD erythrocyte antigen from their father can induce immunization against the RhD+ antigen in their RhD-mother. Sensitization usually occurs at birth when foetal blood cells come into contact with the maternal immune system. In any subsequent pregnancies, maternal anti-RhD antibodies of the IgG type can pass into the placenta and cause severe haemolysis of foetal RhD+ erythrocytes (figure 10.2). Details of blood transfusion reaction and erythroblastosis fetalis has been described in detail in chapter Immunohaematology. Other examples: Drugs (e.g., penicillin) can passively bind to erythrocytes. Antibodies directed against penicillin then lead to lysis of the erythrocytes (figure 10.3). The formation of antibodies directed against the basement membrane (BM) of the glomerulus can develop during the course of kidney inflammation. Lung damage accompanied by pulmonary haemorrhage and renal inflammation (glomerulonephritis) may occur due to cross-reaction of these antibodies with the basement membrane of the lung (Good-pasture's syndrome).

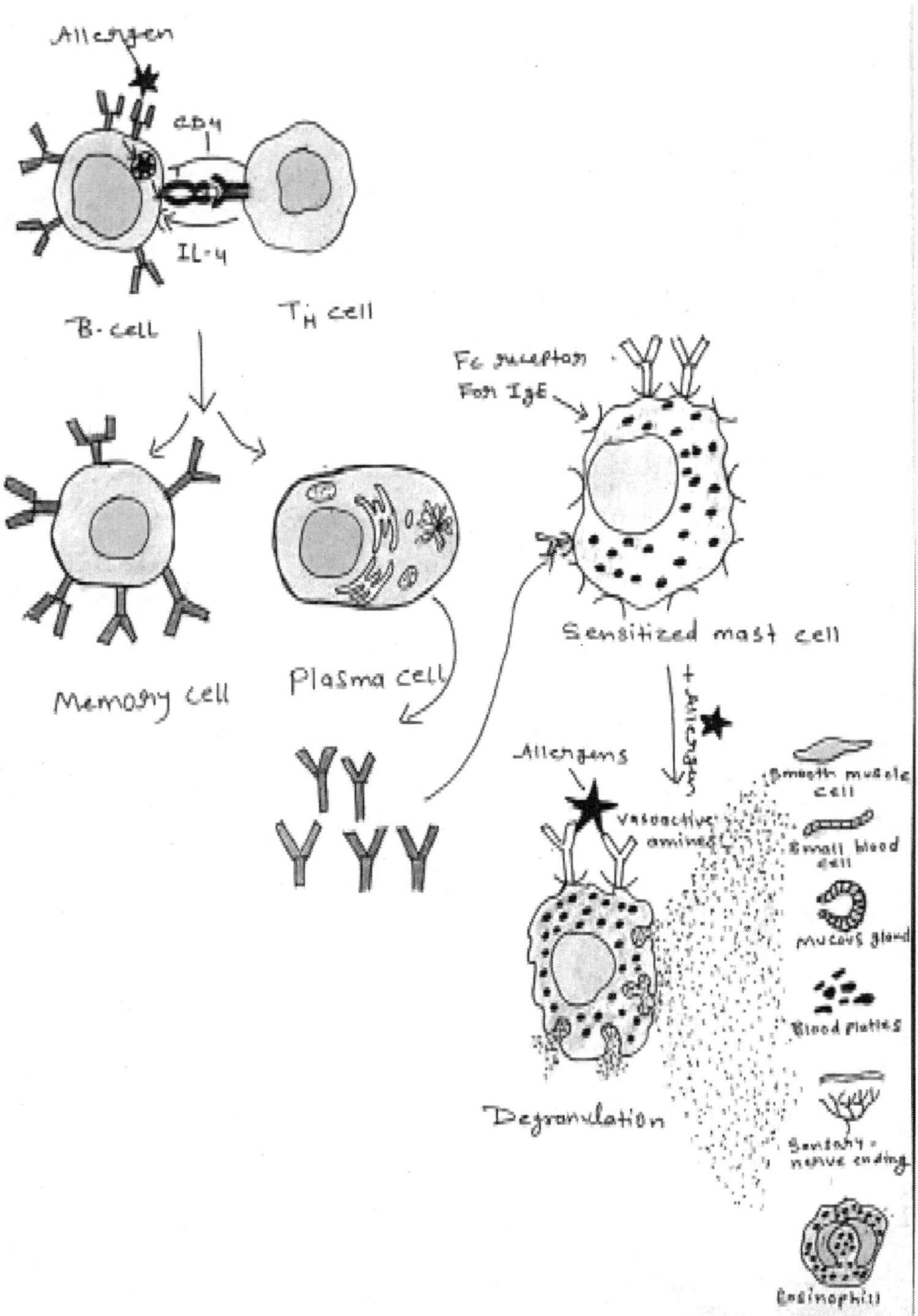

Fig. 10.1 : Type I Hypersensitivity

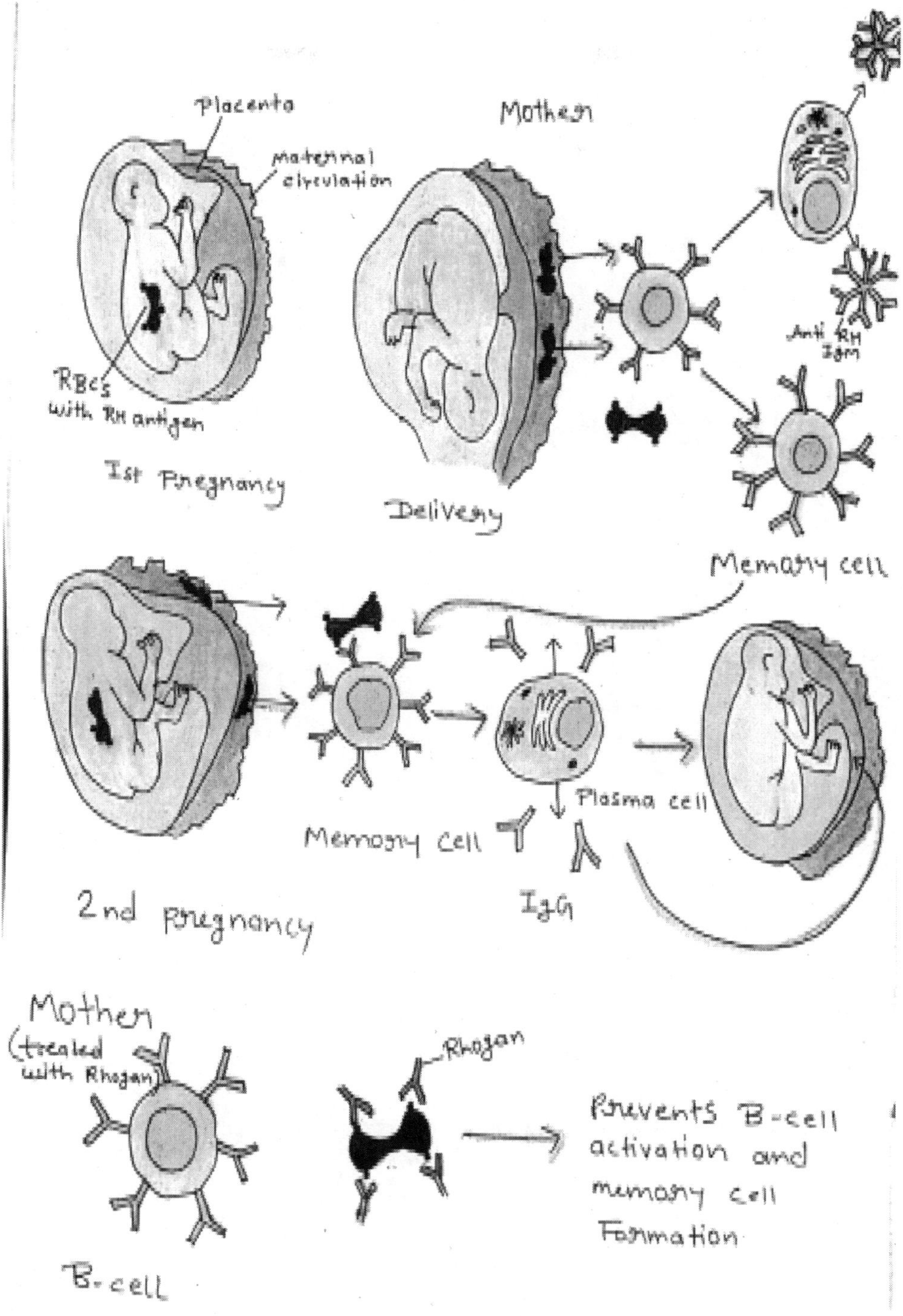

Figure 10.2 – Type II Hypersensitivity (Erythroblastosis fetalis)

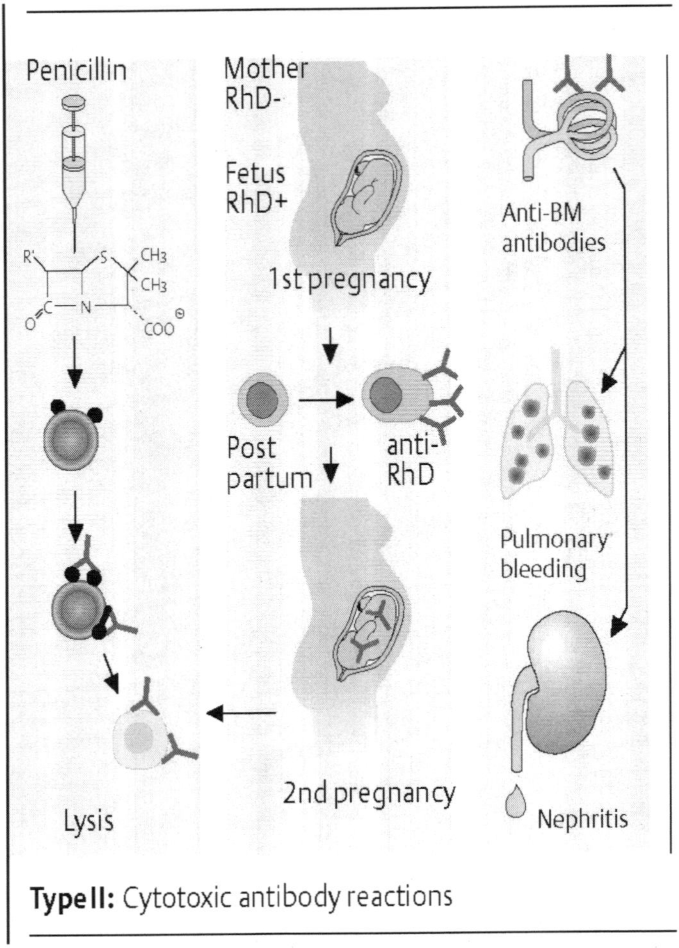

Fig. 10.3 : Penicillin allergy

https://163602-560839-raikfcquaxqncofqfm.stackpathdns.com/wp-content/uploads/2018/03/Type-II-Antibody-mediated-cytotoxic-reaction.jpg

Type III Hypersensitivity

Antibody-antigen complexes (immune complexes) can form during an immune response. Immune complexes can settle in vessel walls, the basement membrane of the lungs and/or kidneys, and in the joints (synovia). They can induce inflammatory processes in these structures by binding complement factors C3a and C5a (anaphylatoxins) (figure 10.4). A particular type III reaction is the Arthus reaction: when an antigen has penetrated the skin of an individual who has preformed IgG antibodies, the immune complexes can bind to Fc receptors of most cells inducing degranulation inflammatory cells are recruited and complement is activated, leading to the release of C5a and local inflammation, platelet accumulation, and eventually to blood vessel occlusion with necrosis (figure 10.5).

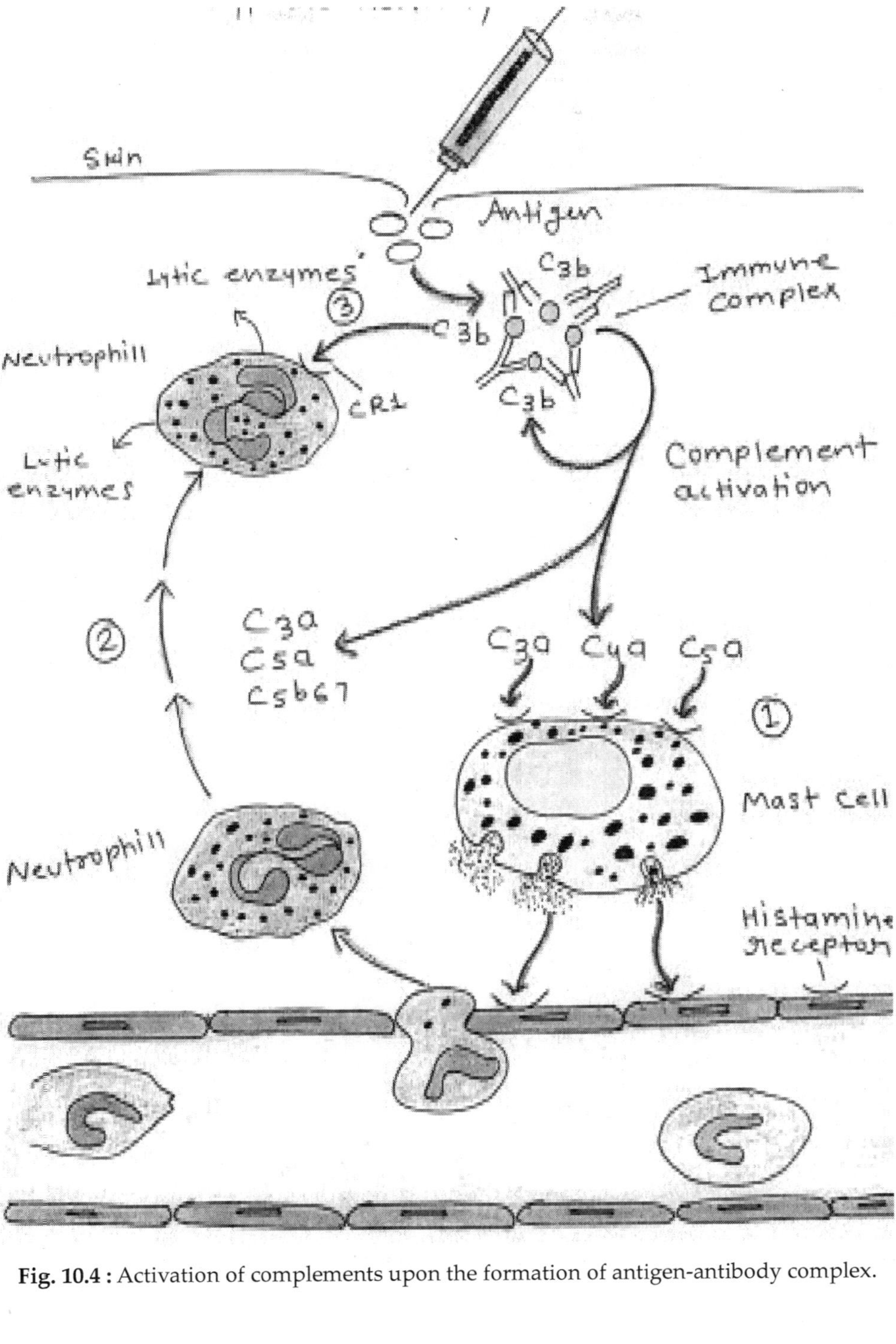

Fig. 10.4 : Activation of complements upon the formation of antigen-antibody complex.

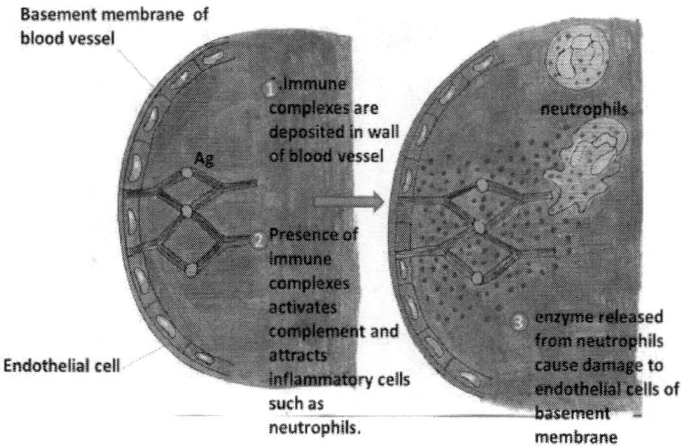

Fig. 10.5 : Type III Hypersensitivity, blood vessel occlusion with necrosis

Type IV Hypersensitivity

Haptens are molecules of very small molecular weight (often < 1 kDa). For example, Pentadecacatechol molecule of poisonous ivy plant. They are too small to function as antigens, but they can penetrate the epidermis and bind to certain proteins in the skin (carrier proteins). Hapten-carrier complexes are bound by antigen-presenting cells of the skin (Langerhans cells) (figure 10.6), which then migrate to regional lymph nodes. T-cell stimulation then occurs at the lymph node. The so-called sensitization phase lasts ca. 10-14 days. If the individual is reexposed to the hapten, antigen-specific T cells migrate to the skin, where they accumulate and proliferate. They also cause edema formation and local inflammation with the help of cytokines. Compounds containing nickel or chrome and chemicals such as those found in rubber are typical triggers of type IV hypersensitivity reactions. Summary of all the types of hypersensitivity is given in figure 10.7.

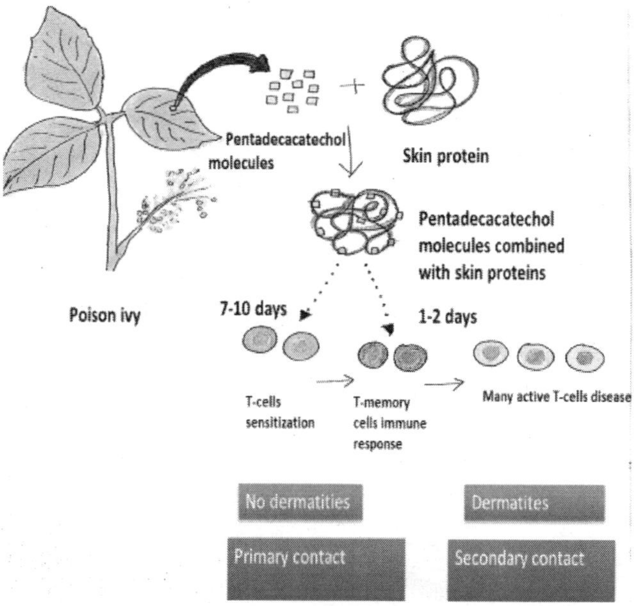

Fig. 10.6 : Type IV Hypersensitivity (Contact Dermatitis)

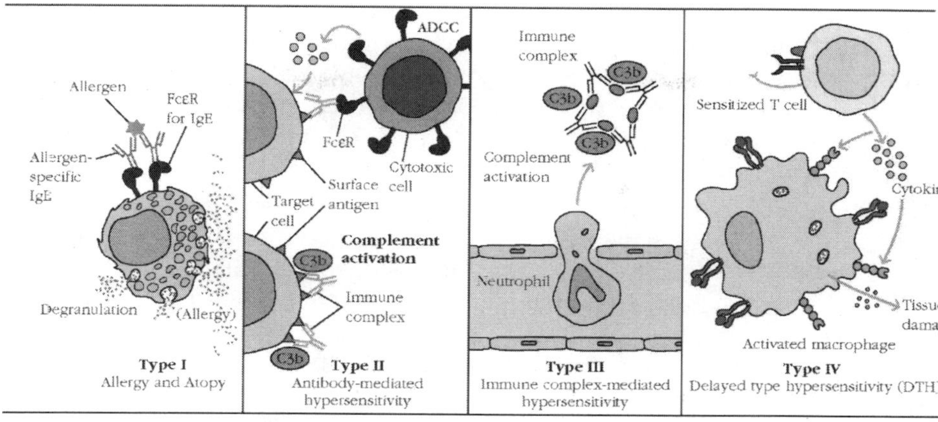

Figure 10.7 : Summary of all types of Hypersensitivities

https://163602-560839-raikfcquaxqncofqfm.stackpathdns.com/wp content/uploads/2018/03/Types-of-Hypersensitivity-Reactions.jpg

Treatment of allergy

Drugs used to treat immediate hypersensitivity act at one of two levels:

1. Inhibitors of the production or release of inflammatory mediators; these include nonsteroidal anti-inflammatory drugs (NSAIDs), such as aspirin and indomethacin, synthetic steroids (glucocorticoids) such as dexamethasone and prednisolone, and the inhibitor of histamine release, cromolyn.
2. Inhibitors of mediator action such as histamine receptor antagonists. Diphenhydramine, chlorphenamine, and cetirizine are representative H_1-blocking agents, which are most useful for relief of the sneezing, rhinorrhea (runny nose) and itching eyes associated with hay fever. They are not useful for bronchial asthma or systemic anaphylaxis, where mediators other than histamine play a more important role. Glucocorticoids also inhibit some of the actions of inflammatory mediators. Other drugs such as epinephrine (adrenaline) and theophyline are used to counteract mediator effect such as low blood pressure and bronchospasm.

More specific treatment involves desensitization that is used to divert the immune response away from a predominantly Th2-driven IgE antibody response and towards a Th1-driven IgG response. This involves injection or ingestion of allergen in low and increasing amounts. Success has been achieved with only a few allergens, for example been venom. A Th1- induced IgG response could have two significant effects. (1) Larger amount of IgG would be produced than IgE and this excess IgG antibody would bind and remove the antigen before it could bind IgE on the mast cell or basophils and trigger degranulation. (2) IgE would also remove antigen before it could bind to and stimulate Th2-drigen IgE-producing B cells, thus decreasing the amount of antigen- specific IgE produced.

Immunotherapy using a monoclonal anti-IgE antibody (omalizumab) has become available for the treatment of asthma and other severe allergic conditions.

This mAb prevents IgE binding to its high- affinity receptor (FceR) on mast cells. Omalizumab is also used in helping to desensitize individuals to insect venoms by allowing increasing concentrations of venom to be used and decreasing the chance of anaphylaxis during desensitizing. Other treatments targeting IL-4 (important for Th2 maturation) or binding IL-4 in situ with recombinant soluble IL-4 receptor (sIL-4R) have shown too little efficacy for patient use.

Future approaches in the treatment of allergy include the involvement of T-regulatory cells. Tregs have been shown to be important in the homeostatic mechanism of the immune system and in the development or prevention of autoimmune disease. Regulation of the immune response is thought in part to be under the control of thymus- derived $CD4^+$ $CD25^+$ Treg cells or $CD4^+$ $CD25^+$ Treg cells that can be induced peripherally from naive T cells. The role of Treg cells in allergy is not understood but would seem important. In experimental models of allergy, $CD4^+$ $CD25^+$ T cells downregulate IgE responses to allergens and, in vitro, suppress the differentiation of Th2 cells from naive CD4 cells. In other in vitro studies of allergy, peripheral blood from atopic individuals has been shown to have reduced suppressive ability in allergen- stimulated T- cell cultures.

Question Bank

1. Very Short Type Answer Questions
   (a) Give full form of ADCC.
   (b) Who gave the term anaphylaxis?
   (c) Who gave the classification of hypersensitivity?
   (d) Which cells are involved in type I hypersensitivity?
   (e) Which cells are involved in type IV hypersensitivity?
   (f) Name the allergens of contact dermatitis
   (g) What is the clinical term for hypersensitivity?
   (h) Name some hypersensitivity reaction.
   (i) Name some vasoactive substances.
2. Short Answer Type Questions
   (a) Define isoimmune.
   (b) Name the substances released during anaphylaxis.
   (c) How to prevent Erythroblastosis fetalis?
   (d) Define serum sickness.
   (e) Define Arthus reaction.
   (f) Define allergy.
   (g) Define hypersensitivity.
   (h) What are the factors that cause hypersensitivity?
   (i) What are the important characteristics of delayed hypersensitivity?
3. Long Answer Type Questions
   (a) Describe in detail the consequences of type I hypersensitivity.
   (b) Describe in detail the consequences of type II hypersensitivity.

(c) Describe in detail the consequences of type III hypersensitivity.
(d) Describe in detail the consequences of type IV hypersensitivity.
(e) Describe in detail the classification of hypersensitivity.
(f) Differentiate between immediate and delayed type hypersensitivity.
(g) Describe in detail contact dermatitis.

Multiple Choice Questions

1. Hypersensitivity is also known as
   (a) Immune Dysfunction
   (b) Allergy
   (c) Immune system gene out of order
   (d) All of the above
2. Hypersensitivity involves
   (a) Humoral Immunity (b) Cell mediated immunity
   (c) Both a and b (d) None of the above
3. Based on the time taken Hypersensitivity is of
   (a) 4 types (b) 3 types
   (c) 2 types (d) 5 types
4. Hypersensitivity is
   (a)beneficial process (b) routine process
   (c) destructive process (d) depends on condition
5. Which of the following is/are hypersensitivity reaction?
   (a) Anaphylaxis (b) Arthus reaction
   (c) Contact dermatitis (d) All of the above
6. Which of the following can cause hypersensitivity?
   (a) Drugs (b) Infectious organisms
   (c) Food Stuffs (d) All of the above
7. Redness of skin due to congestion of capillaries is known as
   (a) Induration (b) Erythema
   (c) Mantoux Rx (d) Erythropoiesis
8. Based on the different mechanism of pathogenesis, hypersensitivity is of
   (a) 2 types (b) 3 types
   (c) 4 types (d) 5 types
9. Which cells are involved in type I hypersensitivity?
   (a) T Cells (b) Null Cells
   (c) Macrophage (d) B Cells
10. Which antibody is involved in anaphylaxis?
   (a) IgD (b) IgE
   (c) IgA (d) IgM

11. Which of the following is true about immediate hypersensitivity?
    (a) At appears and disappears *(b)* Produces Urticaria, Wheal
    (c) Involves T Lymphocytes *(d)* Both a & b are true
12. Mantoux reaction detects the presence of
    (a) Mycobacterium *(b)* Rickettsia
    (c) Streptococcus *(d)* All of the above
13. Which of the following are released during anaphylaxis?
    (a) Histamine *(b)* Serotonin
    (c) PAF *(d)* All Above
14. Arthus reaction is the characteristic of
    (a) Type I Hypersensitivity *(b)* Type II Hypersensitivity
    (c) Type III Hypersensitivity *(d)* Type IV Hypersensitivity
15. Which cells are involved in delayed type hypersensitivity?
    (a) Macrophages *(b)* T Cells
    (c) B Cells *(d)* Null Cells
16. The term anaphylaxis was given by
    (a) Burnet *(b)* Richard Petri
    (c) Richet *(d)* Gell and Coomb
17. Activation of macrophages and release of lytic enzymes by them, takes place in
    (a) Types I Hypersensitivity *(b)* Types II Hypersensitivity
    (c) Types III Hypersensitivity *(d)* Types IV Hypersensitivity
18. Rhogam helps in prevention.
    (a) Types I Hypersensitivity *(b)* Types II Hypersensitivity
    (c) Types III Hypersensitivity *(d)* Types IV Hypersensitivity
19. Insoluble precipitates of immune complex gets attached in and around skin, synovium and choroid plexus in which hypersensitivity?
    (a) Types I Hypersensitivity *(b)*Types II Hypersensitivity
    (c) Types III Hypersensitivity *(d)* Types IV Hypersensitivity
20. When the wrong blood group is transferred, which type of hypersensitivity results?
    (a) Type I *(b)* Type II
    (c) Type III *(d)* Type IV

Answer Key

Question Number	Answer	Question Number	Answer
1.	D	11.	D
2.	C	12.	A
3.	C	13.	D

Question Number	Answer	Question Number	Answer
4.	C	14.	C
5.	D	15.	B
6.	D	16.	C
7.	B	17.	D
8.	C	18.	B
9.	D	19.	C
10.	B	20.	B

References

Alcorn J.F., Crowe C.R. and Kolls J.K. (2010) T_H 17 cells in asthma and COPD. Annual Review of Physiology 72,495-516.

Borish, L. 1999. Genetics of allergy and asthma. Ann. Allergy Asthma Immunol. 82:413.

Broide D.H. (2009) Immunomodulation of allergic disease. Annual Reviws of Medicine 60, 279-291.

Busse, W., and W. Neaville. 2001. Anti-immunoglobulin E for the treatment of allergic disease. Curr. Opin. in Allergy & Immunol.1:105.

Chang, T.W. 2000. The pharmacological basis of anti-IgE therapy. Nat. Biotech. 18:157.

Chapel H., Haney M., Misbah S. and Snowdem N. (2006) Essentials of Clinical Immunology, 5thedn. Blackwell Publishing, Oxford.

Frew A.J. (2008) Sublingual immunotherapy. New England journal of Medicine 358,2259-2264.

Holgate S.T. Church M.K. and Lichtenstein L.M. (2006) Allergy, 3rdedn.Mosdy, London.

Hoyne, G. F., et al. 1995. Peptide modulation of allergen-specific immune responses. Curr. Opin. Immunol. 7:757.

Marsh, D. G., et al. The Collaborative Study on the Genetics of Asthma (CSGA). 1997. A genome-wide search for asthma susceptibility loci in ethnically diverse populations. Nat. Genet. 15:389.

Medoff B.D., Thomas S.Y. and Luster A.D. (2008) T cell trafficking in allergic asthma: the ins and outs. Annual Review Of Immunology 26,205-232.

Metzger, H. 1999. It's spring, and thoughts turn to . . . allergies. Cell 97:287.

Meyer E.H., De Kruyff R.H., and Umetsu D.T (2008) T cells and NKT cells in the pathogenesis of asthma. Annual Reviews of Medicine. 59,281-292.

Novak, N., S. Kraft, and T. Bieber. 2001. IgE receptors. Curr. Opinion in Immunol. 13:721.

Palomares O. at all. (2010) Roll of T regulatory cells in immune regulation of allergic diseases. European Journal of Immunology 40,1232-1240.

Romagnani, S. 2001. T-cell responses in allergy and asthma. Curr. Opin. in Allergy &Clin. Immunol. 1:73.

Rothenberg M.E. and Hogon S.P. (2006) The eosinophil. Annual Review of Immunology 24,147-174.

Sicherer S.H. and Sanpson H.A. (2009) Food allergy: Recent advances in Pathophysiology and treatment. Annual Review of Medicine 60,261-277.

Valenta R. et al (2010) From allergen genes to allergy vaccines. Annual Reviews of Immunology 28,211-241.

Wills-Karp, M., J. Santeliz, and C. L. Karp. 2001. The germless theory of allergic disease: revisiting the hygiene hypothesis. Nature Rev. Immunol. 1:69.

CHAPTER 11

Immunodeficiency Diseases

Introduction

The disease caused by the defects in the immune system is called immunodeficiency disease. Immunodeficiency refers to the defect in the immune system resulting in the depression or hypo function of the immune system. Defects in one or more components of the immune system can result in its failing to recognize and respond properly to antigens. Such immunodeficiencies can make a person more prone to infection than those people capable of a complete and active immune response. Most defects that lead to immunodeficiencies affect either one or the other. The lymphoid cell disorders may affect T cells, B cells, or, in combined immunodeficiencies, both B and T cells. The myeloid cell disorders affect phagocytic function. Most of the primary immunodeficiencies are inherited, and the precise molecular variations and the genetic defects that lead to many of these dysfunctions have been determined.

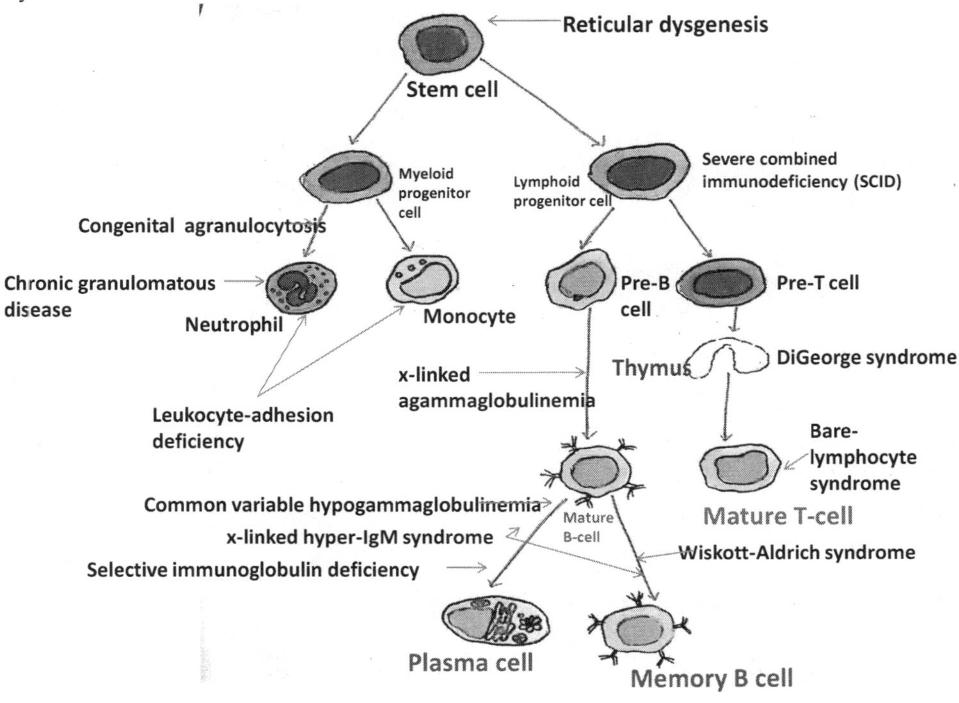

Fig. 11.1 : Immune system cells in various immunodeficiency diseases

The consequences of primary immunodeficiency depend on the number and type of immune system components involved. Defects in components early in the hematopoietic developmental scheme affect the entire immune system. In this category is reticular dysgenesis, a stem-cell defect that affects the maturation of all leukocytes; the resulting general failure of immunity leads to susceptibility to infection by a variety of microorganisms. Reticular dysgenesis is a immunodeficiency disease caused by a defective gene. The defective gene causes stem cell deficiency (figure 11.1). Stem cell deficiency is a defect of haemopoietic origin. In this defect, primordial, stem cell fails to differentiate into mature lymphocyte, macrophages and granulocytes. This disease results in a complete lack of lymphocytes both in the circulation and bone marrow. This disease mainly affects male infants. They are prone to severe infection and they live for not more than 3 days to 3 months. The infection in this disease can be controlled by treating with antibiotics. This disorder may be treated with bone marrow transplantation.

Patients can be immunocompromised by many factors that effects either innate defense mechanism or the adaptive immune system. The immunodeficiency diseases can be classified as either primary - usually congenital (the result of improper development of the innate, and/or cellular immune system), or secondary, that is, acquired (the consequences of other disease, their treatment, or other factors). Primary immune deficiencies are relatively rare diseases. Defects can occur in neutrophil function, the complement system, or in T-or B-lymphocyte function. Chronic granulomatous disease, one of the best-known examples, is due to an impaired ability of neutrophils to kill organisms that have been phagocytosed, rendering patients susceptible to treatment infection with Staphylococcus aureus and other microorganisms. Many other factors such as defects of neutrophil function [e.g. chronic granulomatous disease (CGD)], defects in the complement system, genetic disease altering B or T lymphocyte function [e.g. Severe Combined Immune Deficiency (SCID)] are responsible for primary immunodeficiency (figure 11.1).

1. Primary immunodeficiency

Despite the increase in knowledge of functional derangements and cellular abnormalities in the various immunodeficiency disorders, the fundamental biological errors responsible for them remain largely unknown. To date, most genetic errors associated with these immunodeficiencies are located on the X chromosome and produce primary or congenital immunodeficiency. The depression of immune response causes a number of diseases called immunodeficiency diseases. The defect of the immune system caused by the defective genes is called primary immunodeficiency. Primary immunodeficiency illuminates the importance of individual components of the immune system in combating particular infectious disease. Primary immunodeficiency may be of the following types:

1. T-cell deficiency (table 11.1)
2. B-cell deficiency (table 11.2)
3. Complement deficiency (table 11.3)

4. Phagocyte cell deficiency (table 11.4)
5. Hereditary neutropenia

Table 11.1 : Diseases resulting from T-cell deficiency

Deficiency	Disease
Lack of a thymus	**DiGeorge syndrome** Also known as congenital thymic aplasia, is a defect in thymus embryogenesis leading to incomplete development of the thymus and thus decreased T-cell number. The thymus fails to develop. As thymus is absent, stem cell cannot differentiate to become T cells. The thymus dependent areas of lymph nodes and spleen are devoid of lymphocytes. Cell – mediated immune response is depressed. Parathyroid cardiovascular tissues are also defective. It causes a complex of diseases associated with endocrine and cardiovascular abnormalities such as hypocalcaemic seizures, congenital heart diseases, oesophageal atresia and so on. It occurs in both male and female infants. This developmental defect, which is associated with the deletion in the embryo of a region on chromosome 22, causes immunodeficiency along with characteristic facial abnormalities (photograph 1), hypoparathyroidism, and congenital heart disease. Role of thymus in combating Mycobacterium diseases are researched using mice whose thymus is removed (photograph 2).
Stem cell defect (Photograph 3)	Severe Combined Immunodeficiency disorders (SCID) SCID is primary immunodeficiency disease caused by defective B as well as T-cell. It is a severe congenital disease where death results in one or two years. Humoral and cell–mediated immune responses are depressed. The patient is highly susceptible to infection (photograph 3). Thymus is very small. The patient can be treated with transplantation of bone marrow. SCID occurs due to mutation in the RAG 1 and RAG 2 genes critical to TCR rearrangement, maturation past the pro-T-cell stage does not occur. Null mutation in a number of different genes, including ADA, JAK-3, Artemis and IL-7R α chain result in SCID. There is a complete block in the development of T-cells and thus complete lack of help for B-cells. Depending on the particular gene defect, B-cells and/or NK cells may also be absent. SCID infants suffer from chronic diarrhea, pneumonia, and skin, mouth, and throat lesions as well as a host of other opportunistic infections. The immune system is so compromised that even live attenuated vaccines (such as the Sabin polio vaccine) can cause infection and disease.
Variable T-cell function	**Hereditary ataxia telangiectasia (AT)** Severe sinus/lung infection due to mutations in a DNA-repair gene. Chromosome breaks. It includes deficiency of IgA and sometimes of IgE. The syndrome is characterized by difficulty in maintaining balance (ataxia) and by the appearance of broken capillaries (telangiectasia) in the eyes.

T cells don't help B Cells

Wiscot-Aldrich syndrome (WAS)

The severity of this X-linked disorder increases with age and usually results in fatal infection or lymphoid malignancy. The syndrome includes thrombocytopenia (lowered platelet count; the existing platelets are smaller than usual and have a short half-life), which may lead to fatal bleeding (photograph 4). X-linked mutation in a gene occurs, that encodes adapter proteins sialophorin (CD43). This protein is required for assembly of actin filaments required for the formation of microvesicles.

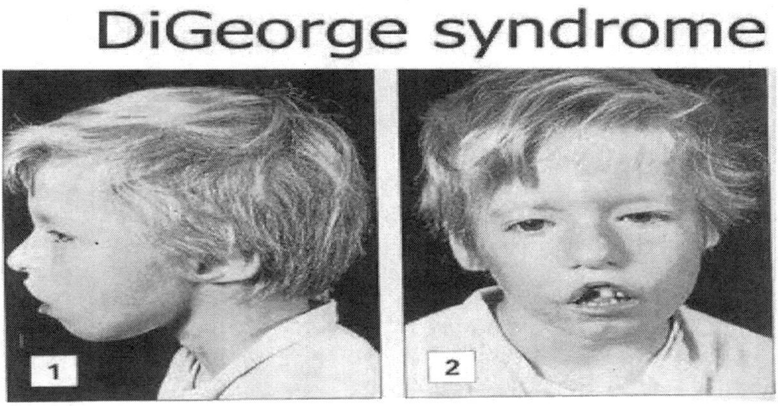

Photograph 1 - DiGeorge syndrome

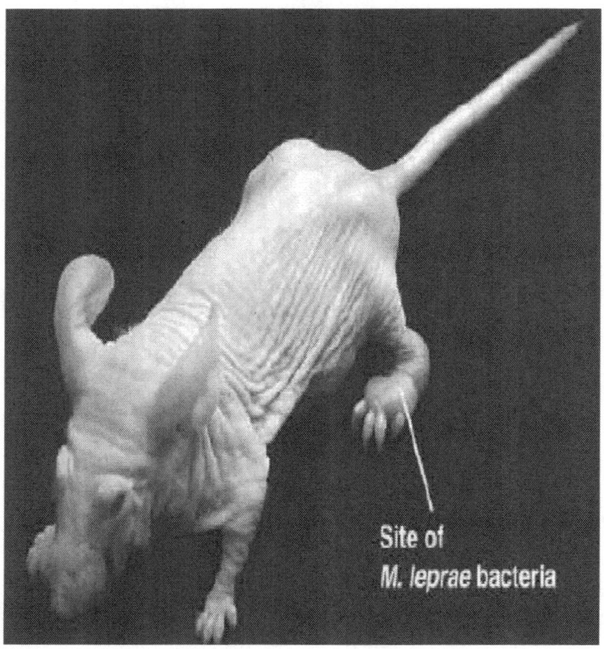

Photograph 2 : Nude Mice with no thymus, employed for Leprosy research

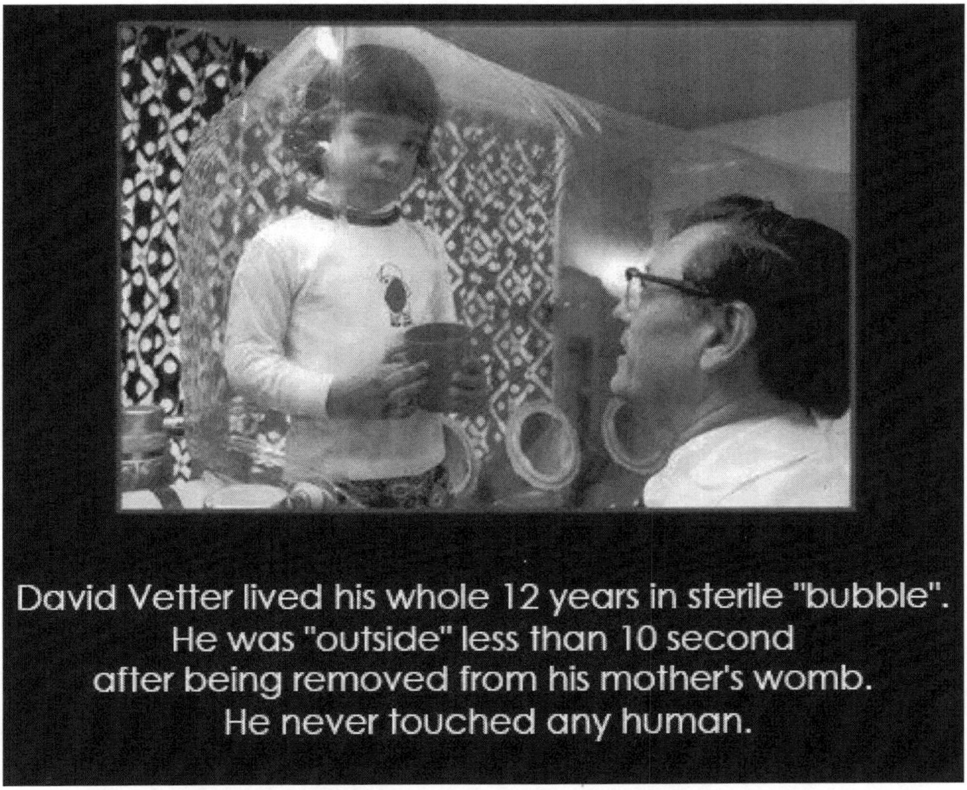

Photograph 3 : Severe Combined Immunodeficiency disorders (SCID)

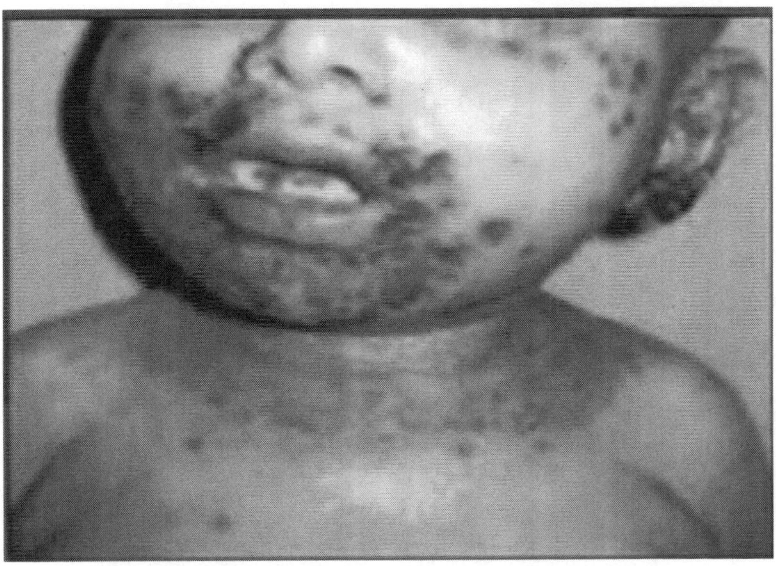

Photograph 4 : Wiscot-Aldrich syndrome (WAS)

Table 11.2 : Diseases resulting from B-cell deficiencies

Stage of differentiation/ maturation	Disease
Lack of development of stem cells into pre-or pro-β cells	**Severe combined immunodeficiency** (SCID) This deficiency is due to ADA/PNP or RAG deficiency; also, effects T-cells development
B cells fail to develop from B-cell precursors	**Bruton's agammaglobulinaemia** It is congenital. Bruton's agammaglobulinaemia is a primary immunodeficiency disease caused by a defective gene characterized by the absence of agammaglobulinaemia (antibodies), mostly X-linked; It is due to a defective gene encoding a tyrosine kinase involved in activation of pre-B cell to immature B cells; T cells are normal. In this disease, B-cells are defective and they fail to differentiate into mature B-cells. Hence B-cells are absent from circulation. Antibodies, especially IgG type, are not produced. Hence humoral immune response is depressed. Plasma cells are not produced. Lymphoid tissues hypoplastic and B-cell dependent areas are poorly developed. This disease mostly affects male infants and the affected infants are subject to repeated infection by pyogenic bacteria – Staph infection by pyogenic bacteria like Staphylococcus aureus, Streptococcus pyogenes, S. pneumonia, Neisseria meningitis, Hemophilus influenza, etc.
B cells do not class switch from IgM	**Hyper- IgM syndrome** It is characterized by increased level of IgM but little or no IgG in the circulation; due to defect in genes encoding CD40L on activated T cells
IgG/IgA deficiency	**Common variable immunodeficiency (CVID)** Defect include inability of B cells to mature into plasma cells and defective T-cell help; IgA deficiency is most common (1 in 700 people)
Antibody deficiency yearly in life	**Transient hypogammaglobulinemia** – It is thought to be the result of intrinsic maturational B cell defect and/or one involving T-helper cells

Table 11.3 : Diseases resulting from Complement deficiencies

Complement deficient	Disease caused/infection
Regulatory components C1q inhibitor	Hereditary angioedema (continuous complement activation and consumption
Decay accelerating factor, DAF, (CD55)	Paroxysmal nocturnal hemoglobulinuria (lysis of blood cells)
Complement components C1, C2, or C4	Immune complex disease, Ag-Ab complexes not removed: C2 deficiency associated with SLE
C3	Most serious; infection with pyogenic bacteria
MAC (membrane attack complex) C5-8, C9	Meningococcal infection, e.g., *Neisseria* Asymptomatic

Table 11.4 : Diseases resulting from phagocytic defects

Defect in	Disease/mechanism
Stem cell differentiation	**Neutropenia** Characterized by too few neutrophils to adequately remove microbes
Adhesion to endothelium for margination	**Leukocyte adhesion deficiency (LAD)** Defective CD18 (due to gene mutation), a critical leukocyte function-associated (LFA) molecule. LAD causes susceptibility to infection with both gram-positive and gram-negative bacteria as well as various fungi. Impairment of adhesion of leukocytes to vascular endothelium limits recruitment of cells to sites of inflammation.
Phagocytosis	**Chediak-Higashi syndrome** It is due to failure of phagolysosome formation and lysosome degranulation caused by a mutation of the LYST (Lysosomal trafficking) gene that encodes a lysosomal trafficking regulator. Accumulation of giant intracytoplasmic granules occurs due to defective migration of the late endosomal/lysosomal compartment within the cell. The patient suffers from sometimes fatal pyogenic infections, particularly with Staphylococcus aureus (photograph 5)
Intracellular killing	**Chronic granulomatous disease (CGD)** In this disease the monocytes, macrophages and neutrophils fail to produce reactive oxygen intermediates (ROIs) due to defect in genes encoding the proteins making up the NADPH (nicotinamide adenine dinucleotide phosphate) oxidase system involved in oxygen-dependent killing within the phagolysosome. CGD sufferers undergo excessive inflammatory reactions that result in gingivitis, swollen lymph nodes, and nonmalignant granulomas (lumpy subcutaneous cell masses); they are also susceptible to bacterial and fungal infection (photograph 6).
IFN γ or IL-12 receptors	Mycobacterial infections; failure to activate NADPH oxidase

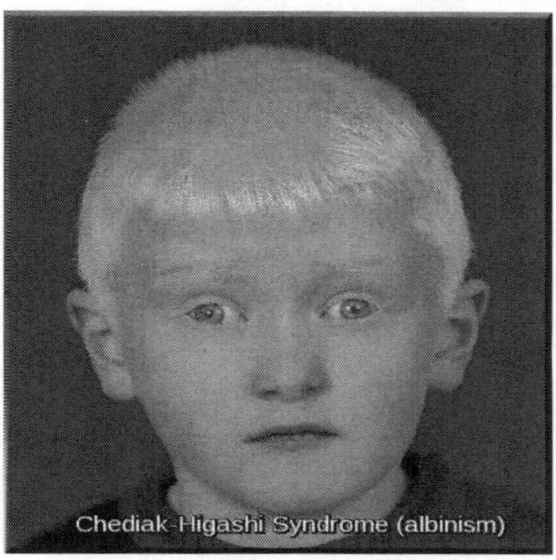

Photograph 5 : Chediak-Higashi syndrome

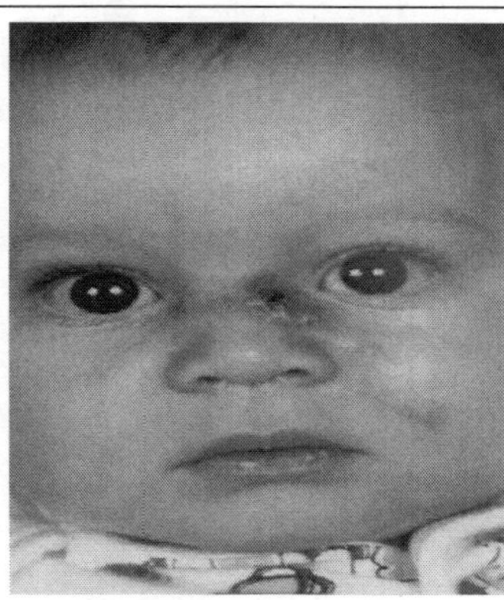

Photograph 6 : Chronic granulomatous disease (CGD)

2. Hereditary neutropenia

It is caused by myeloid cell deficiency. The neutrophils are defective in this disease. The count may be less than 500 per mm^3. This leads to infection with bacteria and inflammation of epithelial surface such as skin. Neutrophils have a short life span, and their precursors must divide rapidly in the bone marrow to maintain levels of these cells in the circulation. For this reason, agents such as radiation and certain drugs (e.g., chemotherapeutic drugs) that specifically damage rapidly dividing cells are likely to cause neutropenia.

There are a variety of causes of neutropenia, but the commonest cause is cancer chemotherapy, particularly for hematological malignancies. The extent and duration of neutropenia vary with the different chemotherapy regimens. The risk of infection is significantly increased when the circulating neutrophil count falls to $< 0.5 \times 10^9$ and is very high with counts $<0.1 \times 10^9$. Infection risks are also related to the duration of neutropenia. For example, the risks of invasive fungal infection particularly increase with neutropenia lasting 14 days.

Patients with neutropenia who develop a temperature are said to have febrile neutropenia. There many causes of febrile neutropenia, but the principal pathogens are gram positive and negative bacteria and fungi. Gram-positive bacteria are common causes of bacteremia in neutropenic patients, with the portal of entry often being an indwelling central venous catheter. Enterococci, including strains that are vancomycin-resistant are also encountered.

Gram-negative bacteria can cause spontaneous septicemia in neutropenic patients, by bacterial translocation from the gastrointestinal tract into the bloodstream. This arise due to -

a) Chemotherapy-induced mucosal damage in the gastrointestinal tract

b) Impaired phagocytosis in the reticuloendothelial system.

Pseudomonas aeruginosa septicemia is associated with a particularly high mortality in this setting. The principal fungal pathogens are Candida species and Aspergillus. Anaerobes are an important cause of preanal infection, and Clostridium tertium is associated with a particular condition.

Microbiological diagnosis of febrile neutropenia is principally by blood cultures, but cultures are negative in a significant proportion of episodes, and the diagnosis of invasive fungal infections is difficult. Treatment of febrile neutropenia is with empiric broad-spectrum antibiotics that include activity against Pseudomonas aeruginosa and other Gram negative bacteria. Antibiotic therapy is adjusted when culture and sensitivity results become available. Patients not respond to the first-line regimen and second-line agents, including antifungal drugs may need to be used.

I. Secondary/ acquired, immunodeficiency

Immune responsiveness can be depressed nonspecifically by many factors. Cell mediated immunity in particular may be impaired in a state of malnutrition, even of the degree which may be encountered in urban areas of more affluent regions of the world. Iron deficiency is particularly important in this respect, as are zinc and selenium deficiencies. Secondary, or acquired, immunodeficiency is by far the most common immunodeficiency and contributes a significant proportion to hospital admission. Secondary immunodeficiency refers to the depression of the immune response, caused by many factors other then genetical. Factors causing secondary immunodeficiency mainly affect phagocytic and lymphocyte functions and include infections (HIV), malnutrition, tumors, cytotoxic, drugs, aging, and trauma.

Factors causing acquired immunodeficiency

1. **Tumors**

   A variety of immunosuppressive molecules, including IL-10, TGFB, vascular endothelial growth factor VEGF, and prostaglandins, produced by tumors. In addition, cells of the adaptive immune system may be induced by tumors to suppress anti-tumor immune responses. These cells include regulatory T (Treg) cells that can mediate immunosuppressive by cell-cell contact or through release of soluble molecules. Cells of the innate immune system, for example myeloid suppressor cells (MSCs), can also be recruited by tumour cells to suppress anti-tumour immunity. Thus, in developing therapeutic approaches to tumor eradication, specially those designed to induce or enhance host immunity to the tumor, consideration must be given to ways of circumventing these tumor-associated immunosuppressive factors.

2. **Therapy using cytotoxic drugs and irradiation**

   Cytotoxic drugs and irradiation that especially target dividing cells are widely used for tumor therapy. Cytotoxic drugs are also used to suppress allogeneic graft rejection in patients receiving kidney or other grafts. These therapies also kill normal immune cells, including stem cells, neutrophil progenitors, and rapidly dividing precursors for all leukocytes, and thus compromise immune defence against pathogens.

3. **Immune senescence: consequences of aging**

   As one ages, changes occur in immune status. Reduce responses to vaccination and increased risk of infectious disease in the elderly are the result of reductions in immune function. The most striking of these changes is the involution of the thymus and the subsequent decrease in T cell education is significantly decreased and the host becomes more dependent on the pool of T cells generated earlier in life.

   As one ages, memory T cells increase and navie cells decrease, resulting in an accumulation of activated T cells and fewer native cells entering the pool. In addition, the ability of T cells from aged individuals to expand is limited, thus further diminishing cell- mediated immune responses. There are also age associated reductions in humoral immunity, at least one part of which results in reduced B-cells development in the bone marrow and thus reduced B cells diversity. This is manifest as a change in the quantity of the antibody response, including a decrease antibody affinity, a diminished response to vaccines, and an increase in auto-antibody production. Overall, the immune system appears to shift with age from one dependent primarily on adaptive immune responses to one somewhat more dependent on innate immunity.

4. **Trauma**

After significant trauma, including that associated with burns or major surgery the immune system seems less able to deal with pathogens. Although the basis for this apparent immunodeficiency is not understood, it is possible that these traumatic events induce release of immunomodulatory factors. E.g. (glucorticoids) which dampen immune responses. Removal of the spleen, the primary organ for removing microbes from the circulation (e.g. after an accident) results in decreased phagocytosis of microbe and thus increased susceptibility to blood-borne infections, especially to infections by encapsulated bacteria, for example Pneumococci.

Recognition of Immunodeficiency

A large number of specific congenital and acquired abnormalities in the immune system have been identified that contribute to patient susceptibility to recurrent infections. These abnormalities range from those that affect the immune system very early in life, and thus compromise immune response to many antigens, to those that effect the final stages of differentiation of particular immune cells and hence lead to very selective abnormalities. A more pathophysiological description characterizes the unspecific immune component that is abnormal by defining qualitative abnormalities of the cells (lymphocytes, phagocytosis) and/or molecules (antibodies, cytokines, complement components) of the immune system. Immunodeficiency can be detected by the following methods:

1. Immunoglobulin deficiency can be tested by the quantitative estimation of antibodies. Levels of 2 g/1 define the lower limit of normal.
2. The deficiency of humoral immune response by inducing active immunization with diphtheria, tetanus, pertussis and killed poliomyelitis vaccines.
3. T - cell deficient patients are unreactive in skin tests to antigens such as tuberculin, Candida, Trichophyton and mumps.

Secondary defects in innate defense mechanism

Many patients are rendered more susceptible to infection through damage to normal intact skin normally provides a very effective barrier to invention of underlying tissues by microorganisms. But this barrier can be damaged in a variety of ways including burns, surgical incision, indwelling intravenous catheters. Burn wounds can be colonized and infected with a variety of bacteria, particularly Staph aureus, B-hemolytic Streptococcus and Pseudomonas aeruginosa. Invasive infection and septicemia may than follow. Infection with B-hemolytic streptococci can also cause damage to skin grafts, and outbreaks may occur in burns units.

Surgical wound infections are a common healthcare associated infection. The principal pathogen Staph aureus, and many of these are now methicillin-resistant.

Infections with B-hemolytic streptococci are less common, but often serious. Polymicrobial wound infection with Coliforms, Enterococci and anaerobes can occur following gastrointestinal or gynecological surgery.

. Indwelling intravenous catheter can allow entry of bacteria and other organisms directly into the bloodstream causing bacteremia. Infection can occur with conventional pathogens but also with more opportunistic pathogens.

A breach of normal mucosal defense can also lead to an increased risk of infection. One of the commonest examples is the increased risk of urinary tract infections in patients with an indwelling urinary catheter. There is also a greatly increased risk of lower respiratory tract infection in patients who are ventilated via an endotracheal tube.

Secondary defects in adaptive immune mechanisms

A wide variety of diseases can impact on the proper functioning of normal immune mechanisms, rendering patients at increased risk of infection. Different patients of infection are associated with each of these factors. Some of these infections also occur in non-immunocompromised hosts, but they occur with a greater frequency in immunocompromised patients. Other infections occur with opportunistic pathogens - microorganisms that are usually harmless to healthy individual, but capable of causing infection in immunocompromised hosts. The range and pattern of opportunistic infection varies according to the nature of the immunocompression, with the widest range of opportunistic pathogens found in the most immunosuppressed patients. AIDS is one such type of secondary immunodeficiency disease.

AIDS is an epidemic viral disease of humane population. It called acquired immune deficiency syndrome. AIDS is caused by the infection of RNA virus on lymphocytes. As a result, the T- helper cells are depressed. This leads to the suppression of the immune system. Hence the name immune deficiency. As the immune system is depressed, the individual is susceptible to infection and a series of disease develops until his death. As the initial infection virus, paves way for the development of a complex of disease, it is called a syndrome. AIDS is caused by an RNA virus called human immune deficiency virus abbreviated as HIV. It is a class of retrovirus and was discovered by Luc Montagnier in 1983. Formerly the HIV was named as LAV (Lymphadenopathy Associated Virus) and IDAV (Immune Deficiency Associated Virus). This virus is also called HTLV-3 (Human T-cell Leukemia Virus-3). The human immunodeficiency virus (HIV) is an RNA virus. HIV belongs to retroviruses. It utilizes reverse transcriptase to convert RNA to DNA. It is spherical in shape. The virus consists of an outer coat called capsid and an inner core. The capsid is a glycoprotein. The core contains two strands of RNA, protein and the enzyme reverse transcriptase (figure 2).

The morphologic structure of HIV-1

HIV-1 viral particles have a diameter of 100 nm and are surrounded by a lipoprotein membrane. Each viral particle contains 72 glycoprotein complexes, which are integrated into this lipid membrane, and are each composed of trimers of an external glycoprotein gp120 and a transmembrane spanning protein gp41.

The bonding between gp120 and gp41 is only loose and therefore gp120 may be shed spontaneously within the local environment. Glycoprotein gp120 can be detected in the serum as well as within the lymphatic tissue of HIV-infected patients. During the process of budding, the virus may also incorporate different host proteins from the membrane of the host cell into its lipoprotein layer, such as HLA class I and II proteins, or adhesion proteins such as ICAM-1 that may facilitate adhesion to other target cells. The matrix protein p17 is anchored to the inside of the viral lipoprotein membrane. The p24 core antigen contains two copies of HIV-1 RNA. The HIV-1 RNA is part of a protein-nucleic acid complex, which is composed of the nucleoprotein p7 and the reverse transcriptase p66 (RT). The viral particle contains all the enzymatic equipment that is necessary for replication: a reverse transcriptase (RT), an integrase p32 and a protease p11(figure 11.2).

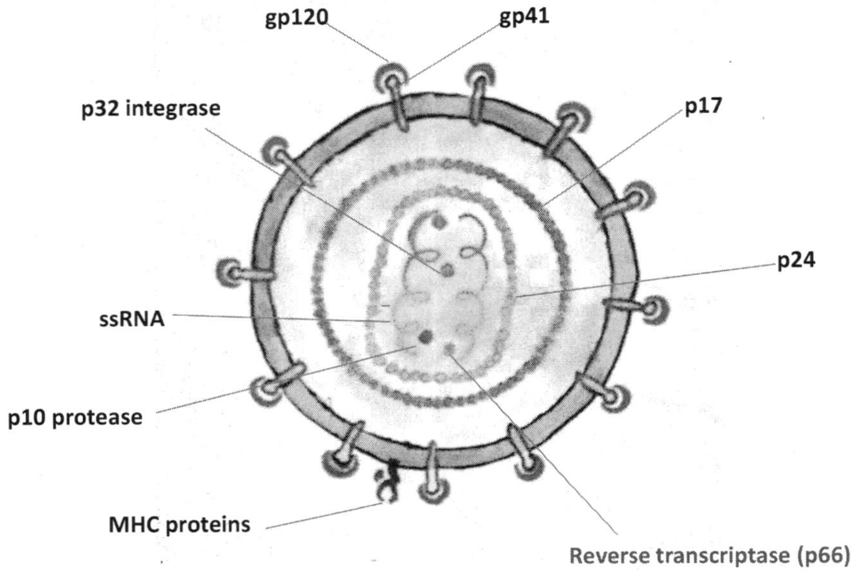

Fig. 11.2 : Structure of HIV I

AIDS results from infection with lentiviruses HIV-1 or HIV-2, with HIV-1 being much more prevalent worldwide. HIV-1 infects $CD4^+$ cells, including $CD4^+$ T-cells, macrophages and dendritic cells. Depletion in $CD4^+$ T-cells, dramatically in primary infection particularly in the gut and then more slowly over a period of years during clinical latency, leads to damage to the immune system, which renders an individual susceptible to opportunistic pathogens. Viral diversity and latency present major challenges to drug therapy but nevertheless drug design has been highly successful and combination drug regimes can hold the virus in check for many years, if not indefinitely. Vaccine design has also struggled with viral diversity and no immunogens that elicit broadly neutralizing antibodies or sufficiently potent T- responses to significantly contain challenges with a wide diversity of HIVs have yet been designed, although effort are intense and there are promising leads.

Infection in patients with HIV

HIV infection causes immunosuppression, principally through depletion of CD4 lymphocytes. This particularly affects the function of the cell mediated immune system. There is a wide variety of infections that can occur in patients with HIV, including a number of opportunistic pathogens (table 11.5). Some of these infections are AIDS- defining illnesses.

Table 11.5 - Common infection in patients with HIV infection

	Organism	Comments
Viruses	Herpes simplex virus (HSV)	Herpes simplex may cause frequent severe recurrent oral or genital herpes-zoster may be life-threatening in an immunosuppressed host
	Cytomegalovirus (CMV)	CMV retinitis and encephalitis can occur in end-stage HIV infection
	Epstein- Barr Virus (EBV)	Lymphoproliferative disorders
	John Cunningham virus (JC virus)	Associated with progressive multifocal leukoencephalopathy, a cause of progressive dementia in HIV patients
Bacteria	Streptococcus pneumonia	Increased incidence of pneumococcal pneumonia in HIV patients
	Mycobacterium tuberculosis	HIV infection is a significant risk factor for tuberculosis
Fungi	Mycobacterium avium intracellular (MAI) complex	Disseminated infection with MAI can occur in end-stage HIV infection
	Candida albicans, Cryptococcus neformans, Pneumocytsis jiroveci	Recurrent mucosal candidiasis is an early marker of immunosuppression in patients with HIV. An important cause of meningitis. PCP (Pneumocystis pneumonia) is the principle AIDS-defining infection
Protozoa	Toxoplasma gondii	Reactivation of toxoplasma cysts can cause encephalitis
	Cryptosporidum parvum	Crytosporidiosis in HIV patients can cause prolonged, serve diarrhea.

Diagnosis and treatment of immunodeficiency

Although there are no cures for immunodeficiency disorders, there are several treatment possibilities. In addition to the drastic option of total isolation from exposure to any microbial agent, treatment options for the immunodeficiencies include:

1. **Family history** - Because defective genes can be inherited, an investigation into the family history is especially important in the diagnosis of the primary immunodeficiency.
2. **Evaluation of specific immune components** - Evaluation of the nature of

immunodeficiency components in a patient is important for determining appropriate treatment. This may be achieved by assay of Ig levels and B-cell numbers for antibody-mediated immunity; T-cell and T-cell subset numbers and their cytokine production for cell-mediated immunity; lytic ability and individual components for complement activity; granulocyte and monocyte counts, their ability to phagocytes and kill bacteria, and their response to various chemotactic and activation signals, for the phagocytic system .

3. **Antibiotics and Antibodies** - Antibiotics therapy is the started treatment for infection. In addition, antibodies from a pool of donors are used for antibody deficiencies.
4. **Bone marrow transplants and gene therapy** - Replacement of faulty cells/organs, with those from normal individuals or with fetal liver or thymus grafts is used when MHC-compatible donors can be found and has been used to reconstitute normal phagocytic function in CGD (chronic granulomatous disease) and B and T cells in SCID. Treatment for genetic defects includes, in some cases, gene therapy, that is, replacing a defective gene with a normal gene.
5.

Question Bank

1. Very short answer type questions
   (a) Give full form of AIDS.
   (b) Give full form of SCID
   (c) Give full form of HIV.
   (d) Which T cell is affected in AIDS?
   (e) Which immune cell becomes deficient in Di-George syndrome?
   (f) Which immune cell becomes deficient in Burton's agammaglobulinemia?
   (g) Which gp of AIDS virus binds with Th cell?
   (h) Name one enzyme found in AIDS virus.
   (i) What is the nature of nucleic acid in AIDS virus?
   (j) Which cancer is associated with AIDS patient?
2. Short answer type questions
   (a) Define immunodeficiency.
   (b) Define primary immunodeficiency.
   (c) Define secondary immunodeficiency.
   (d) Write short note on Reticular dysgenesis.
   (e) Write short note on Burton's agammaglobulinamia.
   (f) Write short note on Di-George syndrome.
   (g) Write short note on severe combined immune deficiency disease.
   (h) Name the factors responsible for secondary immunodeficiency disease.
   (i) Define leucopenia.

(j) Define thrombocytopenia.
(k) Define lymphadenpathy.
(l) Define neutropenia.

3. Long answer type questions
(a) Describe in detail the structure of AIDS virus.
(b) How to control AIDS?
(c) Describe the treatment strategies in AIDS patients.
(d) How to avoid transmission of AIDS?
(e) Describe in detail primary immunodeficiency disease.
(f) Describe in detail secondary immunodeficiency disease.

Multiple Choice Questions

1. Which of the following is true about immunodeficiency?
(a) It is of 2 types
(b) Absence of sufficient immune system
(c) Any cell of immune system may be responsible
(d) All of the above

2. WAS is
(a) X linked disorder (b) Y linked disorder
(c) Cytoplasm disorder (d) Nucleus disorder

3. Defective genes are responsible for
(a) Primary immunodeficiency
(b) Secondary immunodeficiency
(c) Tertiary immunodeficiency
(d) None of the above

4. Thrombocytopenia includes
(a) Lowered platelet count (b) Existing platelets are smaller
(c) Short half- life of platelets (d) All of the above

5. People suffering from DiGeorge's syndrome do not have
(a) Pituitary gland (b) Hypothalamus gland
(c) Adrenal gland (d) Thymus gland

6. Hereditary Ataxia Telangiectasia leads to
(a) Lung infection (b) Deficiency of IgA
(c) Breaks in chromosomes (d) All above are true

7. Lymphoid lineage disorders will lead to the dys-functioning of
(a) T cells (b) B cells
(c) Combined immunodeficiency (d) All above are true

8. Which type of immunity gets depressed in Bruton's agammaglobulinemia?
(a) Humoral (b) CMI
(c) Both a & b (d) None of the above

9. Primary immunodeficiency may result from
   (a) Genetic defect of the immune system
   (b) Developmental defect of the immune system
   (c) Both a & b are true
   (d) None of the above
10. Bruton's Agammaglobulinaemia is
   (a) Congenital disease (b) Primary immunodeficiency
   (c) Affecting B cells (d) All of the above are true
11. Phagocytic function get affected, if there is a disorder in
   (a) Lymphoid lineage (b) Myeloid lineage
   (c) Both a & b (d) None of the above
12. Infections of which agents get prominent in Bruton's agammaglobulinemia
   (a) Mycobacterium leper (b) Mycobacterium tuberculosis
   (c) Virus (d) Streptococcus pyogens
13. AIDS is a________ virus
   (a) DNA (b) RNA
   (c) Both DNA & RNA (d) None of the above
14. Failure of phagolysosome formation is the characteristic of
   (a) SCID (b) HAT
   (c) WAS (d) Chediak-Higashi syndrome
15. Deficiency of which elements leads to secondary immunodeficiency?
   (a) Fe (b) Zn
   (c) Se (d) All of the above
16. Mutation in which gene leads to SCID
   (a) RAG 1 (b) RAG 2
   (c) Both a & b (d) LYST
17. Monocytes, neutrophills & macrophages fails to produce reactive oxygen intermediates in
   (a) CGD (b) SCID
   (c) WAS (d) HAT
18. Secondary immunodeficiency occurs due to
   (a) Malnutrition (b) Tumors
   (c) HIV infection (d) All above are true
19. AIDS virus is also known by the name
   (a) LAV & HTLV-3 (b) IDAV
   (c) HIV (d) All of the above
20. Which cells gets affected in Reticular dysgenesis?
   (a) B cells (b) T cells
   (c) Stem cells (d) All of the above

Answer Key

Question Number	Answer	Question Number	Answer
1	D	11	B
2	A	12	D
3	B	13	B
4	D	14	D
5	D	15	D
6	D	16	C
7	D	17	A
8	A	18	D
9	C	19	D
10	D	20	D

References

Arhel N. & Kirchhoff F. (2010) Host proteins involved in HIV infection: new therapeutic targets. Biochimica et BiophysicaActa 1802, 313-321

Broder S. (2010) The development of antiretroviral therapy & impact on the HIV-1/AIDS pandemic. Antiviral Research 85, 1-18

Buckley,R.H.,2000.Primary immunodeficiency diseases due to defects in lymphocytes. N. Eng. J. Med. 343:1313.

Carpenter, C. J. et al. 2000.Antiretroviral therapy in adults. Updated recommendations of the International AIDS Society— USA Panel. JAMA 283:381.

Cohen,O. J. and A.S.Fauci.2001.Current strategies in the treatment of HIV infection. Adv. in Int. Med. 46:207.

Fischer,A. 2001. Primary immunodeficiency diseases: an experimental model for molecular medicine. The Lancet 357:1863.

Graham, B. 2000. Clinical trials of HIV vaccines. In Human retroviruses and AIDS. Edited by C. Kuiken et al. Los Alamos National Laboratory ,LosAlamos ,NM

Kinter, A., et al. 2000. Chemokines, cytokines, and HIV: a complex network of interactions that influence HIV pathogenesis. Immunol. Rev. 177:88.

Kohn D.B. (2010) Update on gene therapy for immunodeficiencies. Clinical Immunology 135, 247-254

Kohn, D. B. 2001. Gene therapy for genetic haematological disorders and immunodeficiencies. J. Int. Med. 249:379.

Malim M.H. &Emerman M. (2008) HIV-1 accessory proteins – ensuring viral survival in a hostile environment. Cell host & Microbe 3, 388-398.

Mascola, J. R., and G.J.Nabel.2001.Vaccines for the prevention of HIV-1 disease. Curr. Opinion in Immunol. 13:489.

McMichael A.J., Borrow P., Tomaras G.D., Goonetilleke N. & Haynes B.F., (2010) The immune response during acute HIV-1 infection: clues for vaccine development. Nature Reviews Immunology 10, 11-23

Moir, S., et al. 2001. HIV-1 induces phenotypic and functional perturbations of B cells in chronically infected individuals. Proc. Natl Acad Sci. 98:10362.

Notarangelo L.D. et al. (2009) Primary immunodeficiencies:2009 update. International Union of Immunological societies Expert Committee on primary immunodeficiencies. Journal of allergy & clinical immunology.

Richmond, D.D. 2001.HIV chemotherapy. Nature 410:995.

Sharp P.M. & Hahn B.H. (2008) AIDS: prehistory of HIV-1. Nature 455, 605-606

Tilton J.C.& Doms R.W. (2010) Entry inhibitors in the treatment of HIV-1 infection. Antiviral research 85, 91-100

Turvey S.E., Bonilla F.A. & Junker A.K. (2009) Primary immunodeficiency diseases: a practical guide for clinicians. Postgraduates Medical Journal 85, 660-666

Virgin H.W. & Walker B.D. (2010) Immunology & the elusive AIDS vaccine. Nature 464, 224-231

CHAPTER 12

Autoimmune Disease

Introduction

The body is normally able to distinguish its own self-antigens or autoantigens from foreign nonself antigens and does not mount an immunologic attack against the former. This phenomenon is called immune tolerance. The immune system has the capacity to mount an immune response to virtually all molecules and/or cells. Although the capacity to respond to self antigen is present in all us, in most instances we are tolerant or energic to these antigens, indicating that mechanism must exist to prevent or subdue autoimmune responses. Early in the last century, Paul Ehrlich realized that the immune system could go awry and, instead of reacting against foreign antigens, could focus its attack on self-antigens. He termed this condition "horror autotoxicus." While mechanisms of self-tolerance normally protect an individual from potentially self-reactive lymphocytes, there are failures. They result in an inappropriate response of the immune system against self-components termed autoimmunity. It generally leads to the destruction of one's own tissue and cause disease. When the immune cell works against the cell components of the body, it's a problem of self/nonself discrimination. Autoimmunity is defined as humoral or cell mediated immune response against the constituents of the body's own tissues. When the immune system recognizes an antigen of its own body as non-self, the autoimmune response is produced.

It is important to distinguish between autoimmunity and autoimmune disease. Autoimmunity often is benign, whereas autoimmune disease often is fatal. Autoimmunity is characterized only by the presence of serum autoantibodies. It is a normal consequence of aging; is readily inducible by infectious agents, organisms, or drugs; and is potentially reversible (it disappears when the offending "agent" is removed or eradicated).

Moreover, autoreactive T and B cells as well as autoantibodies are found in people who do not have autoimmune diseases, demonstrating that immunological autoreactivity alone is not sufficient for the development of disease. The mechanisms currently thought to prevent/suppress autoimmune responses include inactivation or deletion or autoreactive T and B cells, active suppression by T-reg cells or cytokines, and the immunosuppressive adrenal hormones, the glucocorticoids. When suppressor mechanisms fail or are overridden, a response directed against self-antigen can occur, resulting in autoimmune disease that range from those which are organ-specific (diabetes and thyroiditis) to those which are systemic (non-organ-specific) such as systemic lupus erythematosus (SLE) and rheumatoid arthritis (RA).

Characteristics of Autoimmune Diseases

1. Autoimmune diseases are caused by autoimmune response. The autoantigen which produces autoimmune disease in one individual, will cause the same disease in an experimental animal when the same antigen is injected.
2. The disease can be passively transferred by the transfer of autoantibodies or sensitized lymphocytes.
3. In autoimmune disease, an elevated amount of immunoglobulin is produced.
4. Immunoglobulins or their product are deposited at the site of reaction such as renal glomeruli.
5. Lymphocytes and plasma cells accumulate at the site of lesions.
6. Autoimmune disorders are caused by autoimmune response.

Why does the immune system attack the body?

Doctors don't know exactly what causes the immune-system misfire. Yet some people are more likely to get an autoimmune disease than others. According to a 2014 study, women get autoimmune diseases at a rate of about 2 to 1 compared to men — 6.4 percent of women vs. 2.7 percent of men. Often the disease starts during a woman's childbearing years (ages 15 to 44). Some autoimmune diseases are more common in certain ethnic groups. For example, lupus affects more African-American and Hispanic people than Caucasians. Certain autoimmune diseases, like multiple sclerosis and lupus, run in families. Not every family member will necessarily have the same disease, but they inherit a susceptibility to an autoimmune condition. Because the incidence of autoimmune diseases is rising, researchers suspect environmental factors like infections and exposure to chemicals or solvents might also be involved. A "Western diet" is another suspected risk factor for developing an autoimmune disease. Eating high-fat, high-sugar, and highly processed foods is thought to be linked to inflammation, which might set off an immune response. However, this hasn't been proven. A 2015 study focused on another theory called the hygiene hypothesis. Because of vaccines and antiseptics, children today aren't exposed to as many germs as they were in the past. The lack of exposure could make their immune system prone to overreact to harmless substances.

Spectrum of autoimmune conditions

That autoimmune disease involve immune recognition of specific antigen is evidenced by organ-specific diseases, including thyroiditis, diabetes mellitus, multiple sclerosis (MS), celiac disease (CD), and inflammatory bowel disease, antigens shared by, multiple tissue sites are apparently involved in systemic autoimmunity in disease such as Systemic Lupus Erythematosus (SLE), Rheumatoid Arthritis (RA), systemic vasculitis, and scleroderma . It is also clear that a given individual may develop autoimmune disease of more than one type. For example, thyroid autoimmune disease is sometimes, associated with gastric autoimmunity and the incidence of CD in Sjogren syndrome, type I diabetes, and autoimmune thyroiditis is markedly increased. The pathogenesis associated with autoimmune disease may be mediated primarily by antibody (e.g., hemolytic anemia), by cellular immunity (e.g., MS), or by a combination of antibody and cell-mediated immunity (e.g., RA).

Prevalence

Autoimmune diseases are prevalent in the general population, and it is estimated that approximately 3.5% of individuals are afflicted. The most common are Graves' disease/hyperthyroidism, type I diabetes, pernicious anemia, RA, thyroiditis, CD, vitilligo, MS, and SLE, which together account for 94% of all cases. Overall, women are 2.7 times more likely than men to develop an autoimmune disease, but the female-to-male ratio can be as high as 10:1 in SLE

Factors contributing to the development of autoimmune disease

Following factors can affect gene expression, which directly or indirectly interferes with important immunoregulatory actions.

1. **Autoimmune diseases are multifactorial** - autoimmune diseases arise as the result of a breakdown in self-tolerance factor predisposing and/ or contributing to the development of autoimmune disease include age, genetics, gender infections and the nature of the autoantigen. Combination of these factors are probably important to the development of autoimmune disease.
2. **Age and gender** - autoantibodies are more prevalent in older people and women have a greater risk then man for developing an autoimmune disease. In SLE and Graves' disease, there in a female–to-male bias of 10:1 and 7:1, respectively. A higher incidence in female mice of autoimmune disease is consistence with hormones playing an important role.
3. **Endocrine** - the hormone estrogen promotes autoimmune disease, and androgens act as natural immunosuppressive agents. These physiological modulatory effects of sex hormones acting on normal immune responses partially explain the marked female predominance of autoimmune diseases.
4. **Genetics factors** - Antigen specific-autoimmune phenomena cluster in certain families. Particular HLA genes are associated with certain autoimmune disease and particular HLA haplotype predict the relative risk of developing a particular autoimmune disease. And or mutations also play a role, as evidence by the finding that fas deficiency leads to autoimmune lymphoproliferative syndrome (ALPS) and mutation of the *AIRE* gene expressed by epithelial cell in thymic medulla leads to the development of a rare condition with a range of autoimmune disease. Mutations in gene for certain complement components lead to an increased risk of SLE.
5. **Infection** - many infectious agents (EBV, Mycoplasma, Streptococci, Klebsiella, malaria, etc) have been linked to particular autoimmune disease. Some microbial antigens also have structure similar to self-antigens and induce autoimmune responses through "antigenic mimicry".

6. **Drug and autoimmune reaction** - certain drug can initiate autoimmune reactions by unknown mechanisms. For example, patient receiving procainamide for ventricular arrhythmias, nearly 10% develop SLE-like symptoms and have antinuclear antibodies that disappear following discontinuation of the drug.
7. **Psychoneuroimmunological factor** - that is, the influence of stress and neurochemicals on the immune response.
8. **Immunodeficiency** - A deficient immune response may allow persistence of infection or inflammation, which can lead to an increased incidence of autoimmune disease. For example, patient deficient in the complement components C2, C4, C5, or C8 have increased incidence of autoimmune disease, perhaps because of inefficient clearance of immune complexes.

Autoimmune diseases-mechanisms of development

- **Breakdown of self-tolerance** - The mechanisms that lead to autoimmunity are unclear but may include molecular mimicry, defective regulation of the anti-self response through Th1, Th2, and treg cells, polyclonal activation, modification of self-antigens through microbes and drugs, and availability of normally sequestered self-antigen.
- **Molecular mimicry and T-cell bypass** - An immune response may be generated against an epitope that is identical, or nearly identical, in both a microbe and host tissue, resulting in attack on host tissue by the same effector mechanisms activated to eliminate the pathogen. For example, a cross-reactive antigen between heart muscles and group A Streptococci predisposes to the development of rheumatic fever as a result of inducing autoantibodies to heart muscle.
- **Defective regulation mediated via Th cells** - Microbial infection induces primarily either Th1 or Th2 cytokines. The Th1 response leads to the production of the pro-inflammatory cytokines, while the Th2 response occurs in some autoimmune diseases, and changes in the relative contribution of these subsets (e.g., as seen in pregnancy) can influence disease activity in RA and SLE.
- **Polyclonal activation via microbial antigens** - some microbes or their product activate lymphocytes independently of their antigenic specificity, that is, are polyclonal activators (e.g., LPS and EBV). Patients with infectious mononucleosis produce only IgM antibodies to several autoantigens, including DNA. Since a switch to production of IgG autoantibodies (which requires Th cells) does not occur, T cells are probably not involved or are inhibited in their action.
- **Modification of cell surfaces by microbes and drugs** - Foreign antigens, for example viruses and drugs, may become adsorbed onto the surfaces of cells or react chemically with surface antigens in a hapten-like manner to alter their immunogenicity. For example, thrombocytopenia is also common in children following viral infections, and may involve association of viral antigen or immune complexes with the surface of platelets.

- **Availability of normally sequestered self-antigen** - because tolerance induction occurs mainly during embryonic development, antigens which are absent or automatically separated (sequestered) from the immune system during this period are not recognized as self. Such antigens include the proteins of the eye, and molecules associated with the central nervous system, the thyroid, and testes.
- **Defective regulatory T cells (Tregs)** - Tregs play in important role in the maintenance of self-tolerance. Decrease Treg numbers and/or function have been described in several human autoimmune diseases, suggesting a breakdown in tolerance.

Classification of Autoimmune Diseases

1. Hemolytic Autoimmune Disease

Hemolytic autoimmune disease is a clinical disorder resulting in the destruction of the components of blood. Here autoantibodies are formed against one's own RBCs or platelets or leucocytes. E.g. Hemolytic anemia, leucopenia, thrombocytopenia, etc.

2. Localized / organ-specific Autoimmune Disease

In localized autoimmune. Disease a particular organ is affected due to autoantibodies, Hence, it is also called organ-specific autoimmune disease. E.g. Thyrotoxicosis, Addison's disease, Myasthenia gravis, etc.

3. Systemic / Non-organ specific Autoimmune Disease

Systemic autoimmune disease affects the whole body or many organs. Hence it is also called non-organ specific autoimmune disease. E.g. Lupus erythematosus, rheumatoid arthritis, etc. Table 12.1 depicts various organ-specific diseases and non-organ specific diseases, and the antigens where auto-antibodies bind themselves in these diseases.

Table 12.1 : Antigens target in autoimmune disease

Organ-specific diseases		Non-organ specific diseases	
Diseases	**Antigen (s)**	**Diseases**	**Antigen(s)**
Addison's disease	Adrenal cortical cells*	Ankylosing spondylitis	Vertebral
Autoimmune Hemolytic anemia	RBC membrane Antigens	Chronic active hepatitis	Nuclei, DNA
Graves' diseases	TSH receptor	Multiple sclerosis	Brain/myelin basic protein
Guilliabarre' syndrome	Peripheral nerves (gangliosides)	Rheumatoid arthritis	IgG (rheumatoid factor) Connective tissues
Hashimoto's Thyroiditis	Thyroid peroxidase Thyroglobulin/T4	Scleroderma	Nuclei, elastin. Nucleoli Centromeres, Topoisomerase

Organ-specific diseases		Non-organ specific diseases	
Diseases	**Antigen (s)**	**Diseases**	**Antigen(s)**
Insulin-dependent Diabetes mellitus	β cells in the pancreas (GAD, tyrosine phosphate)	Sjogren syndrome	Exocrine glands, kidney, liver, thyroid
Pemphigus	Desmosal antigens in keratinocytes	Systemic lupus erythematosus	Double-stranded DNA, Nuclear antigens
Pernicious anemia	Intrinsic factor	Wegener's Granulomatosis	Proteinase 3
Polymyositis	Muscle (histidine tRNA synthesis)	Celiac disease	Small intestine

This section will elaborate various autoimmune diseases, based on upper classification mentioned.

1. Hemolytic Autoimmune Disease

a) Autoimmune Hemolytic Anemia

Autoimmune anemias include pernicious anemia, autoimmune hemolytic anemia, and drug-induced hemolytic anemia. Pernicious anemia is caused by auto-antibodies to intrinsic factor, a membrane-bound intestinal protein on gastric parietal cells. Intrinsic factor facilitates uptake of vitamin B12 from the small intestine. Binding of the auto-antibody to intrinsic factor blocks the intrinsic factor–mediated absorption of vitamin B12. In the absence of sufficient vitamin B12, which is necessary for proper hematopoiesis, the number of functional mature red blood cells decreases below normal. Pernicious anemia is treated with injections of vitamin B12, thus circumventing the defect in its absorption.

Autoimmune hemolytic anemia is a clinical disorder where there is a reduction below normal of the number of RBCs or quantity of hemoglobin. The reduction in RBC number is caused by the destruction or lysis of RBCs and this process is called hemolysis (figure 12.1). The lysis of RBCs is due to the production of autoantibodies against antigens present on the RBCs. It is an antibody mediated autoimmune disease. It is type 2 hypersensitivity reaction which damage to the membrane of the cell (RBC) occur. The half-life of normal RBC is about 21 days. But in autoimmune hemolytic anemia, the half-life of RBC is less than 7 days. Autoimmune hemolytic anemia is also caused by drug- therapy, secondary to infection or disease of the lymphoid tissue. Drug-induced hemolytic anemia occurs when certain drugs such as penicillin or the anti-hypertensive agent methyldopa interact with red blood cells, the cells become antigenic.

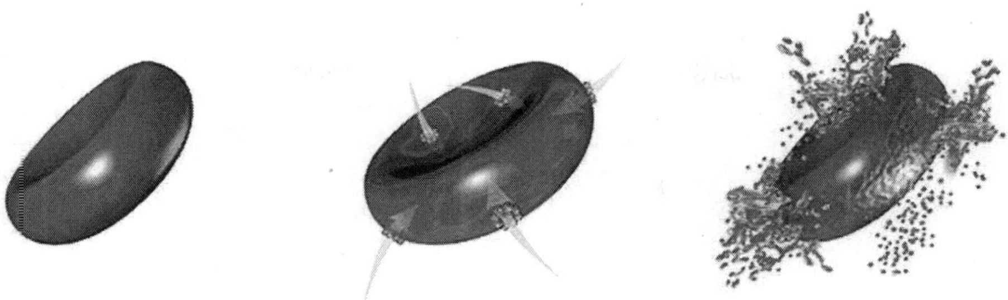

Fig. 12.1 : Haemolytic anaemia

b) Leucopenia

Leucopenia is a decrease in the number in the number of white blood cells found in the blood. It is not actually a disease, rather it's a condition that increases the chances of getting affected by several disease.

c) Thrombocytopenia

It is an autoimmune disease characterized by low platelet count. It is due to the production of antiplatelet antibodies of the type IgG. The antiplatelet antibody production is due to a new antigen formed by the interaction between heptenic component of a therapeutic agent and cell surface antigen of the platelets. The antibody production may also be induced by a complex formed by drug in association with some protein that can nonspecifically be absorbed on the surface to cause damage to platelets. An interaction of antibody with bound drug or new antigen can cause intravascular agglutination of platelets or lysis in the presence of complement components and can be engulfed and eliminated by phagocytic cells. It is an antibody – mediated autoimmune disease. Thrombocytopenia causes deficiency of platelets in the blood. This causes bleeding into tissues, bruising and slow blood clotting after injury (figure 12.2).

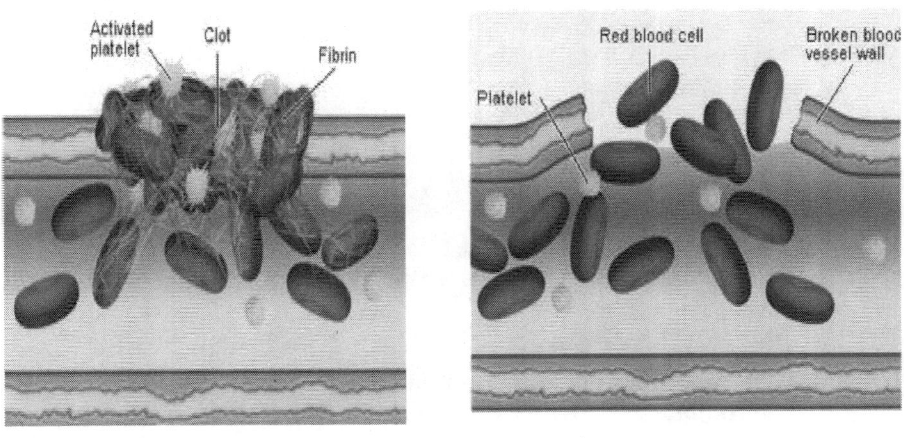

Fig. 12.2 : Normal thrombocyte population Thrombocytopenia

2. Localized Autoimmune Disease

a) Addison's Disease

Addison's disease is due to adrenocortical damage and hence insufficient secretion of adrenocortical hormones. The tissue damage is caused by autoantibodies against zona glomerulosa cells of adrenal cortex (figure 12.3). Addison disease is a disorder in which the adrenal glands do not produce enough steroid hormones. It results when the adrenal glands are damaged, producing insufficient amount of hormone cortisol and often aldosterone.

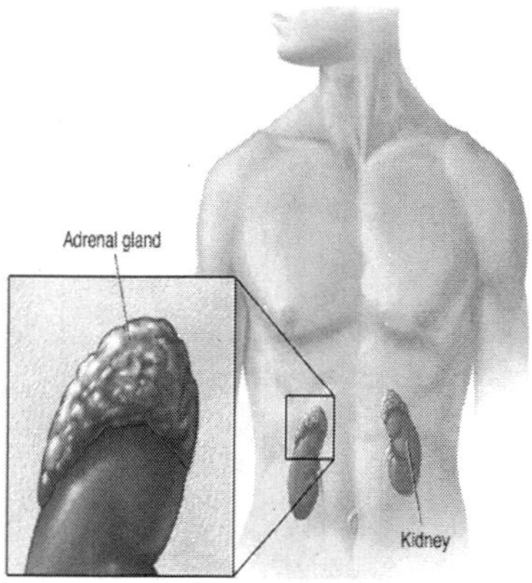

Fig. 12.3 : Location of Adrenal gland

b) Grave's Diseases

The production of thyroid hormones is carefully regulated by thyroid-stimulating hormone (TSH), which is produced by the pituitary gland. Binding of TSH to a receptor on thyroid cells activates adenylate cyclase and stimulates the synthesis of two thyroid hormones, thyroxine and triiodothyronine. A patient with Grave's disease produces auto-antibodies that bind the receptor for TSH and mimic the normal action of TSH, activating adenylate cyclase and resulting in production of the thyroid hormones (figure 12.4). Unlike TSH, however, the autoantibodies are not regulated, and consequently they over stimulate the thyroid. For this reason, these auto-antibodies are called long-acting thyroid-stimulating (LATS) antibodies. The LATS is an IgG type antibody. The LATS is a stimulating molecule. It is shown to activate the adenocylase 4 present in the thyroid cell membrane. Thus, it is considered that LATS has a complementary site similar to thyroid stimulating hormone. It is type V hypersensitivity reaction.

Grave's disease is an autoimmune disease that leads to an overactive thyroid gland. It is due to an abnormal immune response that causes the thyroid gland to produce too much thyroid hormone. Grave's disease is also known as toxic diffuser goiter. A swelling of the neck and protrusion of the eyes results from an overactive thyroid gland (figure 12.5). Thyrotoxicosis is a condition of hyperthyroidism, over secretion of thyroxine, resulting in exophthalmos and goiter.

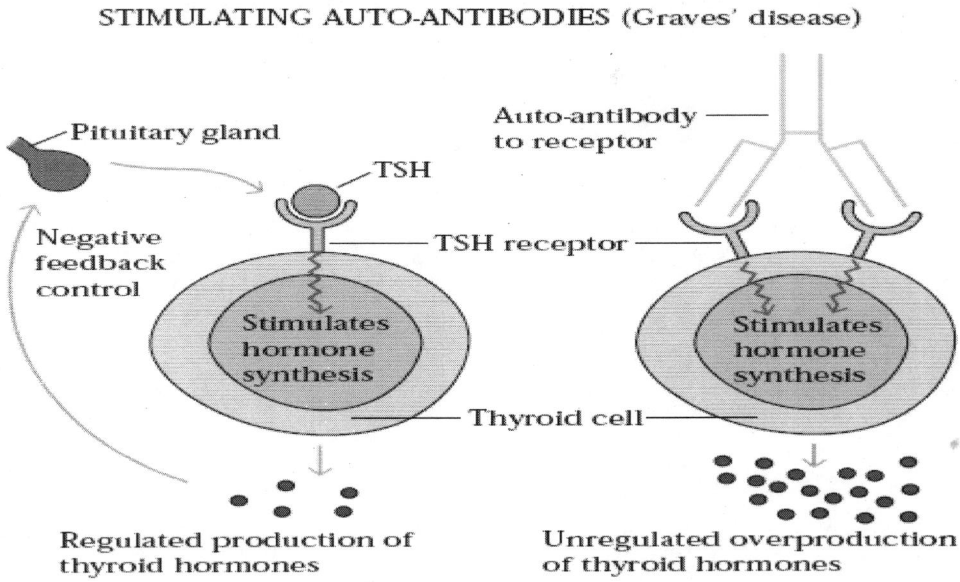

Fig. 12.4 : In Grave's disease, binding of auto-antibodies to the receptor for thyroid-stimulating hormone (TSH) induces unregulated activation of the thyroid, leading to overproduction of the thyroid hormones

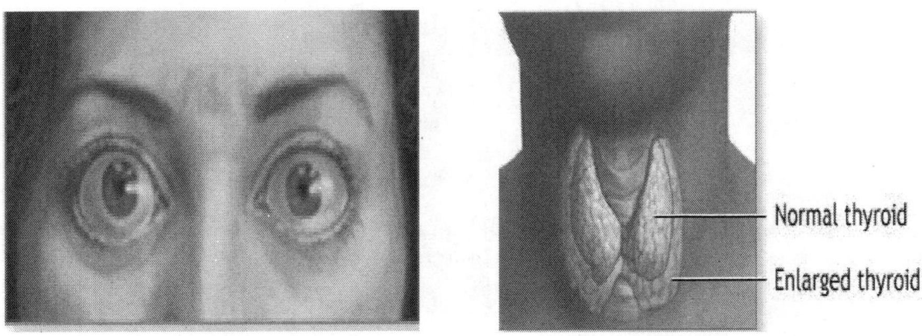

(a) Exophthalmos (bulging eyes) (b) Diffuse thyroid

Fig. 12.5 : Symptoms of Grave's disease

c) Myasthenia gravis

Myasthenia gravis is the prototype autoimmune disease mediated by blocking antibodies. A patient with this disease produces auto-antibodies that bind the acetylcholine receptors on the motor end-plates of muscles, blocking the normal binding of acetylcholine and also inducing complement mediated lysis of the cells. The neuromuscular junction is severely affected in these patients. When autoantibodies against acetylcholine receptor antigen are produced, acetylcholine cannot get attached with these receptors. Hence the nerve impulse cannot be transmitted from the nerves to the muscles. Ultimately, the antibodies destroy the cells bearing the receptors (figure 12.6).

The early signs of this disease include drooping eyelids and inability to retract the corners of the mouth, which gives the appearance of snarling. Myasthenia gravis is a disease of skeletal muscle characterized by gradually increasing weakness of muscles that make one easily fatique. In this disease, speaking, eating and walking become tiredsome. Without treatment, progressive weakening of the muscles can lead to severe impairment of eating as well as problems with movement. However, with appropriate treatment, this disease can be managed quite well and afflicted individuals can lead a normal life.

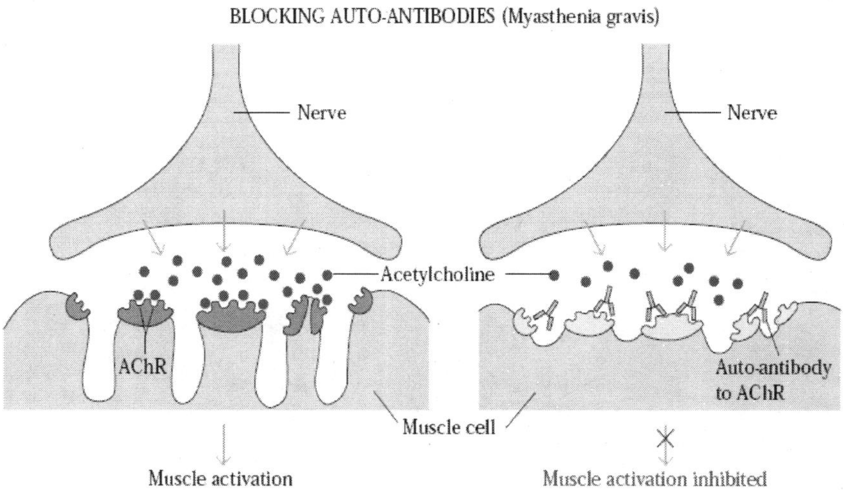

Fig. 12.6 : In myasthenia gravis, binding of auto-antibodies to the acetylcholine receptor (*right*) blocks the normal binding of acetylcholine (burgandy dots) and subsequent muscle activation (*left*). In addition, the anti-AChR auto-antibody activates complement, which damages the muscle end-plate; the number of acetylcholine receptors declines as the disease progresses. AChR = acetylcholine receptor.

3. Systemic Autoimmune Disease

a) Lupus Erythematosus

Lupus erythematosus is an autoimmune disease. It is a skin disease affecting mostly women than man. It is characterized by the appearance of blood-red spots over the bridge of nose and cheeks. The lesions take the shape of a butterfly (figure 12.7). It is an immune – complex mediated autoimmune disease. The primary cause for this disease is the formation of autoantibodies to the nuclear factors (ANF) or antinuclear autoantibodies. Affected individuals may produce autoantibodies to a vast array of tissue antigens, such as DNA, histones, RBCs, platelets, leukocytes, and clotting factors; interaction of these auto-antibodies with their specific antigens produces various symptoms. Auto-antibody specific for RBCs and platelets, for example, can lead to complement-mediated lysis, resulting in hemolytic anemia and thrombocytopenia, respectively. It is a systemic disease affecting the whole body. In addition, it can affect other organ in the body such as kidneys, lungs, heart and brain. Most patient feel fatigue, have rashes, swollen joints and fever.

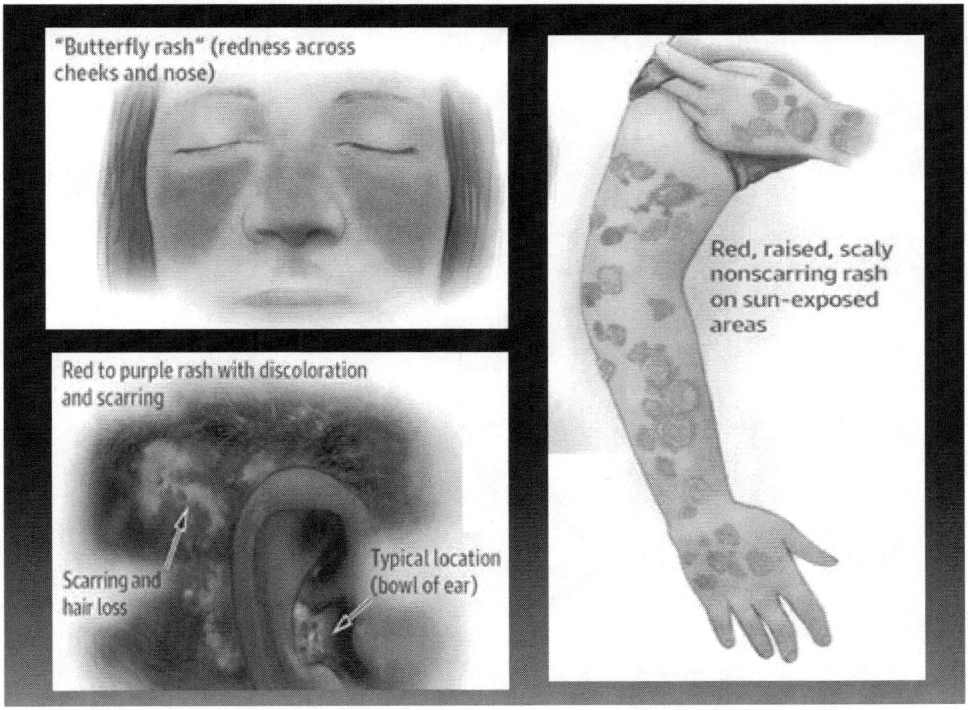

Fig. 12.7 : Symptoms of systemic lupus erythematosus

Laboratory diagnosis of SLE focuses on the characteristic antinuclear antibodies, which are directed against double stranded or single-stranded DNA, nucleoprotein, histones, and nucleolar RNA. Indirect immunofluorescent staining with serum from SLE patients produces various characteristic nucleus-staining patterns.

b) Rheumatoid Arthritis

Rheumatoid arthritis is a common autoimmune disorder, most often affecting women from 40 to 60 years old. It is triggered by a faulty immune system and affects the wrist and small joints of the hand, including knuckles and middle joints of the finger. It is a chronic systemic disease of the joints marked by inflammatory changes in the synovial membrane and articular structures and by atrophy of bones (figure 12.8). In later stage deformity and ankylosis develop. The major symptom is chronic inflammation of the joints, although the hematologic, cardiovascular, and respiratory systems are also frequently affected. If inflammation goes unchecked, it can damage cartilage, the elastic tissue that covers the ends of the bone in a joint. Over time, there is a loss of cartilage and the joint spacing become smaller. Joints can lose, unstable, painful and lose their mobility. The synovial fluid of these patients contains increased number of T-cells, and macrophages. This disease is caused by autoantibodies of the type IgM and hence they are called *rheumatoid factors* that are reactive with determinants in the Fc region of IgG. The classic rheumatoid factor is an IgM antibody with that reactivity. Such auto-antibodies bind to normal circulating IgG, forming IgM-IgG complexes that are deposited in the joints. These immune complexes can activate the complement cascade, resulting in a type III hypersensitive reaction, which leads to chronic inflammation of the joints.

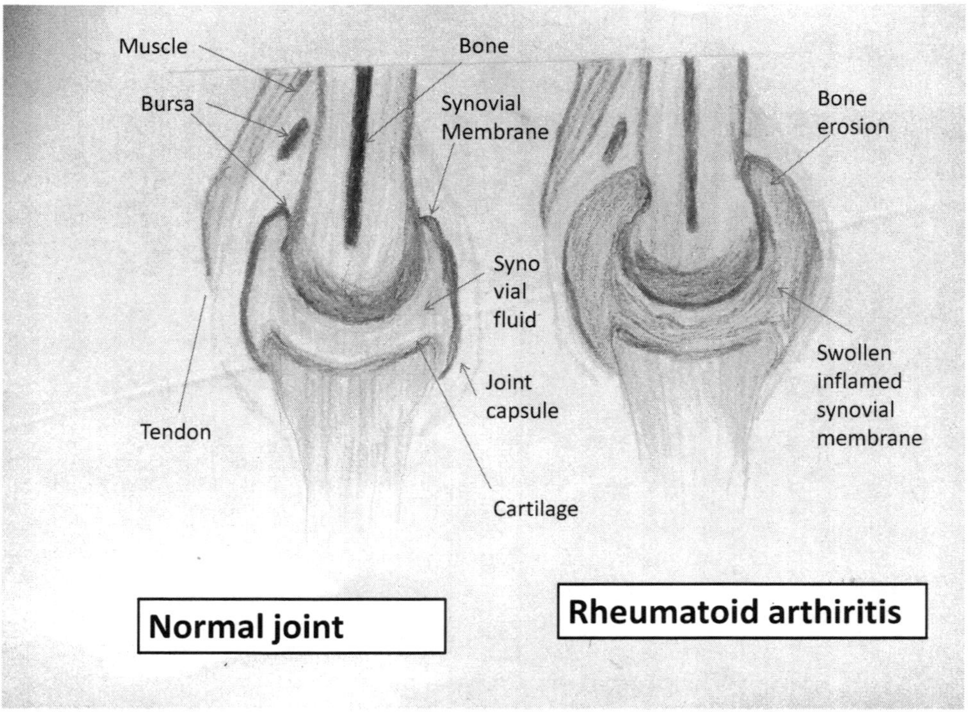

Fig. 12.8 : Difference between a normal joint and Rheumatoid arthiritis

c) Scleroderma

Scleroderma or systemic sclerosis, is a chronic connective tissue disease. This disease has been called 'progressive systemic sclerosis'. Sclero means hard and derma means skin. Hardening of the skin in most visible manifestation of the disease (figure 12.9). The symptoms vary greatly for each person and the effect can range from very mild to life threatening. Proper diagnosis may minimize the symptoms and reversible damage.

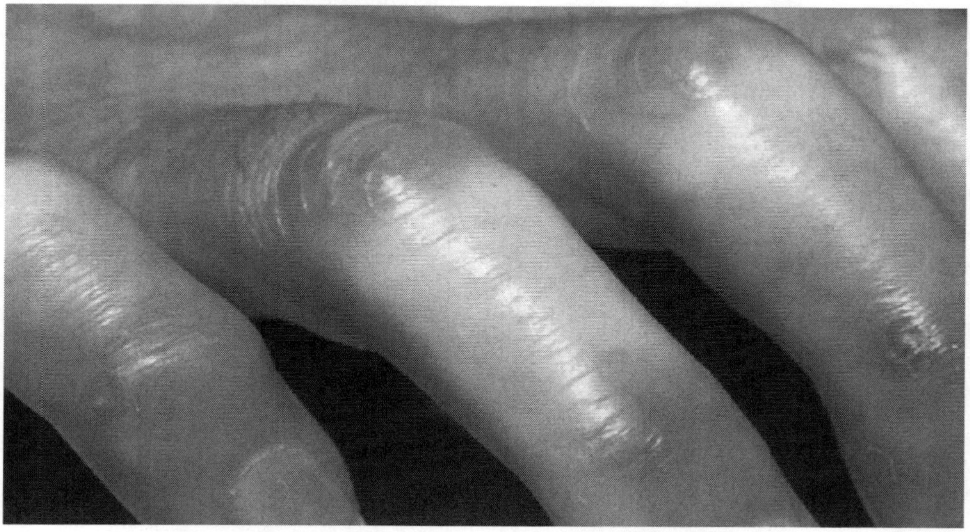

Fig. 12.9 : Symptoms of Scleroderma (Hardening of skin)

Diagnosis of Autoimmune Diseases

Diagnosis of autoimmune disease is through clinical and laboratory criteria that differ for each disease. Autoantibodies to variety of autoantigens are detected using immunofluorescence on tissue section and ELISA techniques. These techniques allow the detection of the IgG Abs to double-stranded DNA that are characteristic of SLE, IgA antibodies to tTG that are diagnostic of celiac disease, rheumatoid factor (IgM) found in Rheumatoid arthritis patients, and a variety of other autoantigens. Following tests are performed to diagnose autoimmune diseases-

1. **ANA (Antinuclear Antibody) Test**

An ANA test looks for antinuclear antibodies in blood. If the test finds antinuclear antibodies in blood, it may mean person has an autoimmune disorder. An antinuclear antibody attacks our own healthy cells. It's called "antinuclear" because it targets the nucleus (center) of the cells. An ANA test is used to help diagnose autoimmune disorders, including: Systemic lupus erythematosus (SLE), Rheumatoid arthritis, Scleroderma and Sjogren's syndrome.

2. **C-Reactive Protein (CRP) Test**

A c-reactive protein test measures the level of c-reactive protein (CRP) in blood. CRP is a protein made by liver. It's sent into bloodstream in response to inflammation. Inflammation is body's way of protecting tissues that have been injured or have an infection. It can cause pain, redness, and swelling in the injured or affected area. Some autoimmune disorders and chronic diseases can also cause inflammation. Normally, we have low levels of c-reactive protein in our blood. High levels may be sign of a serious infection or other disorder. A CRP test may be used to find or monitor conditions that cause inflammation and an autoimmune disorder such as lupus or rheumatoid arthritis

3. **Erythrocyte Sedimentation Rate (ESR)**

An erythrocyte sedimentation rate (ESR) is a type of blood test that measures how quickly erythrocytes (red blood cells) settle at the bottom of a test tube that contains a blood sample. Normally, red blood cells settle relatively slowly. A faster-than-normal rate may indicate inflammation in the body. Inflammation is part of our immune response system. It can be a reaction to an infection or injury. Inflammation may also be a sign of a chronic disease, an immune disorder, or other medical condition. An ESR test can help determine if we have a condition that causes inflammation. These include arthritis, vasculitis, or inflammatory bowel disease. An ESR may also be used to monitor an existing condition.

4. **Immunofixation (IFE) Blood Test**

An immunofixation blood test, also known as protein electrophoresis, measures certain proteins in the blood. There are two main types of proteins in the blood: albumin and globulin. The test separates these proteins into subgroups based on their size and electrical charge. The subgroups are: Albumin, Alpha-1 globulin, Alpha-2 globulin, Beta globulin and Gamma globulin. Measuring the proteins in each subgroup can help diagnose a variety of diseases.

5. **Complete blood count** - Measures the number of red & white blood cell in the body, when the immune system is actively fighting something, the numbers vary from the normal.

Treatment of autoimmune disease

The current approach in autoimmune can be broadly categorized into two categories: (1) symptomatic or replacement therapy (a conservative approach) and (2) the immunosuppressive or immune-modulation therapy (aggressive therapy). Autoimmune thyroid disease is the best example, which is predominantly managed either by reducing the thyroxin production at the time of hyperfunctioning or by replacing the hormone once the gland is damaged, whereas in systemic diseases like SLE which targets vital organs such as kidney, etc. the primary treatment is to use immunosuppressive to prevent further organ damage. Other approaches include-

1. **Replacement therapy**

In some cases, critical self-antigens are compromised by the autoimmune process and may need to be replaced. In thyroid autoimmunity, the patient is treated with thyroid hormones. In myasthenia gravis, inhibitors of enzymes which breakdown acetylcholine are used. In diabetes, insulin is given to replace that lost by damage to islet cells.

2. **Suppression of the autoimmune process** and drug therapy

Current treatments are aimed at nonspecific suppression of the autoimmune inflammatory process. These include nonspecific aspirin-like drugs (non-steroidal anti-inflammatory drugs; NSAIDs) or glucocorticoids, used to dampen inflammation, and plasmapheresis to remove antibodies. Cytotoxic drugs, cyclosporine, and monoclonal antibodies to T or B cells are also used to modulate or eliminate autoreactive lymphocytes. Drugs targeting cytokines (or their receptors) are used to treat a number of autoimmune diseases.

3. **Syndromic Approach**

The drug therapy used despite different definition of autoimmune syndromes in the end drugs used are combinations of different immunosuppressive drugs or modulators. Researchers find few of the drugs being effective in majority of autoimmune diseases, such as steroids, and some of the immunosuppressive, while only few of them are disease specific. For example, anti-TNF drugs work in diseases like RA, ankylosing spondylitis and related arthritis, psoriatic arthritis, and inflammatory bowel disease. In the same group of anti-TNF (Tumor necrosis factor) strategies, anti-TNF receptor do not help in Crohn's disease while Infliximab works well. Some of the drugs like methotrexate, azathioprine, and mycophenolate have been found to be useful in much wider autoimmune diseases. The responses do vary between syndromes, but this variation occurs even within the same syndrome. For instance, in RA only 70% of patients showed significant response to methotrexate. Thus, the disease classification based on immune pathogenesis may help more to device the treatment protocols in contrast to the syndromic approach.

Haemolytic anaemia can be treated with vitamin B12. Myasthenia gravis can be treated with cholinesterase inhibitors. Rheumatoid arthritis can be treated with anti-inflammatory drugs. Lupus Erythematosus can be treated with immunosuppressive or antimitotic drugs such as corticosteroid, cyclophosphamide and azathioprine. Mode of action of various drugs are mentioned in table 12.2.

Table 12.2 : Therapy of autoimmune diseases and mode of action

Replacement of targeted antigen	**For example, thyroid hormone for thyroid autoimmune disease, insulin for type 1 diabetes**
Nonsteroidal anti-inflammatory drugs (NSAIDs), e.g., aspirin, ibuprofen	Inhibit prostaglandins: RA and other
Corticosteroids, e.g., prednisone cytotoxic drugs	Anti-inflammatory
Azathioprine	Inhibits cell division, suppresses T cells
Cyclophosphamide	Blocks cell division, inhibits antibody production

Replacement of targeted antigen	**For example, thyroid hormone for thyroid autoimmune disease, insulin for type 1 diabetes**
Cyclosporine (ciclosporin)	Inhibits T-cell cytokine IL-2 production
Monoclonal antibodies to CD20	In drugs-resistant Rheumatoid Arthritis
Inhibitors of TNAα	In drugs-resistant Rheumatoid Arthritis
Inhibitors of inflammatory cytokine	Psoriasis, Rheumatoid Arthritis
Molecule involved in T-lymphocyte traffic	Treatment of Multiple Sclerosis
Experimental – not yet approved	Treatment of Rheumatoid Arthritis
Collagen	Treatment of Multiple Sclerosis
Small peptides from myelin basic protein	

Question Bank

1. Very short answer type questions
   (a) Give one example of sequestered antigen
   (b) Give one example of cross-reactive antigens
   (c) Give 2 example of hemolytic autoimmune
   (d) Give 2 example of localized autoimmune disease
   (e) Give 2 example of systemic autoimmune disease
   (f) Which hormones becomes deficient in Hasimoto's disease.
   (g) Name the autoantibodies produced in systemic Lupus erythematosus?
   (h) What is the other name of grave disease?
2. Short answer type questions
   (a) Define auto antigens
   (b) Define auto antibodies.
   (c) What are sequestered antigens?
   (d) Write short note an autoimmune Hemolytic anemia
   (e) Write short note on thrombocytopenia
   (f) Write short note on Grave disease
   (g) Write short note on Addison's disease.
   (h) Write short note on Myasthenia Gravis
   (i) Write short note on Lupus erythematosus.
   (j) Write short note on Rheumatoid arthritis
   (k) Write short note on Hasimoto's disease
3. Long answer type questions
   (a) Describe in detail the characteristics of autoimmune disease.
   (b) Describe in detail the causes of autoimmune disease.
   (c) Describe in detail the classification of autoimmune disease.
   (d) Describe in detail the localized autoimmune disease.
   (e) Describe in detail the systemic autoimmune diseases.

Multiple Choice Questions

1. Self antigens are also known as
   (a) Fetal Antigen (b) Neoantigen
   (c) Auto-antigen (d) None of the above
2. "Horror Autotoxicus" term was given by
   (a) Donath (b) Landsteiner
   (c) Metchnikoff (d) Paul Ehrlich
3. Which is organ specific autoimmunity?
   (a) Diabetes (b) Thyroiditis
   (c) Both a & b (d) Rheumatoid Arthritis
4. Which is systemic autoimmunity?
   (a) Rheumatoid Arthritis (b) Systemic Lupus erythematosus
   (c) Both a and b (d) Grave's disease
5. Which of the following is true for autoimmune disease?
   (a) Elevated amount of immunoglobulin is produced.
   (b) The disease can be passively transferred.
   (c) Immunoglobulins or their products are deposited at the site of reaction.
   (d) All of the above.
6. An autoimmune disorder may result in
   (a) The destruction of body tissue.
   (b) Abnormal growth of an organ.
   (c) Change in organ function.
   (d) All of the above.
7. In hemolytic autoimmune disorder, auto-antibodies are formed against one's own
   (a) RBCs (b) Platelets
   (c) Both a and b (d) T cells
8. Leucopenia is a condition in which WBC number
   (a) Increases (b) Decreases
   (c) May vary from time to time (d) None of above
9. Deficiency of platelets in the blood is known as
   (a) Leucopenia (b) Thrombocytopenia
   (c) Leukemia (d) None of the above
10. Which gland gets affected in Addison's disease?
    (a) Pituitary gland (b) Islet of Langerhans
    (c) Thymus glands (d) Adrenal glands
11. Production of which hormone gets affected in Graves' disease?
    (a) Insulin (b) Cortisone
    (c) Aldosterone (d) Thyroid hormone

12. Joints get affected in
    (*a*) Addison's disease (*b*) Grave's disease
    (*c*) Rheumatoid Arthritis (*d*) None of the above
13. Acetylcholine receptors get affected in
    (*a*) Myasthenia gravis (*b*) Addison's disease
    (*c*) Hashimoto thyroiditis (*d*) All of the above
14. Antinuclear autoantibodies are produced in which autoimmune disease?
    (*a*) Hashimoto thyroiditis (*b*) Myasthenia gravis
    (*c*) Addison's disease (*d*) Lupus Erythematosus
15. Loss of cartilage and the joint spacing becomes smaller in
    (*a*) Addison's disease (*b*) Hemolytic anemia
    (*c*) Rheumatoid arthritis (*d*) Diabetes Mellitus
16. Which of the following can be used for diagnosis of autoimmunity?
    (*a*) CRP (*b*) ESR
    (*c*) Autoantibody test (*d*) All of the above
17. The tissue damage is caused by autoantibodies against zona glomerulosa cells of adrenal cortex in
    (*a*) Addison's disease (*b*) Grave's disease
    (*c*) Myasthenia gravis (*d*) Lupus Erythematosus
18. Rheumatoid factor in the name given to which antibody?
    (*a*) IgG (*b*) IgM
    (*c*) IgE (*d*) IgD
19. When the synovial fluid of person contains increased number of T cells and macrophages, that person is suffering from
    (*a*) Rheumatoid Arthritis (*b*) Grave's disease
    (*c*) Leucopenia (*d*) Thrombocytopenia
20. In SLE, antinuclear antibodies are directed against
    (*a*) DNA (*b*) Nucleoprotein
    (*c*) Histones (*d*) All of the above

Answer Key

Question Number	Answer	Question Number	Answer
1	C	11	D
2	D	12	C
3	C	13	A
4	C	14	D
5	D	15	C
6	D	16	D
7	C	17	A

Question Number	Answer	Question Number	Answer
8	B	18	B
9	B	19	A
10	D	20	D

References

Benoist, C., and D. Matis. 2001. Autoimmunity provoked by infection: how good is the case for T cell epitopemimicry? Nat Immunol. 2:797.

Cunningham M.W. (2009) Molecular mimicry. In Encyclopedia of Life Sciences. John Wiley & Sons, Ltd, Chichester http://www.els.net/ DOI:10.1002/9780470015902.a0000958.pub2

Eizirik D.L., Colli M.L. & Ortis F. (2009) The role of inflammation on insulitis and β-cell loss in type 1 diabetes. Nature Reviews Endocrinology 5, 219-226.

Guilherme L. & Kalil J. (2010) Rheumatic fever and rheumatic heart disease: cellular mechanisms leading to autoimmune reactivity and disease. Journal of Clinical Immunology 30, 17-23.

Levin, M. C., et al. 2002. Autoimmunity due to molecular mimicry as a cause of neurological disease. Nat Med. 8:509.

Liblau, R. S., S. M. Singer, and H. O. McDevitt. 1995. TH1 and TH2 CD4+ T cells in the pathogenesis of organ-specific autoimmune diseases. Immunol. Today 16:34.

Lockshin,M. D. 1998.Why women? J. Am. Med.Womens Assoc. 53:4.

Marsh S.G. et al. (2010) Nomenclature for factors of the HLA system, 2010. Tissue antigens 75, 291-455.

Masters S.L., Simon A., Aksentijevich I. &Kastner D.L. (2009) Horror autoinflammaticus: the molecular pathophysiology of autoinflammatory disease. Annual Review of Immunology 27, 621-668.

O'Garra, A., L. Steinman, and K. Gijbels. 1997. CD4+ T-cell subsets in autoimmunity. Curr. Opin. Immunol. 9:872.

Oh. S., Rankin A.L. &Caton A.J. (2010) CD+CD25+ regulatory T cells in autoimmune arthritis. Immunological Review 233, 97-111.

Pascual V., Chaussabel D. & Banchereau J. (2010) A genomic approach to human autoimmune disease. Annual Review of Immunology 28,535-571.

Rahman A. & Isenberg D.A. (2008) Systemic lupus erythematosus. The New England Journal of Medicine 358, 929-939.

Rose, N. R. 1998. The role of infection in the pathogenesis of autoimmune disease. Semin. Immunol. 10:5.

Silverstein, A. M., and N. R. Rose. 1997. On the mystique of the immunological self. Immunol. Rev. 159:197.

Streilein, J.W., M. R. Dana, and B. R. Ksander. 1997. Immunity causing blindness: five different paths to herpes stromal keratitis. Immunol. Today 18:443.

Theofilopoulos, A. N. 1995. The basis of autoimmunity. Part I: Mechanisms of aberrant self-recognition. Immunol. Today16:90.

Zenewicz L.A., Abraham C., Flavell R.A. & Cho J.H. (2010) Unraveling the genetics of autoimmunity. Cell 140, 791-79

CHAPTER 13

Immunity Against Microorganisms

Introduction

The survival of the human species is dependent on its ability to defend itself against the constant threat from microbial infections. Infection refers to the invasion of harmful microorganisms into the body causing diseases. Infectious disease cause approximately 25 percent of all deaths in the world but in low income countries this can rise to 45 percent.

Microorganisms such as viruses, bacteria, etc virtually live everywhere in the environment. They exist in our food, in the water, on our utensils and on our bed sheets. They inhabit the surfaces of living human and animal bodies and grow abundantly in the mouth and intestinal tract. But the human body resists and there is a continuous war between the microbes and the body. In this war, if our body succeeds, the microbes are killed and the person remains healthy without any infectious diseases. If our body fails in the war, microbes invade the internal organs and cause diseases. All the organs such as circulatory system, respiratory system, nervous system, excretory system, etc, are the sterile and free from microbes in a healthy man. Microorganisms are kept out of the body by the skin, the secretion of mucus, ciliary action, the lavaging action of bactericidal fluids (e.g. tears), gastric acids and microbial antagonism. At every moment, the microbes try to invade the internal organs. If penetration occurs, bacteria are destroyed by soluble pattern recognition molecules such as lysozyme and complement, as well as by phagocytosis followed by intracellular digestion. Immunity plays an important role in protecting life from these deadly microorganisms. Immunity is of two types viz.

1. Humoral immunity

Humoral immunity refers to the resistance developed by man against microbes by the production of chemical substances called antibodies. Hence it is called antibody- mediated immunity. Here the antibodies are produced in the humors (body fluids) and hence this immunity is called humoral immunity.

The bacteria, after entry into the human body, release toxins. The toxins are of two types, namely endotoxins and exotoxins. Endotoxins are released as a result of the death of gram negative bacteria. They are lipopolysaccharides. The exotoxins are released by living gram positive bacteria. They are composed of proteins. Both endotoxins and exotoxins are antigenic and they function as antigens. In response to these antigens, the human body produces antibodies. These antibodies are called anti- toxin antibodies. The antitoxin antibodies neutralize the toxins. The diphtheria and tetanus infections are prevented by the action of antitoxin antibodies. The whole bacteria entering the body are clumped by specific antibodies produced against the bacterium. These antibodies are called anti- bacterial antibodies. These antibodies attach with the bacteria and bacteria are clumped and immobilized. Opsonization is a phenomenon of coating an antigen with substances such as an antibody or an activated complement component to increase the susceptibility of the antigen to phagocytosis. Opsonin is an antibody which renders bacteria and other cells susceptible to phagocytosis. The antibody which functions as the opsonin belongs to the class of IgG. When the bacteria enter the human body, IgG antibodies are produced. These antibodies coat the surface of bacteria. The phagocytes have receptors for IgG antibodies, the phagocytes migrate towards the antibody- coated bacteria and are eaten by phagocytosis. Bacteria with a capsule are disposed by the method of opsonization. Examples includes Stereptococcus aureus, Bacillus anthrax, Haemophilus influenza, etc.

2. Cell- mediated immunity

The resistance against infection produced by the sensitized lymphocytes is called cell- mediated immunity. Here antibodies are not produced, but specific lymphocytes are triggered against microbes and the microbes are disposed. Cell-mediated immunity gives adequate protection against viruses, fungi, protozoa, and certain bacteria. It does not give protection against cocci. When a microbe enters the body, it is processed by a macrophage. While processing, macrophage prepares the cell for immunogenicity and it retains antigen (of the microbe) on its surface membrane. The macrophage than presents the microbe to the T-cell. The T-cell recognizes the microbe, when a cell to cell contact between T-cell and antigen- macrophage complex is made. This recognition activates a population of T-lymphocytes. These activated T-cells release certain chemical substances called lymphokines. The lymphokines mediate the immune response. The lymphokines recruit and draw macrophages to the site of infection and the microbe is destroyed by the macrophages.

Many microorganisms live inside the host cells where humoral antibody can't reach. Such intracellular microbes are killed by cell mediated immunity. Viruses replicate only inside cells. Similarly, Leishmania, Trypanosoma cruzi and certain bacteria like Mycobacterium tuberculosis, M. leprae, etc. thrive inside the macrophages after their uptake by phagocytosis. These microbes are killed by cell mediated immunity. The macrophages, containing intracellular parasites, deposit on their surface some antigenic substances of the parasites. T-helper cells (a sub–population of T-lymphocytes) recognize the antigen present on the macrophages. These T-helper cells bind to the antigen. The T-helper cells are triggered and they produce lymphokines. The lymphokines activate the microbicidal mechanisms of the macrophage and bring about the death of the intracellular microbes.

Role of Innate and adaptive immune responses

Immunity—the state of protection from infectious disease—has both a less specific and more specific component. The less specific component, innate immunity, provides the first line of defense against infection. Most components of innate immunity are present before the onset of infection and constitute a set of disease-resistance mechanisms that are not specific to a particular pathogen but that include cellular and molecular components that recognize classes of molecules peculiar to frequently encountered pathogens. Phagocytic cells, such as macrophages and neutrophils, barriers such as skin, and a variety of antimicrobial compounds synthesized by the host all play important roles in innate immunity (figure 13.1).

The innate immune system is also comprised of a soluble factors and cells that detect and responds to infectious agents through binding to relatively non specific structures like pathogen-associated molecular patterns (PAMPs) common to many pathogens. Innate responses are initiated through detection of pathogen-associated molecular patterns (PAMPs) representing nonself or danger-associated molecular patterns (DAMPs) that represent hidden self. Pattern recognition receptor molecules (PRRs), which can be either soluble (humoral) or cell-associated, are used by immune system to detect the presence of PAMPs or DAMPs. PRR engagement leads to a diversity of responses that are aimed at directly killing or engulfing microorganisms via phagocytosis, and also results in amplification of immune responses through release of a range of messenger molecules such as cytokines and chemokines.

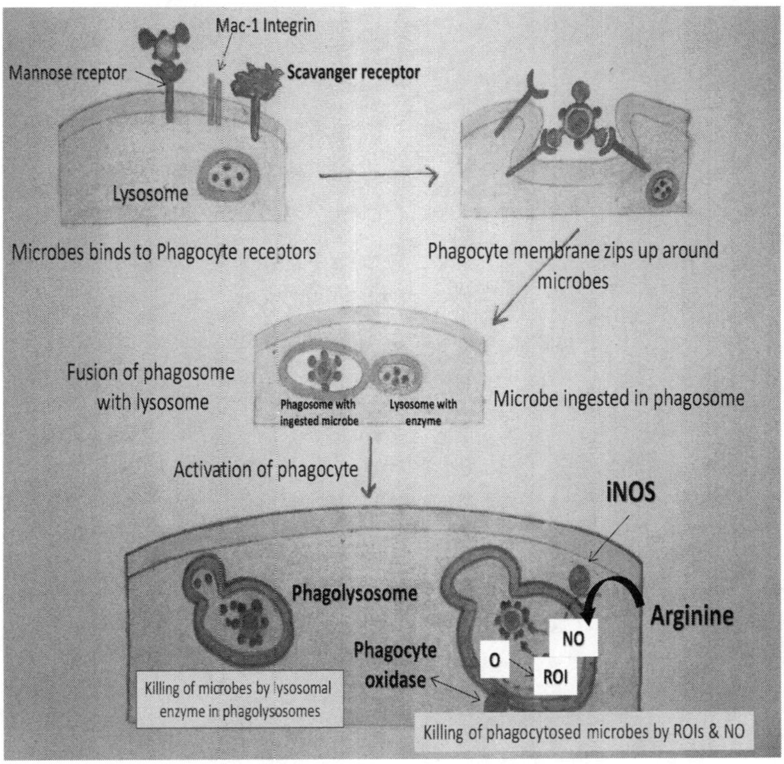

Fig. 13.1 : Process of phagocytosis

Inflammation is the term used to describe the series of events that surround an immune response and includes local swelling (due to recruitment of phagocytes and plasma protein from blood), redness, pain and temperature elevation. The products of activated mast cells and complement activation collectively promote inflammation. Following the activation of complement with the ensuing attraction and stimulation of neutrophils, the activated phagocytes bind to the C3b-coated microbe by their surface C3b receptors and may then ingest them. The influx of polymorphs and the increase in vascular permeability constitute the potent antimicrobial acute inflammatory response. Inflammation can also be initiated by tissue macrophages that subserve a similar role to the mast cell, as signaling by bacterial toxins, C5a- or iC3b- coated bacteria adhering to surface complement receptors causes release of neutrophil chemotactic and activating factors (figure 13.2).

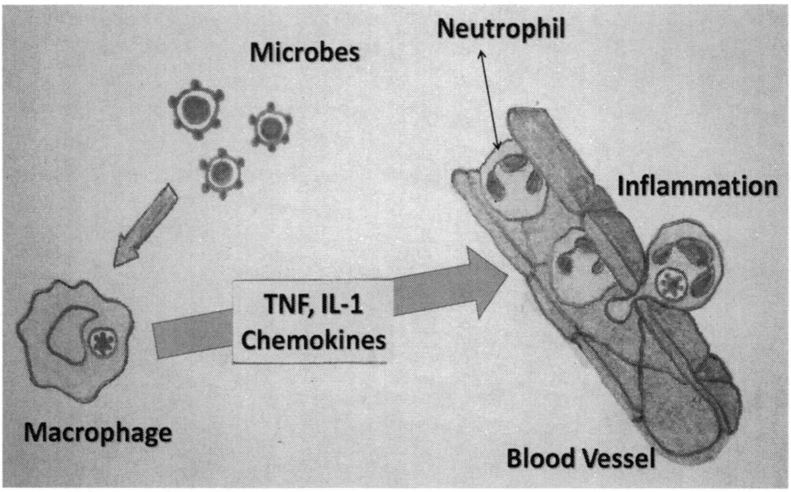

Fig. 13.2 : Process of Inflammation.

Innate and adaptive immune responses are interdependent and cooperate to kill infectious agents. The adaptive immune system is comprised of T- and B- lymphocytes that recognize highly specific structures (antigens) on microorganisms via highly diverse membrane receptors that are generated randomly and are uniquely tailored to individual pathogens. Adaptive immune responses exhibit four immunologic attributes: specificity, diversity, memory, and self/nonself recognition. The high degree of specificity in adaptive immunity arises from the activities of molecules (antibodies and T-cell receptors) that recognize and bind specific antigens. Antibodies recognize and interact directly with antigen. T cell receptors recognize only antigen that is combined with either class I or class II major histocompatibility complex (MHC) molecules. The two major subpopulations of T lymphocytes are the$CD4^+$ T helper (TH) cells and $CD8^+$ T cytotoxic (TC) cells.TH cells secrete cytokines that regulate immune response upon recognizing antigen combined with class II MHC. TC cells recognize antigen combined with class I MHC and give rise to cytotoxic T cells (CTLs), which display cytotoxicability. Exogenous (extracellular) antigens are internalized and degraded by antigen-presenting cells (macrophages, B cells, and dendritic cells); the resulting antigenic peptides complexed with class II MHC molecules are then displayed on the cell surface. Endogenous (intracellular) antigens (e.g., viral and tumor proteins produced in altered self-cells) are degraded in the cytoplasm and then displayed with class I MHC molecules on the cell surface.

Immunity to Bacteria

There are four primary steps in bacterial infection:

- Attachment to host cells
- Proliferation
- Invasion of host tissue
- Toxin-induced damage to host cells

Host-defense mechanisms act at each of these steps, and innate immune responses form the initial defense against pathogens. These include physical barriers, such as skin, as well as the nonspecific production of complement components and certain cytokines in response to infection by various pathogens. The primary defense against microbial infection are the natural physical barriers such as the skin, mucous membrane, tears, earwax, mucus and stomach acid. The immunological defenses are provided by the innate and adaptive immune systems.

Humoral immunity appears to be more important than cell mediated immunity in the defense against most bacterial pathogens. Defense against bacterial infections requires many and varied strategies. These include circulating protein such as complement that can directly destroy some bacteria through lytic activity or engulfment and killing by phagocytic cells that can recognize PAMPs through their pattern recognition receptors (PRRs). Alternatively bacteria may be opsonized by acute phase reactants, C- reactive protein and serum amyloid P, or by specific antibodies and engulfed by phagocytes express receptors for IgG as well as IgA. Inflammatory cytokines such as IFNy can dramatically upregulate expression of these receptors and improve the efficiency of killing by these effector cells. In addition, the Toll Like Receptors (TLRs) expressed by macrophages and dendritic cells are important in cytokine production and initiating responses against bacteria by the adaptive immune system, whose primary aim is to produce appropriate specific antibody responses and to provide memory against future infections.

The immune response to extracellular bacterial infections is generally mediated by antibody. Antibody can induce localized production of immune effector molecules of the complement system, thus facilitating development of an inflammatory response. Antibodies and complement attack pathogens in many ways. IgG, and the C3b and C4b components of complement are opsonins. That is, they aid in the phagocytosis of bacteria by macrophages and granulocytes through the process called opsonization (figure 13.3). Antibody can also activate complement-mediated lysis of the bacterium, neutralize toxins, and serve as an opsonin to increase phagocytosis. IgM and IgG will agglutinate bacterial pathogens, thus limiting their spread and enhancing the efficiency of phagocytosis.

Antibodies can trigger complement attack on the wall of gram-negative bacteria by the classical pathway. Once this pathway is activated, it forms a C5b-9 membrane attack complex that forms channel or pore in the bacterial cell, leading to lyses. Complement C3a, C5a, and C5b67 also attract neutrophils and macrophages to a site of infection. Antibodies called antitoxins bind to bacterial exotoxins and block their action (neutralization). Some bacteria secrete protease enzymes that cleave IgA dimers, thus reducing the effectiveness of IgA in the mucous secretions. Other bacteria escape phagocytosis by producing surface capsules or proteins that inhibit adherence to phagocytes, by secreting toxins that kill phagocytes, or by their ability to survive within phagocytes.

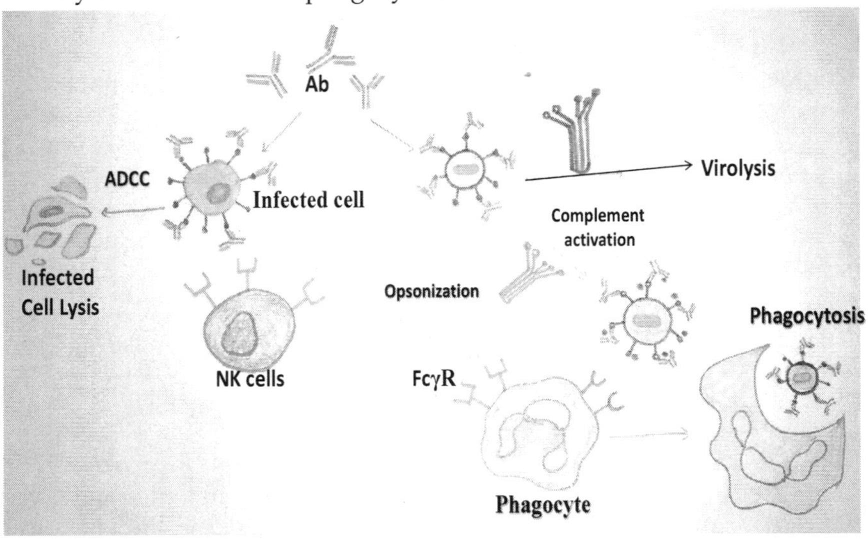

Fig. 13.3 : Process of Opsonization

Some bacteria invade host cells and survive in them, including TB bacilli, Listeria monocytogenes, Salmonella typhi, and Brucella species. These intracellular bacteria evade the immune system counteracts them by mounting a cell- mediated immune response to the infection. Cells involved in the CMI response include Th1 and Th2 CD4+ T cells, CD8+ T cells, monocytes/macrophages, and NK cells. Cell-mediated immune responses by activated macrophages and T-cells are important, particularly in resisting intracellular bacterial pathogens. Activated T cells secrete several cytokines, which have a variety of effects. Th1 cells release IFNy, which makes monocyte/macrophages more potent at killing intracellular bacteria and also enhances their antigen–presenting capabilities. Interleukin-2 (IL-2) stimulates the proliferation of activated T cells to increase the population of cells involved in the cell-mediated immune response. It also increases the effectiveness of cytotoxic T cells and NK cells by promoting the synthesis of immune interferon (γ interferon) by T cells. The macrophage activating factor stimulates macrophages to become "angry" macrophages and more effectively phagocytose and destroy pathogens. Interferon-γ is a major macrophage activating factor. The macrophage chemotactic factor and migration inhibition factor attract more macrophages and keep them in the area of infection after arrival. The CMI response is important in the protection against not only diseases such as TB but also some viral and fungal infections. Host defense against intracellular bacteria depends largely on CD4+ T-cell–mediated responses.

Examples of modes of infection and immunity to specific microbes:

1. **Staphylococcus aureus**

   Staphylococcus aureus is a gram-positive coccus that is present in the skin and mucous membranes of the gastrointestinal and genitourinary tracts of humans. It is very common microbe found in the anterior nasal passages of 15 to 30% of adults and attaches to skin and mucosal surfaces through several adhesion molecules. It is only when there is damage to these epithelia burns, traumatic wounds, surgical incisions, ulceration, viral skin lesions and so forth, that infection can take place. Infection is more common in individuals with reduced host resistance that is patients with cystic fibrosis or diabetes mellitus and those undergoing immunosuppression. Normally invasion by S. aureus is prevented through an intact barrier and the production of antimicrobial peptides such as α- defensins and cathelicidin by the epithelial cells. Once through the epithelial barrier, neutrophils also produce these antimicrobials, but the microbe secretes substances to inactivate them. In addition, complement mediated neutrophil chemotaxis and phagocytosis is suppressed. In fact, multiple mechanisms are used by S. aureus to evade the immune system. It is envisaged that tissue damage through exotoxins released by S. aureus results in acute inflammation and that macrophages and dendritic cells process and present microbial antigen to T cells and B cells in draining lymph nodes, giving rise to some neutralizing antibodies. Even the IgG antibodies are blocked by staphylococcus A protein released by the microbe, resulting in the inhibition of opsonization. Entry of S. aureus into the blood stream can lead to seeding and infection of many organs, including the heart, lungs, bones and joints. Pneumonia may result if bacteria reach the lungs, while acute and chronic osteomyelitis or septic arthritis can also occur. Eventually, sufficient neutralizing antibody is produced but generally antibiotic therapy is required for systemic infections. The development of methicillin-resistant S. aureus is still a major public health problem.

2. **Human Leprosy**

   Human Leprosy presents as a spectrum ranging from the tuberculoid form, with lesions containing small numbers of viable organisms, to the lepromatous form, characterized by an abundance of Mycobacterium leprae within the macrophage. CMI rather than humoral immunity is important for control of the leprosy bacillus. Although the tuberculoid state is associated with good cell mediated dermal hypersensitivity reactions and a bias towards Th 1-type responses, these are still not good enough to eradicate the bacilli completely. In the lepromatous form, there is poor T-cell reactivity to whole bacilli and poor lepromin dermal responses, although there are numerous plasma cells that contribute to a high level of circulating antibody and indicate a more prominent Th2 activity. Leukocyte Ig-like receptor- A2 (LILRA2) expression is increased in lesions of lepromatous patients, causing a block in TLR-directed anti-microbial activity and reduced production of proinflammatory IL-2, but enhanced secretion of immunosuppressive IL-10, by monocytes.

Immunity to Virus

Virus is a particle on all types of organisms. They are living or non- living organisms. Outside the living cell viruses remain inactive. They infect animals, plants, bacteria, algae, insects etc. They are unique group infection agent. They are especially small, filterable and obligate intracellular parasites requiring a living host for its multiplication. Virus occur on very wide host such as plants (angiosperms, ferns, algae, fungi) and animals (fish, birds, mammals, human).

The immune response to viral infections involves both humoral, interferon sensitization of host cells and cell-mediated components. Antibodies are particularly effective in protecting against infection if they are localized at the site of viral entry into the body. Antibodies enhance phagocytosis and destruction of viruses in much the same way as for bacteria. Most viruses express surface receptor molecules that enable them to initiate infection by binding to specific host-cell membrane molecules. For example, influenza virus binds to sialic acid residues in cell membrane glycoproteins and glycolipids; rhinovirus binds to intercellular adhesion molecules (ICAMs); and Epstein-Barr virus binds to type 2 complement receptors on B cells. Antibody to a viral receptor can block viral infections of host cells. Antibodies can neutralize viruses by combining with them and interfering with their adsorption and entrance into cells. However, a number of viruses, including influenza, are able to mutate their receptor molecules and thus evade the humoral antibody response. Since viruses require attachment to host cells before they can replicate and cause infection, antibodies to the virus that prevent attachment represent an important mechanism that protects against viral infection. These protective antibodies may be IgG or IgA as in the case of polio prevention. Once a viral infection has been established, cell-mediated immunity appears to be more important than humoral.

Natural immunity to viral infections is associate (especially INFα and INF β), so called because of their interference with viral replication. IFNAγ is probably more effective in protecting against extracellular bacteria through its ability to enhance immune-mediated mechanisms. Interferons are important in resistance when the target cell is reached immediately as in the case of colds and influenza. Interferon-stimulated cells shut down protein synthesis and destroy viral mRNA. Some interferon also stimulates the activity of T cells and natural killer cells, thus accelerating the immune response to a viral infection. The innate immune response to viral infection is primarily through the induction of type I interferons (IFN-α and IFN-β) and the activation of NK cells. Double stranded RNA (ds RNA) produced during the viral life cycle can induce the expression of IFN-α and IFN- β

by the infected cell. Macrophages, monocytes, and fibroblasts also are capable of synthesizing these cytokines, but the mechanisms that induce the production of type I interferons in these cells are not completely understood. IFN-α and IFN- β can induce an antiviral response or resistance to viral replication by binding to the IFN α/ β receptor. Once bound, IFN-α and IFN- β activate the JAK-STAT pathway, which in turn induces the transcription of several genes. One of these genes encodes an enzyme known as 2′-5′-oligo-adenylate synthetase [2-5(A) synthetase], which activates a ribonuclease (RNAse L) that degrades viral RNA. Other genes activated by IFN- α / β binding to its receptor also contribute to the inhibition of viral replication. For example, IFN- α / β binding induces a specific protein kinase called dsRNA-dependent protein kinase (PKR), which inactivates protein synthesis, thus blocking viral replication in infected cells. The binding of IFN- α and IFN- β to NK cells induces lytic activity, making them very effective in killing virally infected cells. The activity of NK cells is also greatly enhanced by IL-12, a cytokine that is produced very early in a response to viral infection.

The virally infected cells are killed by antibody dependent cell mediated cytotoxicity (ADCC). ADCC is a form of lymphocyte mediated cytotoxicity in which an effector cell kills an antibody coated target cell. The virally infected cells are deposited with surface antigens of the virus. In response to the virus antigen, the human body produces antibodies. These antibodies coat the virus infected cells. The natural killer cells have specific receptors for these antibodies. These antibodies will bring the NK cell very closer to the virally infected cell and a bridge id formed between the antibody and NK cell. When the NK cell is complexed with the antibody, the NK cell is activated. The activated NK cell is able to kill the virally infected cell by its extracellular mechanism.

Cell-mediated immunity to viruses is a major resistance mechanism when enveloped viruses modify host cell membranes and bud off from the surface (e.g., herpesvirus, poxvirus, influenza, mumps, measles, rabies, and rubella viruses). Because viruses replicate in cell where they are no longer exposed to circulating antibodies, their eradication depends upon killing the infected host cells. This of course would require a CTL response. CTLs destroy virus-infected cells through FasL, and the production of granzymes and perforin that form channels through the plasma membrane of infected cells causing apoptosis and cytolysis. The class I MHC proteins are involved in T-cell recognition of infected cells. Cells displaying both viral antigen sand the proper class I MHC will be destroyed. CTLs are also involved in the destruction of cancer cells (immune surveillance). Activated lymphocytes can recognize and destroy virus-infected cells because the target cell's plasma membrane has been altered. As virally infected cells usually express viral peptides in MHC class 1 on their surface, they become susceptible to killing by NK cells and NKT cells. Natural killer cells (NK cells) are non B, non T lymphocytes that are active without any prior antigen exposure. Interferon and antibodies, however, will stimulate them to greater activity. They also are capable of destroying virus-infected and cancer cells. They are components of innate immunity and possess no antigen receptors. In this way viral replication is prevented and the viral infection eliminated.

Examples of modes of infection and immunity to specific microbes:

1. **The influenza virus**

   Influenza A is an RNA virus that is associated with seasonal outbreaks of infection. The influenza virus infects the upper respiratory tract and major central airways in human, horses, birds, pigs and even seals. Up to 10% of the population can be infected, leading to increases in hospital admissions and Influenza related deaths. In 1918-19 an influenza pandemic killed more than 20 million people, a toll surpassing the no of casualties in world war 1. Some areas, such as Pacific Islands, lost more than half of their population during that pandemic. Influenza virus particles or virions are roughly spherical or avoid in shape, with a average diameter of 90-100mm. The virions are surrounded by an outer envelope a lipid bilayer acquired from the plasma membrane. Of the infected host cell during the process of budding. Inserted into the envelop are 2 glycoproteins, hemagglutinin (HA) and neuraminidase (NA), which form radiating projections that are visible in electron micrographs. It enters the body via the nasal or oral mucosal epithelium and through its hemagglutinin (HA) binds to the surface of the respiratory epithelial cells through cell surface receptors. The virus enters the host cell uncoats, and replicates and new virion are released by the infected cells through budding at the plasma membrane of the host cell. Humoral antibody specific for the HA molecule is produced during influenza infection.

   Humoral antibody specific for the HA molecule is produced during an influenza infection. This antibody confers protection against influenza, but its specificity is strain-specific and is readily bypassed by antigenic drift. Antigenic drift in the HA molecule results in amino acid substitutions in several antigenic domains at the molecule's distal end (figure 13.4). Two of these domains are on either side of the conserve disialic-acid–binding cleft, which is necessary for binding of virions to target cells. Serum antibodies specific for these two regions are important in blocking initial viral infectivity. These antibody titers peak within a few days of infection and then decrease over the next 6 months; the titers then plateau and remain fairly stable for the next several years.

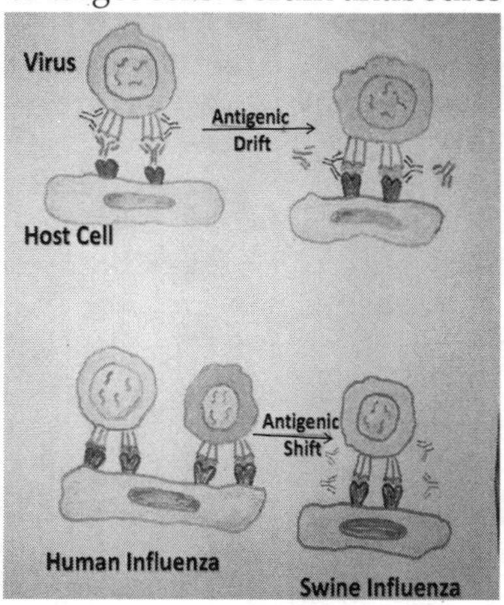

Fig. 13.4 : Antigenic drift and antigenic shift in Influenza virus

2. **The Human immunodeficiency virus**

   HIV can enter the body through the sexual organ, the blood stream and the mouth. Many people experience a flu like illness a few weeks after being exposed to HIV. The seroconversion illness may be accompanied by rash, ulcers in the mouth, severe headaches, diarrhea, fevers and pains and swollen glands. The illness is followed by the development of antibodies to HIV, and the immune system brings HIV under control. Not everyone experiences such as illness, but within a few months after becoming infected everyone produce antibodies to HIV. The immune system is gradually disrupted. HIV kills cells in the lymph nodes (clusters of immune cells that trap foreign organisms) and throws the immune system out of balance. The CD4 lymphocytes gradually decline in number because they are killed by HIV and are killed rapider as HIV levels increase. HIV destroys the immune systems memory. Most people infected with HIV will mount an effective immune response to the virus during the 1st few months of infection. However, over time this response will prove in effective. The response comes in 2 forms- cellular and humoral. The cellular response refers to the activity of CD4 and CD8 T cells the latter known as cytotoxin lymphocytes. The humoral response refers to antibody production and activity. In the 1st few weeks after infection, the no of CD8 T cells increases to upto 20 fold above the normal range, whilst CD4 T cell numbers fall sharply. Six months after infection CD4 T cell function improves except in relation to HIV specific antigen. The few people who maintain strong HIV specific CD4 T cell responses have lower viral loads than people with poor responses. CD8 T- cells play a crucial role in HIV replication during the early phase of infection. HIV specific CD8 cells are targeted at the dominant viral variant and their immergence. CD8 T cells appear to act against HIV in two ways during primary infection: by killing HIV infected cells and by secreting chemokines. HIV specific CD8 T cells recognize a specific gene sequence of HIV and are primed to copy themselves if this sequence is encountered again in the future. Structure of HIV is depicted in figure 13.5.

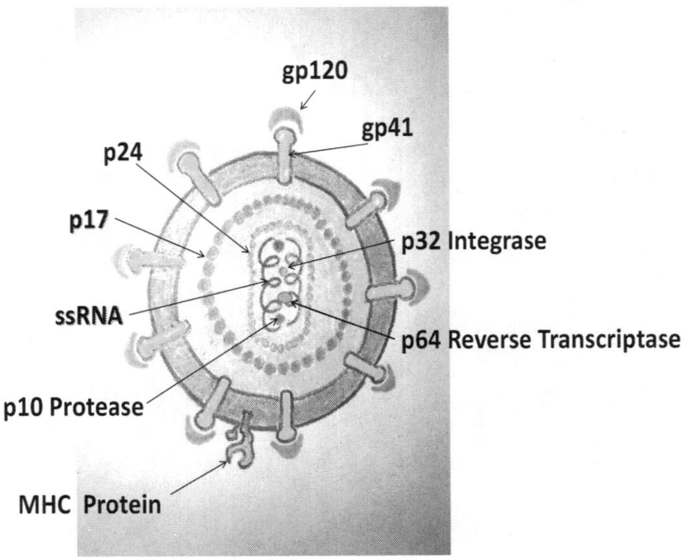

Fig. 13.5 : Structure of HIV

Immunity to Fungi

Although hundreds of thousands of fungal species are found in the environment, only about 50 can produce disease in humans. Medical mycology is the discipline that deals with the fungi that causes human disease. These fungal diseases, known as mycoses [mycosis; Greek *mykes,* fungus], are divided into five groups according to the type of infected tissue in the host: superficial, cutaneous, subcutaneous, systemic, and opportunistic mycoses. Most fungi, such as Histoplasma capsulatum (figure 13.6), Aspergillus species, Cryptococcus neoformans and Candida albicans, are ubiquitous in the environment. Fungal diseases (mycoses) are common but are problematic when associated with immunocompromised individuals. It should be noted that the importance of opportunistic fungal pathogens is increasing because of the expansion of the immunocompromised patient population. Superficial mycoses are caused by dermatophytes like Microsporium, Epidermiphyton and Trichophyton (figure 13.6).

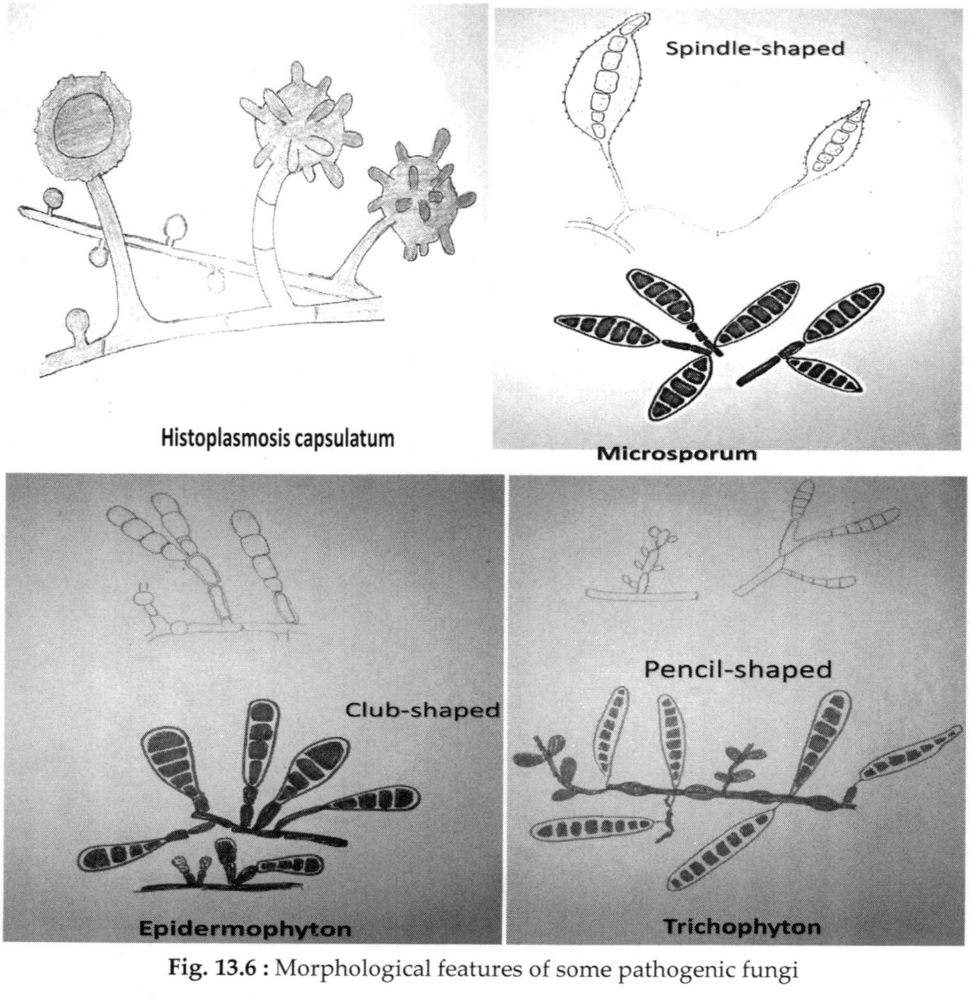

Fig. 13.6 : Morphological features of some pathogenic fungi

In the hospital setting, blood-borne fungal infections are the forth most important cause of septicemia. Although the immune response to fungal infections is not fully understood both the innate and adaptive arms of the immune system are important to eradicate or keep these infections under control. It also seems clear that protective immunity is principally cellular, especially in those infections deep within the body. This is particularly evidenced by studies of acquired immune deficiency syndrome (AIDS) patients, where low T-cell counts are commonly associated with fungal infections. A number of cell wall components of fungi may act through distinct TLRs on macrophages and dendritic cells activating essential components of the immune system. Dendritic cells are uniquely efficient at presenting fungal antigens to the adaptive immune system as are NKT cells acting through the CD1 family of glycoprotein receptors in responses to glycolipids expressed by fungi. In the past, the immunopathogenesis of fungal infections was explained primarily on the basis of Th1/Th2 responses. Th1 responses are associated with protection and eradication while increased Th2 type cell responses are associated with severity of disease. Although the Th1 axis driven by IL12 and IFNγ is still central to protection against fungi, patients with inborn deficits of the IL2/IFNγ loop do not have increased susceptibility to fungal infections. More recently Th17 cells have been shown to have important implications for failure to remove pathogens and resolve chronic inflammation in fungal disease. Inflammation previously attributed to Th1 cells would appear to be a product of dysregulation of these cells. Although IL-17, a Th 17-cell product, is important for neutrophil mobilization and eradication of some fungal infections such as candidiasis, in other fungal infections Th17 cells were associated with defective pathogen clearance and failure to resolve inflammation. Moreover, in murine studies of pulmonary aspergillosis, neutralization of IL-17 greatly ameliorates the disease. Thus, Th17 cells appear to have important connections between the failure to resolve inflammation, lack of fungal immune resistance, and susceptibility to chronic fungal infections. Finally, fungal infection represents a paradox to the immune system: whereas a severe inflammatory response may be detrimental to the host, corticosteroids may be ameliorating and protective.

Opportunistic fungal infections often become established in immunocompromised hosts or when the normal commensal flora is upset by prolonged administration of broad-spectrum antibiotics. Phagocytosis, particularly following Th1- cell mediated activation of macrophages by IFN-γ and TNF, plays a major role in dealing with fungal infections. Reactive oxygen intermediates are fungicidal for most species (for Histoplasma capsulatum, that reside in macrophages) by inducing protein modifications, damaging nucleic acid and causing lipid peroxidation. Following inhalation of Aspergillus fumigatus the alveolar macrophages phagocytose and destroy conidia (spores), although fungal protease may help protect the spores from such activities. In the lungs the conidia can germinate into branching hyphae, which are probably dealt with by the release of oxidants and fungicidal granule contents from neutrophils (figure 13.7).

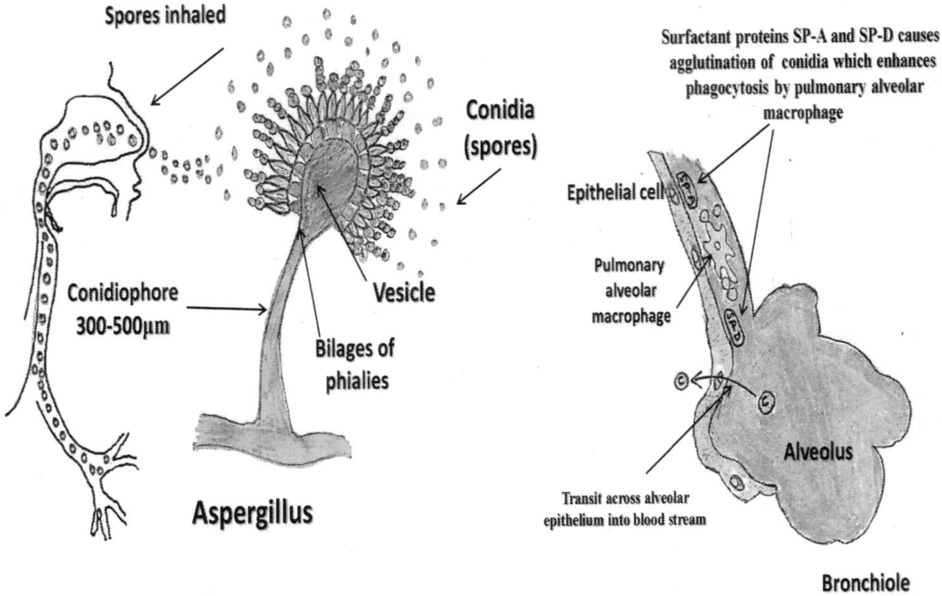

Fig. 13.7 : Immunity against Aspergillus spores in lungs

NK cells have been shown to have constitutive antifungal activity against this organism needs to be induced in CTL. In the case of A. fumigatus the adaptive immune response becomes activated following uptake of conidia and hyphae by local dendritic cells and subsequent presentation to T-cells in the draining lymph nodes. Fungal cell wall components can signal dendritic cells through a number of pattern recognition receptors, resulting in release of IL-12, which drives a Th1 response

Mannose binding protein is able to agglutinate Candida albicans and subsequently activate the complement system. Adhesins on the fungal surface also behave as virulence factors as their neutralization by antibody variable region fragment can block infection in an animal model of vaginal candidiasis.

Re-emergence of Infectious Agents

Several times a year, it seems, we hear about a new virus or bacterium that arises in a particular location and causes severe illness or death in a population. The major causes of death in the developing world are diarrheal diseases, HIV/AIDS, pneumonia, and TB. In the developing world the young child dies every 3 seconds from an infectious disease. People have to bear a huge economic burden due to the high annual incidence of various diseases. Approximately 40 million people are infected with HIV/AIDS, with approximately 2.5 million new cases added each year. In other instances, diseases that were no longer causing widespread infection suddenly began to infect an ever-larger number of individuals. These are referred to as "re-emerging" infectious diseases. Bacteria can adapt to living in almost any environment hence the re-emergence of these diseases should not be surprising. If they can adapt to living at the high temperatures of the thermal vents deep within the oceans, it is near possible that they can evolve to evade antimicrobial drugs.

Tuberculosis, once thought to be under control, kills 2 million people each year and even more if complicated with HIV/AIDS. It is estimated that approximately one third of the world population has latent TB is not as rampant, it is making progressive inroads into society and requires constant vigilance, especially with the increase of infections with multi-drug resistant strains. Tuberculosis is a well-known re-emerging disease. Fifteen years ago, public health officials were convinced that tuberculosis would soon disappear as a major health consideration in the United States. Then, because of a number of events, including the AIDS epidemic, thousands of infected individuals developed TB strains resistant to the conventional battery of antibiotics. These individuals then passed on the newly emerged, antibiotic-resistant strains of *M. tuberculosis* to others. While the rate of infection with *M. tuberculosis* in the United States increased sharply during the early part of the 1990s, by 1995 the incidence had begun to decline again. However, the worldwide incidence of the disease is still increasing, and the World Health Organization predicts that, between 1998 and 2020, one billion more people will become infected and over 70 million will die from this disease if preventive measures are not adopted.

In the past, plagues and large epidemics have changed social structures and behaviors. It is estimated that the 1918 flu pandemic killed between 40 and 100 million people. This was a usually severe form of flu caused by a virus subtype of H1N1. It had an infection rate greater than 50% severe symptoms, in part, suspected to be attributable to the immune system (cytokine storms). Between 2 and 20% of those infected died, in contrast to normal flu epidemics where the mortality rates are about 0.1%. As well as the infectious diseases listed above new and emerging infectious diseases such as severe acute respiratory syndrome (SARS), Clostridium difficile infection, Legionnaires disease, Lyme disease, and disease caused by hantavirus, present new challenges to the immune system.

Question Bank

1. Very short answer type questions
   (a) Name two toxins produced by bacteria.
   (b) Which class of antibody helps is opsonization?
   (c) Name few bacteria that are disposed by opsonization.
   (d) Name few microorganism that thrives inside cells.
   (e) Give the full form of PAM.
   (f) Give the full form of DAMP.
   (g) Give the full form of PRR.
   (h) Give the full form of TLR.
   (i) Give the full form of CTLs.
   (j) Give the full form of ADCC.
   (k) Name two opportunistic fungi.

2. Short answer type questions
   (a) Define humoral immunity.
   (b) Define cell mediated immunity.
   (c) Define opsonization.
   (d) Define exotoxin.
   (f) Define inflammation.
   (g) What are the steps in bacterial infections?
   (h) What is the role of interferons in immunity?
   (i) Define mycoses.
   (j) Define opportunistic infections.
3. Long answer type questions
   (a) Describe is detail the role of innate and adaptive immune responses.
   (b) Describe in detail the mode of infections of any bacteria and its immunity.
   (c) Describe in detail the role of interferon in combating with virus.
   (d) Describe in detail the immunity to virus with suitable examples.
   (e) Describe in detail the immunity to fungal infection.

Multiple Choice Questions - Immunity against bacteria

1. Pathogenicity of Staphylococci is because of
   (a) Lecithinase *(b)* Coagulase
   (c) M protein *(d)* Cell wall
2. Staphylococcal toxin syndrome is due to
   (a) Enterotoxin A *(b)* Enterotoxin D
   (c) Enterotoxin E *(d)* Enterotoxin F
3. Staphyloccocal food poisoning include the following features
   (a) Incubation period of 24 hours *(b)* Requires immediate antibiotics
   (c) Common with dairy products *(d)* Heat labile enterotoxin
4. Staphylococcus does not causes
   (a) Osteomyelitis *(b)* Abscess
   (c) Scarlet fever *(d)* Bronchopneumonia
5. Lancefield's classification of β-hemolytic streptococcus is based on
   (a) M protein *(b)* Polysaccharide C antigen
   (c) Type of lipid in cell membrane *(d)* Biochemical properties
6. Which toxin of streptococcus causes hemolysis?
   (a) Streptolysin O *(b)* Streptolysin S
   (c) Streptodomanase *(d)* Hyaluronidase
7. Antistreptolysin O test is diagnostic in
   (a) Acute rheumatic fever *(b)* SLE
   (c) SBE *(d)* Rheumatoid arthritis

8. Neonatal meningitis acquired passage through birth canal is due to
(*a*) Streptococcus agalactiae (*b*) Streptococcus equisimilis
(*c*) Streptococcus pyogens (*d*) Pneumococci

9. Dental caries is due to
(*a*) Streptococcus sanguis (*b*) Streptococcus mitis
(*c*) Streptococcus mutans (*d*) Streptococcus salivarius

10. The factor which promotes virulence of M tuberculosis is
(*a*) Wax D (*b*) Cord factor
(*c*) Muramyl dipeptide (*d*) Mycolic acid

11. Mycobacterium TB can be differentiated from other mycobacteria by
(*a*) Production of niacin (*b*) Aryl sulphate test
(*c*) Coagulation test (*d*) Bile solubility test

12. Rapid diagnosis of tuberculosis is possible with
(*a*) Ziehl-Neelsen stain (*b*) Kin-Young stain
(*c*) Auramine-Rhodamine stain (*d*) Giema stain

13. Positive tuberculin test indicates
(*a*) Exposure to TB (*b*) Sensitivity to tuberculin protein
(*c*) Tuberculin infection (*d*) Fulminant tuberculosis

14. Tuberculin test positivity depends on
(*a*) Erythema (*b*) Nodule formation
(*c*) Induration (*d*) Ulcerative change

15. Tuberculin unit is
(*a*) 0.00002 mg of PPD-S (*b*) 0.00001 mg of PPD-S
(*c*) 1 cc of BCG (*d*) 1cc of PPD-S

16. The only known toxin secreted by mycobacterium species is secreted by
(*a*) M tuberculosis (*b*) M kansasii
(*c*) M avium (*d*) M ulcerans

17. Cutaneous lesions may be produced by all the following mycobacteria EXCEPT
(*a*) M. intracellulare (*b*) M. leprae
(*c*) M. marinum (*d*) M. tuberculosis

18. Leprosy bacilli can be grown in
(*a*) Foot pad of nine-branded armadillo
(*b*) Tail of guinea pig
(*c*) Testes of albino rats
(*d*) Hansen's media

19. Neurological involvement is pronounced in which type of leprosy?
(*a*) Tuberculoid (*b*) Lepromatous
(*c*) Boderline (*d*) Indeterminate leprosy

20. Leprous bacilli are transmitted from person to person by all EXCEPT
(*a*) Discharge from nasal mocosa (*b*) Through open sore
(*c*) Through intact skin (*d*) Through breast milk

Answer Key

Question Number	Answer	Question Number	Answer
1	B	11	A
2	D	12	C
3	C	13	B
4	C	14	C
5	B	15	A
6	B	16	D
7	A	17	A
8	A	18	A
9	C	19	A
10	B	20	D

Multiple Choice Questions - Immunity against Fungi

1. Which dermatophyte infects hair, nails and skin?
   (a) Trichosporum (b) Trichophyton
   (c) Microsporium (d) Epidermophyton
2. Candida is the etiological agent in all of the following EXCEPT
   (a) Endocarditis (b) Mycetoma
   (c) Meningititis (d) Oral thrush
3. Which of the following is an endogenous disease in origin?
   (a) Aspergillosos (b) Candidiasis
   (c) Phycomycosis (d) All of the above
4. Which of the following is true regarding fungal infections?
   (a) Dermatophyte infections are exclusively from humans to animals
   (b) Rhinosporidiumseeberi causes deep infection in humans
   (c) Candida albicans is not pathogenic to laboratory animals
   (d) Candida infection is usually endogenous
5. Which of the following is false about Candida albicans?
   (a) Yeast-like fungus
   (b) Forms chlamydospores
   (c) Blastomeres seen in isolates
   (d) Causes meningitis in immunocompromised
6. The fungal nucleolus
   (a) Contains true chromosomes
   (b) Contains DNA fragments
   (c) Differs from the bacterial nucleus
   (d) All of the above
7. Asexual spores of fungi are following EXCEPT
   (a) Arthrospores (b) Chlamydospores
   (c) Blastospores (d) Ascospores
8. Which of the following is produced sexually
   (a) Ascospore (b) Conidium
   (c) Oidium (d) Yeast buds
9. The culture media used for cultivation of fungus is
   (a) Tellurite medium (b) NNN medium
   (c) Chocolate agar medium (d) Sabouraud's medium
10. A sporangium contains
    (a) Spherules
    (b) Sporangiospores
    (c) Chlamydospores
    (d) Oidia

11. Sclerotic bodies measuring 3-15μ in size, multiseptate, chestnut brown colour (sclerotic cells) are seen in
    (a) Rhinosporidiosis (b) Chromblastomycosis
    (c) Phacohypomycosis (d) Histoplasmosis
12. Asteroid bodies are cigar-shaped globi may be produced by
    (a) Sporothrix (b) Sporothrichosis
    (c) Phialophora (d) Aspergillus
13. Non-cultivable fungus is
    (a) Rhinosporodium (b) Candida
    (c) Sporothrix (d) Penicillium
14. The only deep mycosis common in India is
    (a) Cryptococcosis (b) Blastomycosis
    (c) Coccidiodomycosis (d) Histoplasmosis
15. Which of the following is false about C neoformans?
    (a) Grows at 37°C (b) Grows on Sabouraud's agar
    (c) Polysaccharide capsule (d) Urease negative
16. Which of the following stains is used for Cryptococcus ?
    (a) Negative India ink (b) Giemsa
    (c) Albort (d) Gram
17. Coccidiodes immitis is identified in tissues on the basis of which of the following ?
    (a) Budding yeast cells with pseudohyphae
    (b) Yeast-like forms with very large capsules
    (c) Arthrospores
    (d) Endosporulating spherules
18. Aspergilloma has
    (a) Septate hyphae
    (b) Pseudo hyphae
    (c) Metachromatic hyphae
    (d) No hyphae
19. Actinomycetes is
    (a) Gram-positive bacteria
    (b) Gram-negative bacteria
    (c) Fungus
    (d) A yeast-like form
20. Farmer's lung is caused by
    (a) Micromonospore faenia
    (b) Aspergillosis
    (c) Histoplasma capsulatum
    (d) All of the above

Answer Key

Question Number	Answer	Question Number	Answer
1	B	11	B
2	B	12	B
3	B	13	A
4	D	14	A
5	C	15	D
6	D	16	A
7	D	17	D
8	A	18	A
9	D	19	A
10	B	20	A

Multiple Choice Questions - Immunity against virus

1. Cytokines
   (a) Are polypeptides
   (b) Act on surface receptors
   (c) Take part in intrinsic enzymatic reactions
   (d) Are chemotactic
2. Interleukin-1 is produced by
   (a) T-helper cells (b) B-helper cells
   (c) Monocytes (d) None
3. Interleukin-1 primarily acts on
   (a) Lymphocytes (b) Macrophages
   (c) Neutrophils (d) Erythrocytes
4. Which of the following is true about influenza?
   (a) Large epidemics is due to antigenic drift
   (b) Has double-stranded RNA
   (c) Nucleocapsid is protective
   (d) Neuraminidase and hemagglutination are specific
5. Which of the following is false about HIV?
   (a) It is a DNA virus
   (b) It attacks CD4 cells
   (c) Macrophages are the reservoir
   (d) It reverses CD4:CD8 ratio
6. During the window period of patients with AIDS
   (a) ELISA is negative
   (b) Western blot is negative
   (c) Both ELISA & Western blot are negative
   (d) PCR is negative
7. All the following are characteristic opportunistic infections in AIDS EXCEPT
   (a) Cryptosporidium (b) Kaposi sarcoma
   (c) M avium intracellulare (d) Aspergillosis
8. The best laboratory method to diagnose AIDS infection is
   (a) RIA (b) ELISA
   (c) Western blot test (d) Complement fixation test
9. The approximate chance of infection per exposure is less in the case of
   (a) Blood transfusion (b) Tissue or organ donation
   (c) Sexual contact (d) Transplacental transmission
10. An example of an artificial virus is
    (a) Vaccinia virus (b) Rabies virus
    (c) Mumps virus (d) Reovirus

11. Inclusion bodies of vaccinia are known as
    (a) Guarnieri bodies (b) Negri bodies
    (c) Asteroid bodies (d) Schuffner dots
12. Which of the following virus does not belong to the herpes family?
    (a) Varicella (b) Herpes simplex
    (c) CMV (d) Hepatitis B
13. Epstein-Barr virus causes all the following EXCEPT
    (a) Burkit's lymphoma (b) Infectious mononucleosis
    (c) Nasopharyngeal carcinoma (d) Cervical carcinoma
14. Paul-Bunnell test is done in
    (a) Malta fever (b) Enteric fever
    (c) Infectious mononucleosis (d) Typhus fever
15. The most definitive diagnostic method for polio is
    (a) Virus isolation from blood
    (b) Virus isolation from CSF
    (c) Virus isolation from feces or throat
    (d) Serological diagnosis
16. Oral polio vaccine is preferred over Salk's killed polio vaccine in epidemics for
    (a) Easy administration
    (b) Development of local immunity
    (c) Passive immunisation of fellow children in community
    (d) All of the above
17. The virus which does cause hemagglutination of human erythrocytes is
    (a) Myxovirus
    (b) Rubella
    (c) Enterovirus
    (d) Revovirus
18. Plaque test is used routinely in virology labs
    (a) To identify viral disease
    (b) To separate specific clone of virus
    (c) To maintain certain viral culture
    (d) To prepare vaccines
19. One virus species preventing multiplication of a second virus is called
    (a) Viral interference (b) Mutation
    (c) Supervision (d) Permutation
20. Interferon is a
    (a) Protein (b) Lipid
    (c) Polysaccharide (d) All of the above

Answer Key

Question Number	Answer	Question Number	Answer
1	A	11	A
2	C	12	D
3	A	13	D
4	D	14	C
5	A	15	C
6	C	16	D
7	B	17	B
8	C	18	A
9	C	19	A
10	A	20	A

References

Alcami A., Hill A.B. & Koszinoski U.H. (2006) Viral interference with the host immune response. In Topley& Wilson's Microbiology & microbial infection 10thedn. Pp. 617-644. Wiley-Blackwell, Oxford.

Berg D.E.& Kalia A. (2011) Pathogen evolution in adaptive landscapes. Annual Review of Microbiology 65.

Black R.E., Cousens S., Johnson H.L. et al. (2010) Global, regional, and national causes of child motality in 2008: A systematic analysis. The Lancet 375,1969-1987.

Blue C.E., Spiller O.B. & Blackbourn D.J. (2004) The relevance of complement to virus biology. Virology 319,176-184.

Flannagan R.S., Cosio G. & Grinstein S. (2009) Antimicrobial mechanisms of phagocytes and bacterial evasion strategies. Nature Reviews Microbiology 7.355-366.

Goering R. et al. (2007) Medical Microbiology, 4thedn. Mosby, London.

Hansen T.H. & Bouvier M. (2009) MHC class I antigen presentation: learning from viral evasion strategies. Nature Reviews Immunology 9,503-513.

Lambris J.D., Ricklin D. & Geisbrecht B.V. (2008) Complement evasion by human pathogens. Nature reviews Microbiology 6, 132-142.

Lewis D.B. (2006) Avian flu to human influenza. Annual Review of Medicine 57, 139-154.

Lloyd-Smith J.O. et al. (2009) Epidemic dynamics at the human-animal interface. Science 326 1362-1367,

Papayannopoulos V. & Zychlinsky A. (2009) NETs: a new strategy for using old weapons. Trends in Immunology 30, 513-521.

Romani L. (2004) Immunity to fungal infections. Nature Reviews Immunology 4, 1-23.

Schmid-Hempel P. (2009) Immune defense, parasite evasion strategies and their relevance for 'macroscopic phenomena' such as virulence. Philosophical Transactions of the royal society B 364, 85-98.

Templeton T.J. (2009) The varieties of gene amplification, diversification and hypervariability in the human malaria parasite, Plasmodium falciparum. Molecular & biochemical parasitology 166, 109-116.

The following website of the Centers for Disease Control and Prevention contain a large body of information:

http://www.cdc.gov/DiseaseConditions/ ,

Parasitic diseases: http://www.cdc.gov/parasites/

Glossary

Antibody (immunoglobulin) - A glycoprotein made by plasma cells (mature B cells) in response to the introduction of an antigen. The antibody-binding region of an antibody molecule assumes a final configuration that is the three-dimensional mirror image of the antigen that stimulated its synthesis. Thus, the antibody can bind to the antigen with exact specificity.

Antibody affinity - The strength of binding between an antigen and an antibody.

Antibody-dependent cell-mediated cytotoxicity (ADCC) - The killing of antibody-coated target cells by cells with Fc receptors that recognize the Fc region of the bound antibody. Most ADCC is mediated by NK cells that have the Fc receptor or CD16 on their surface.

Antibody titer - An approximation of the antibody concentration required to react with an antigen.

Antigen-binding fragment (Fab) - "Fragment antigen binding." A monovalent antigen-binding fragment of an immunoglobulin molecule that consists of one light chain and part of one heavy chain, linked by interchain disulfide bonds.

Antigen processing - The hydrolytic digestion of antigens to produce antigen fragments. Antigen fragments are often collected by the class I or class II MHC molecules and presented on the surface of a cell. Antigen processing can occur by proteasome action on antigens that entered a cell by means other than phagocytosis. This is known as endogenous antigen processing. Antigen processing can also occur during phagocytosis as antigens are degraded within the phagolysosome. This is known as exogenous antigen processing.

Antigenic determinant site (epitope) - The molecular configuration of the variable region of an antibody molecule that interacts with the epitope of an antigen.

Antigenic drift - A small change in the antigenic character of an organism that allows it to avoid attack by the immune system.

Antigenic shift - A major change in the antigenic character of an organism that makes it unrecognized by host immune mechanisms.

Antigen-presenting cells Antigen-presenting cells (APCs) - are cells that take in protein antigens, process them, and present antigen fragments to B cells and T cells in conjunction with class II MHC molecules so that the cells are activated. Macrophages, B cells, dendritic cells, and Langerhans cells may act as APCs.

Artificially acquired active immunity - The type of immunity that results from immunizing an animal with a vaccine. The immunized animal now produces its own antibodies and activated lymphocytes.

Artificially acquired passive immunity - The type of immunity that results from introducing into an animal antibodies that have been produced either in another animal or by in vitro methods. Immunity is only temporary.

Antiserum - Serum containing induced antibodies.

Antitoxin- An antibody to a microbial toxin, usually a bacterial exotoxin, that combines specifically with the toxin, in vivo and in vitro, neutralizing the toxin.

Avidity - The combined strength of binding between an antigen and all the antibody-binding sites.

Autoimmune disease - A disease produced by the immune system attacking self-antigens. Autoimmune disease results from the activation of self-reactive T and B cells that damage tissues after stimulation by genetic or environmental triggers.

Autoimmunity is a condition characterized by the presence of serum autoantibodies and self-reactive lymphocytes. It may be benign or pathogenic. Autoimmunity is a normal consequence of aging; is readily inducible by infectious agents, organisms, or drugs; and is potentially reversible in that it disappears when the offending "agent" is removed or eradicated.

Basophil - A white blood cell in the granulocyte lineage. It is weakly phagocytic. Importantly, it synthesizes and stores vasoactive molecules (e.g., histamine) that are released in response to external triggers (see mast cell).

B cell - also known as a B lymphocyte A type of lymphocyte derived from bone marrow stem cells that matures into an immunologically competent cell under the influence of the bursa of Fabricius in the chicken and bone marrow in nonavian species. Following interaction with antigen, it becomes a plasma cell, which synthesizes and secretes antibody molecules involved in humoral immunity.

B-cell receptor (BCR) - A transmembrane immunoglobulin complex on the surface of a B cell that binds an antigen and stimulates the B cell. It is composed of a membrane-bound immunoglobulin, usually IgD or a modified IgM, complexed with another membrane protein.

Bronchial-associated lymphoid tissue (BALT) - The type of defensive tissue found in the lungs. Part of the nonspecific (innate) immune system.

Cell-mediated immunity - The type of immunity that results from T cells coming into close contact with foreign cells or infected cells to destroy them; it can be transferred to a nonimmune individual by the transfer of cells.

Cluster of differentiation molecules (CDs) - Functional cell surface proteins or receptors that can be measured in situ from peripheral blood, biopsy samples, or other body fluids. They can be used to identify leukocyte subpopulations. Some examples include interleukin-2 receptor (IL-2R), CD4, CD8, CD25, and intercellular adhesion molecule-1 (ICAM-1).

Communicable disease - A disease associated with a pathogen that can be transmitted from one host to another.

Cytotoxic T lymphoryte (CTL) - A type of T cell that recognizes antigen in class I MHC molecules, destroying the cell on which the antigen is displayed. Also called CD8cell.

Double diffusion agar assay (Öuchterlony technique) - An immunodiffusion reaction in which both antibody and antigen diffuse through agar to form stable immune complexes, which can be observed visually.

Disease - A deviation or interruption of the normal structure or function of any part of the body that is manifested by a characteristic set of symptoms and signs.

Enterotoxin - A toxin specifically affecting the cells of the intestinal mucosa, causing vomiting and diarrhoea.

Enzyme-linked immunosorbent assay (ELISA) - A serological assay in which bound antigen or antibody is detected by another antibody that is conjugated to an enzyme. The enzyme converts a colorless substrate to a colored product reporting the antibody capture of the antigen.

Eosinophil - A polymorphonuclear leukocyte that has a two-lobed nucleus and cytoplasmic granules that stain yellow-red. A mobile phagocyte that is highly antiparasitic.

Epidemic - A disease that suddenly increases in occurrence above the normal level in a given population.

Epidemiologist - A person who specializes in epidemiology.

Epidemiology - The study of the factors determining and influencing the frequency and distribution of disease, injury, and other health-related events and their causes in defined human populations.

Food-borne infection - Gastrointestinal illness caused by ingestion of microorganisms, followed by their growth within the host. Symptoms arise from tissue invasion and/or toxin production.

Food intoxication - Food poisoning caused by microbial toxins produced in a food prior to consumption. The presence of living bacteria is not required.

Food poisoning - A general term usually referring to a gastrointestinal disease caused by the ingestion of food contaminated by pathogens or their toxins.

Hapten - A molecule not immunogenic by itself that, when coupled to a macromolecular carrier, can elicit antibodies directed against itself.

Human immunodeficiency virus (HIV) - A lentivirus of the family Retroviridae that is the cause of AIDS.

Human leukocyte antigen complex (HLA) - The major histocompatibility protein antigens on the surface of cells of human tissues and organs is recognized by the immune system cells and therefore is important in the regulation of the immune response and graft rejection. This is the same as MHC class II. Also see major histocompatibility complex.

Humoral (antibody-mediated) immunity - The type of immunity that results from the presence of soluble antibodies in blood and lymph; also known as antibody-mediated immunity.

Hypersensitivity - A condition of increased immune sensitivity in which the body reacts to an antigen with an exaggerated immune response that usually harms the individual. Also termed an allergy.

Idiotype - A set of one or more unique epitopes in the variable region of an immunoglobulin that distinguishes it from immunoglobulins produced by different plasma cells.

IgA Immunoglobulin A - the class of immunoglobulins that is present in dimeric form in many body secretions (e.g., saliva, tears, and bronchial and intestinal secretions) and protects body surfaces. IgA also is present in serum.

IgD Immunoglobulin D - the class of immunoglobulins found on the surface of many B lymphocytes; thought to serve as an antigen receptor in the stimulation of antibody synthesis.

IgE Immunoglobulin E - the immunoglobulin class that binds to mast cells and basophils, and is responsible for type I or anaphylactic hypersensitivity reactions such as hay fever and asthma. IgE is also involved in resistance to helminth parasites.

IgG Immunoglobulin G - the predominant immunoglobulin class in serum. Has functions such as neutralizing toxins, opsonizing bacteria, activating complement, and crossing the placenta to protect the fetus and neonate.

IgM Immunoglobulin M - the class of serum antibody first produced during an infection. It is a large, pentameric molecule that is active in agglutinating pathogens and activating complement. The monomeric form is present on the surface of some B lymphocytes.

Immune complex - The product of an antigen-antibody reaction, which may also contain components of the complement system.

Immune surveillance - The process by which cells of the immune system police the host for nonself antigens.

Immune system - The defensive system in a host consisting of the nonspecific (innate) and specific(adaptive) immune responses. It is composed of widely distributed cells, tissues, and organs that recognize foreign substances and microorganisms and acts to neutralize or destroy them.

Immunity - Refers to the overall general ability of a host to resist a particular disease; the condition of being immune.

Immunization - The deliberate introduction of foreign materials into a host to stimulate an adaptive immune response.

Immunodeficiency - The inability to produce a normal complement of antibodies or immunologically sensitized T cells in response to specific antigens.

Immunodiffusion – A technique involving the diffusion of antigen and/or antibody within a semisolid gel to produce a precipitin reaction where they meet in proper proportions. Often both the antibody and antigen diffuse through the gel; sometimes an antigen diffuses through a gel containing antibody.

Immunoelectrophoresis - The electrophoretic separation of protein antigens followed by diffusion and precipitation in gels using antibodies against the separated proteins.

Immunofluorescence - A technique used to identify particular antigens microscopically in cells or tissues by the binding of a fluorescent antibody conjugate.

Immunology - The study of host defences against invading foreign materials, including pathogenic microorganisms, transformed or cancerous cells, and tissue transplants from other sources.

Immunopathology - The study of diseases or conditions resulting from immune reactions.

Immunoprecipitation - A reaction involving soluble antigens reacting with antibodies to form a large aggregate that precipitates out of solution.

Inflammation - A localized protective response to tissue injury or destruction. Acute inflammation is characterized by pain, heat, swelling, and redness in the injured area

Infection - The invasion of a host by a microorganism with subsequent establishment and multiplication of the agent. An infection may or may not lead to overt disease.

Influenza or flu - An acute viral infection of the respiratory tract, occurring in isolated cases, epidemics, and pandemics. Influenza is caused by three strains of influenza virus, labeled types A, B, and C, based on capsid antigens.

Interferon (IFN) - A glycoprotein that has nonspecific antiviral activity by stimulating cells to produce antiviral proteins, which inhibit the synthesis of viral RNA and proteins. Interferons also regulate the growth, differentiation, and/or function of a variety of immune system cells. Their production may be stimulated by virus infections, intracellular pathogens (chlamydiae and rickettsias), protozoan parasites, endotoxins, and other agents.

Interleukin - A glycoprotein produced by macrophages and T cells that regulates growth and differentiation, particularly of lymphocytes. Interleukins promote cellular and humoral immune responses.

Isotype - A variant form of an immunoglobulin (e.g., an immunoglobulin class, subclass, or type) that occurs in every normal individual of a particular species. Usually the characteristic antigenic determinant is in the constant region of H and L chains.

J chain A polypeptide present in polymeric IgM and IgA that links the subunits together.

Leukemia - Aprogressive, malignant disease of blood-forming organs, marked by distorted proliferation and development of leukocytes and their precursors in the blood and bone marrow. Certain leukemias are caused by viruses (HTLV-1, HTLV-2).

Leukocidin - A microbial toxin that can damage or kill leukocytes.

Lymph node - A small secondary lymphoid organ that contains lymphocytes, macrophages, and dendritic cells. It serves as a site for (1) filtration and removal of foreign antigens and (2) the activation and proliferation of lymphocytes.

Lymphocyte - A nonphagocytic, mononuclear leukocyte (white blood cell) that is an immunologically competent cell, or its precursor. Lymphocytes are present in the blood, lymph, and lymphoid tissues.

Major histocompatibility complex (MHC) - A chromosome locus encoding the histocompatibility antigens. Class I MHC molecules are cell surface glycoproteins present on all nucleated cells; class II MHC glycoproteins are on antigen-presenting cells. Class I MHC glycoproteins present endogenous antigens to CD8T cells. Class II MHC glycoproteins present exogenous antigens to CD4T cells.

Medical mycology - The discipline that deals with the fungi that cause human disease.

Membrane attack complex (MAC) - The complex complement components (C5b–C9) that create a pore in the plasma membrane of a target cell and leads to cell lysis. C9 probably forms most of the actual pore.

Monoclonal antibody (mAb) - An antibody of a single type that is produced by a population of genetically identical plasma cells (a clone); a monoclonal antibody is typically produced from a cell culture derived from the fusion product of a cancer cell and an antibody-producing cell (a hybridoma).

Monocyte - A mononuclear phagocytic leukocyte that circulates briefly in the bloodstream before migrating to the tissues where it becomes a macrophage.

Mycologist - A person specializing in mycology; a student of mycology.

Mycology - The science and study of fungi.

Natural killer (NK) - cell A type of white blood cell that has a lineage independent of the granulocyte, B cell, and T-cell lineages. It is often called a non-B, non-T lymphocyte because it does not make antibody; nor does it make cytokines associated with T cells. NK cells are part of the innate immune system, exhibiting MHC-independent cytolytic activity against virus-infected and tumor cells.

Naturally acquired active immunity - The type of active immunity that develops when an individual's immunologic system comes into contact with an appropriate antigenic stimulus during the course of normal activities; it usually arises as the result of recovering from an infection and lasts a long time.

Naturally acquired passive immunity - The type of temporary immunity that involves the transfer of antibodies from one individual to another.

Mucosal-associated lymphoid tissue (MALT) - Organized and diffuse immune tissues found as part of the mucosal epithelium. It can be specialized to the gut (GALT), the bronchial system (BALT), or skin (SALT).

Parasite - An organism that lives on or within another organism (the host) and benefits from the association while harming its host. Often the parasite obtains nutrients from the host.

Passive immunization - The induction of temporary immunity by the transfer of immune products, such as antibodies or sensitized T cells, from an immune vertebrate to a nonimmune one.

Pathogen-associated molecular pattern (PAMP) - Conserved molecular structures that occur in patterns on microbial surfaces. The structures and their patterns are unique to particular microorganisms and invariant among members of a given microbial group.

Pathogenicity - The condition or quality of being pathogenic, or the ability to cause disease.

Polymorphonuclear leukocyte - A leukocyte that has a variety of nuclear forms.

Precipitation (or precipitin) reaction - The reaction of an antibody with a soluble antigen to form an insoluble precipitate.

Precipitin - The antibody responsible for a precipitation reaction.

Radioimmunoassay (RIA) - A very sensitive assay technique that uses a purified radioisotope-labelled antigen or antibody to compete for antibody or antigen with unlabelled standard and samples to determine the concentration of a substance in the samples.

Serology - The branch of immunology that is concerned with in vitro reactions involving one or more serum constituents (e.g., antibodies and complement).

Serotyping - A technique or serological procedure used to differentiate between strains (serovars or serotypes) of microorganisms that have differences in the antigenic composition of a structure or product.

Serum - The clear, fluid portion of blood lacking both blood cells and fibrinogen. It is the fluid remaining after coagulation of plasma, the noncellular liquid fraction of blood.

Systemic lupus erythematosus - An autoimmune, inflammatory disease that may affect every tissue of the body.

Symptom - A change during a disease that a person subjectively experiences (e.g., pain, bodily discomfort, fatigue, or loss of appetite). Sometimes the term symptom is used more broadly to include any observed signs

TB skin test - Tuberculin hypersensitivity test for a previous or current infection with Mycobacterium tuberculosis.

T cell or T lymphocyte - A type of lymphocyte derived from bone marrow stem cells that matures into an immunologically competent cell under the influence of the thymus. T cells are involved in a variety of cell-mediated immune reactions.

T-cell antigen receptor (TCR) - The receptor on the T cell surface consisting of two antigen-binding peptide chains; it is associated with a large number of other glycoproteins. Binding of antigen to the TCR, usually in association with MHC, activates the T cell.

T-dependent antigen - An antigen that effectively stimulates B-cell response only with the aid of T helper cells that produce interleukin-2 and B-cell growth factor.

TH 1 - cell A CD4 T-helper cell that secretes interferon-gamma, interleukin-2, and tumor necrosis factor, influencing phagocytic cells.

TH 2 - cell A CD4T-helper cell that secretes interleukin (IL)-4, IL-5, IL-6, IL-9, IL-10, and IL-13, influencing growth and differentiation of lymphocytes.

TH 0 - cell A CD4T cell that secretes cytokines of TH1 and TH2 cells, implicating them as precursors to TH1 and TH2 cells.

Toll-like receptor (TLR) - A type of pattern recognition receptor on phagocytes such as macrophages that triggers the proper response to different classes of pathogens. It signals the production of transcription factor NF B, which stimulates formation of cytokines, chemokines, and other defence molecules.

Toxoid - A bacterial exotoxin that has been modified so that it is no longer toxic but will still stimulate antitoxin formation when injected into a person or animal.

Tuberculoid (neural) leprosy - A mild, nonprogressive form of leprosy that is associated with delayed-type hypersensitivity to antigens on the surface of Mycobacterium leprae. It is characterized by early nerve damage and regions of the skin that have lost sensation and are surrounded by a border of nodules.

Tuberculosis (TB) - An infectious disease of humans and other animals resulting from an infection by a species of Mycobacterium and characterized by the formation of tubercles and tissue necrosis, primarily as a result of host hypersensitivity and inflammation. Infection is usually by inhalation, and the disease commonly affects the lungs (pulmonary tuberculosis), although it may occur in any part of the body.

Tumor necrosis factor (TNF) - A cytokine produced by activated macrophages. Originally named for its cytotoxic effect on tumor cells, TNF has activities similar to those of interleukin-1, such as inducing inflammation, lipid metabolism, and coagulation.

Type I hypersensitivity - A form of immediate hypersensitivity arising from the binding of antigen to IgE attached to mast cells, which then release anaphylaxis mediators such as histamine. Examples: hay fever, asthma, and food allergies.

Type II hypersensitivity - A form of immediate hypersensitivity involving the binding of antibodies to antigens on cell surfaces followed by destruction of the target cells (e.g., through complement attack, phagocytosis, or agglutination).

Type III hypersensitivity – A form of immediate hypersensitivity resulting from the exposure to excessive amounts of antigens to which antibodies bind. These antibody-antigen complexes activate complement and trigger an acute inflammatory response with subsequent tissue damage.

Type IV hypersensitivity – A delayed hypersensitivity response (it appears 24 to 48 hours after antigen exposure). It results from the binding of antigen to activated T lymphocytes, which then release cytokines and trigger inflammation and macrophage attacks that damage tissue. Type IV hypersensitivity is seen in contact dermatitis from poison ivy, leprosy, and tertiary syphilis.

Vaccine - A preparation of either killed microorganisms; living, weakened (attenuated) microorganisms; or inactivated bacterial toxins (toxoids). It is administered to induce development of the immune response and protect the individual against a pathogen or a toxin.

Virus - An infectious agent having a simple acellular organization with a protein coat and a nucleic acid genome, lacking independent metabolism, and reproducing only within living host cells.

Virusoid - An infectious agent that is composed only of single-stranded RNA that encodes some but not all proteins required for its replication; can be replicated and transmitted to a new host only if it infects a cell also infected by a virus that serves as a helper virus.

Vaccine - A preparation of either killed microorganisms; living, weakened (attenuated) microorganisms; or inactivated bacterial toxins (toxoids). It is administered to induce development of the immune response and protect the individual against a pathogen or a toxin.

Widal test - A test involving agglutination of typhoid bacilli when they are mixed with serum containing typhoid antibodies from an individual having typhoid fever; used to detect the presence of Salmonella typhi and S. paratyphi.

Xenograft - A tissue graft between animals of different species.

Books Referred

1. N. Arumugam, Dulsy Fatima. Immunology. Saras Publication. ISBN 9789382459880
2. Jenni Punt, Sharon Stranford, Patricia Jones, Judy Owen . Kuby Immunology Eighth Edition. W. H. Freeman; Eighth edition. ISBN 978-1464189784
3. Peter J Delves. Roitt's Essential Immunology. John Wiley; 13th edition. ISBN 9781118415771
4. Peter Lydyard, Alex Whelan and Michael W Fanger. BIOS Instant Notes in Immunology. Garland Science, Taylor & Francis Group; Third edition. ISBN 978-0-4156-0753-7
5. Lansing M. Prescott, John P. Harley, Donald A. Klein. Microbiology (Fifth Edition) Fifth Edition. McGraw-Hill Higher Education; Fifth edition. ISBN-13: 978-0072320411
6. Richard A. Goldsby, Thomas J. Kindt, Janis Kuby, Barbara A. Osborne Immunology, Fifth Edition. W. H. Freeman; 5th edition (November 29, 2002). ISBN-13: 978-0716749479
7. William L. Irving, Dlawer A. A. Ala'Aldeen, Tim Boswell. Medical Microbiology
8. Garland Science, Taylor & Francis Group 2005. ISBN 1-8599-6254-8

Index